Cell, Tissue and Disease

The Basis of Pathology

Commissioning Editor: Timothy Horne
Project Development Manager: Sarah Keer-Keer
Project Controller: Frances Affleck
Designer: Erik Bigland

Cell, Tissue and Disease

The Basis of Pathology

Professor Neville Woolf

Faculty Tutor
Royal Free and University College Medical School of University College London

PhD, MMed(path), FRCPath

THIRD EDITION

W. B. SAUNDERS COMPANY LTD

EDINBURGH LONDON NEW YORK PHILADELPHIA ST LOUIS SYDNEY TORONTO 2000

W.B. SAUNDERS
An imprint of Harcourt Publishers Limited

© Harcourt Publishers Limited 2000

⟨※⟩ is a registered trademark of Harcourt Publishers Limited

First edition 1977
Second edition 1986
Third edition 2000

ISBN 0 7020 2478 3

British Library Cataloguing in Publication Data
A catalogue record for this book is available from the British Library

Library of Congress Cataloging in Publication Data
A catalog record for this book is available from the Library of Congress

Note
Medical knowledge is constantly changing. As new information becomes available,
changes in treatment, procedures, equipment and the use of drugs become necessary. The
author and the publishers have, as far as it is possible, taken care to ensure that the
information given in this text is accurate and up-to-date. However, readers are strongly
advised to confirm that the information, especially with regard to drug usage, complies
with the latest legislation and standards of practice.

The
publisher's
policy is to use
paper manufactured
from sustainable forests

Printed in China

Preface

A considerable period has elapsed since the last edition of this book appeared. Its gratifying reception and the continuing sales suggest general acceptance of its approach to the learning of the processes involved in disease. Nevertheless the advance of knowledge in this field dictates the need for a new updated version of both text and illustrations. Most of the text has been rewritten and several new sections have been inserted.

In relation to the illustrations, the decision has been taken to omit the photographic examples of pathological lesions and, instead, to increase greatly the number of line diagrams. It is intended that these should constitute an integral part of the book, rather than acting merely as decoration, and should, in themselves, be a useful learning and revision aid. Thus the diagrams make use of a limited number of visual patterns which students can adapt for themselves for use in contexts not dealt with in this book.

As before, the text is intended to be a bridge between laboratory-based biological science and disease as it appears to patients and their carers. It provides an appropriate body of factual knowledge but emphasizes the importance of understanding and the ability to use knowledge in a number of disparate contexts. It emphasizes the use of certain contextual paradigms of which 'things are more the same than they are different' is perhaps the most important. Since the reaction patterns of cells and tissues are finite, knowledge gained in one context may be equally usefully applied in another. Thus, for example, familiarity with the biological processes involved in wound healing equips one to understand what occurs in the formation of the connective tissue 'cap' of an atherosclerotic plaque, the scarring which occurs in interstitial lung disease and the formation of the connective tissue stroma in certain neoplasms.

I hope that this third edition will prove as useful to students of the health sciences as its predecessors.

December 1999   *Neville Woolf*

Preface

Contents

1 The nature of pathology

Pathology is the bridge between the basic biological sciences and the practice of medicine. It is the study of the changes in structure and function that are produced either by injury, in its broadest sense, or by inborn errors.

The reactions of cells and tissues are finite. Thus identical structural features may be found in both normal and disease states, and altered structure alone may be an unreliable marker of the presence of disease. For instance, the smooth muscle cells of the uterus increase enormously in size during pregnancy – a perfectly physiological, indeed essential, change. However, if, for example, some obstruction to the normal outflow of urine were to occur, the smooth muscle cells of the bladder wall would also increase greatly in size, providing a clear indication of dysfunction in the lower urinary tract.

Even cell death can be a physiological as well as a pathological phenomenon; programmed cell death (apoptosis) is an important process in events as diverse as morphogenesis in the embryo, or surveillance against the development of cancer by removing cells with particular mutations in DNA. The local tissue responses elicited by 'pathological' cell injury may occur also under physiological circumstances. For example, the structural changes characteristic of acute inflammation are the inevitable consequences of a wide range of injuries, but inflammation may also occur in such physiological events as the shedding of the endometrial lining of the uterus at the end of a menstrual cycle.

THE CONCEPT OF DISEASE

What is disease? Some define it as the condition in which the normal function of some part or organ of the body is disturbed. Others maintain that disease does not exist except as a **reaction to injury**. These definitions are both valid and in no way mutually exclusive. One easy way of looking at a disease is to think of it in terms of simple set theory, as the common set of a

1

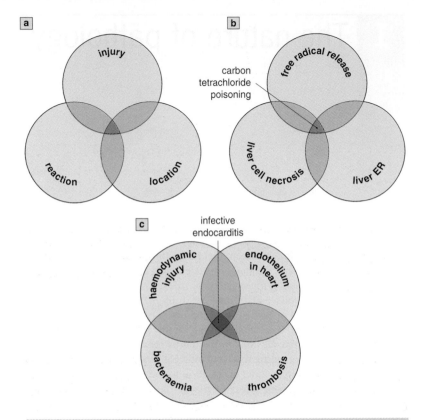

Fig. 1.1 Use of set theory to categorize disease.

The chosen sets in this instance are shown in **a** and are the type of injury, its location and the type of local reaction. In example **b**, carbon tetrachloride initiates free radical release in the endoplasmic reticulum (ER) of the liver cells and this leads to lipid peroxidation and liver cell necrosis. In example **c**, a haemodynamic injury to the endothelium within the heart, such as might occur with a scarred mitral or aortic valve, will, in the presence of microorganisms in the blood, give rise to infected thrombi on the heart valve surface (infective endocarditis).

number of sets, most notably **type of injury**, **type of reaction** and the **location of injury** (*Fig. 1.1*). This simple concept can be extended to cover situations in which cells, tissues or organs are acted upon unfavourably either by injurious agents or by inborn errors acting alone, or in conjunction with environmental circumstances. The sequence of events that follows may be dominated by the direct effects of the injurious agent on the cell (as in certain chemical injuries). Alternatively it may be a combination of these direct effects and the local and general cell and tissue reactions that may be elicited.

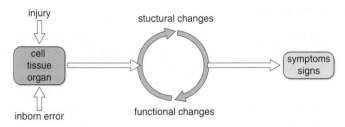

Fig. 1.2 Signs and symptoms.

Injury or inborn error may lead to functional and then structural disturbances within cells and tissues. These are expressed as the 'symptoms' experienced by the patient and the 'signs' observed by the physician.

The functional disturbances produced by injury to cells are often mirrored by structural changes (a lesion), just as, in turn, structural damage may be followed by loss or alteration of some normal function. The sum of these effects finds its expression in the symptoms experienced by the patient and the signs observed by the physician (*Fig. 1.2*).

Severe functional disturbances need not be accompanied by significant structural changes

Disordered function does not always lead to disordered structure; the former may be very severe without any significant structural changes being present. A striking example of this is the serious diarrhoeal disease, **cholera**. Cholera, which has killed millions, is caused by *Vibrio cholerae*, an organism that can neither destroy the lining cells of the gut wall nor even penetrate between them. There is no microscopic evidence that the organism damages any tissue. However, if untreated, more than half of those infected will die from the dehydration and electrolyte disturbances that result from the profuse watery diarrhoea caused by *V. cholerae*. This diarrhoea occurs because the epithelial lining cells of the intestine respond to a toxin secreted by the organism. The toxin behaves in the same way as a normal hormonal regulatory signal in that when food is delivered to the small intestine, a peptide binds to a receptor site on the luminal membrane of the small intestinal epithelial cell and stimulates the adenylate cyclase system, with the result that about 2 litres of alkaline fluid are pumped into the small intestine (see pp. 19–21).

Morphological change can occur without significant functional disturbance

In other situations a considerable degree of morphological alteration may be present as, for instance, in some large benign neoplasms, but functional disturbance may be slight or absent.

GENERAL PATHOLOGY

General pathology is the study of the functional and structural changes occurring in cells and tissues as a result of direct damage by, or reactions to, a wide range of unfavourable circumstances. While our knowledge is still incomplete, it is probably true to say that the number of responses of the mammalian cell is finite. These responses represent either an increase or a reduction (or loss) in some of the components of a large, but not infinite, number of normal cell processes.

This general principle holds good only so long as **no change has taken place in the genome** of the target cell or in the transcription of its genetic information. If such changes have occurred, then a new phenotype and new responses that are uncharacteristic of this cell (at least in its adult or fully differentiated form), may be acquired. The words 'adult or fully differentiated' should be stressed because the acquisition of apparently new functions (such as the secretion of fetal antigens by the cells of some tumours) may be the expression of functions that were normal and appropriate at an earlier stage of the organism's embryological development.

Characteristics of a disease

How one regards any individual disease process depends largely on one's point of view. The patient will wish to know whether he or she will recover or not (i.e. the **prognosis**); the clinician wants to know the diagnostic features and the best mode of treatment; and the histopathologist will tend to classify the disease on the basis of its morphological features. All should want to know the basic cause (or **aetiology**) because only in the light of this knowledge can diseases be avoided.

Another concept of importance is the **pathogenesis** of a disease. Many people tend to confuse the terms aetiology and pathogenesis. Pathogenesis refers not to the actual cause of the disease but to the **sequence of events** that occurs from the initial injury to the time when the disease expresses itself in functional and structural terms. Full understanding of pathogenesis is important because it may provide a number of novel therapeutic targets that may lead to a beneficial alteration in the natural history of a given disease.

An example of the pathogenesis of a common and serious disease may be found in the natural history of coronary artery atherosclerosis, the complications of which are responsible for approximately 25% of adult male deaths in the UK. Atherosclerosis is characterized by focal thickenings of the intima of large elastic and muscular arteries. These thickenings consist of a combination of proliferated connective tissue forming a 'cap' to the lesion, and a basal accumulation of lipid and tissue debris. As these plaque-like foci increase in thickness, they may result in significant narrowing of the vessel lumen. This may lead areas of the heart muscle to receive an insufficient blood supply, and the patient may experience chest pain provoked by exercise or cold and relieved by rest or vasodilator (**stable angina**). Not infrequently, the plaque softens as its constituents undergo necrosis. This may be followed by splitting of the connective tissue cap and exposure of the subendothelial elements of the plaque. This in turn leads to adherence and aggregation of platelets, and within a very short time the mass of platelets and fibrin (a **thrombus**) may block the lumen of the artery. The segment of ventricular wall supplied by this artery will thus be deprived totally of its arterial blood supply. In clinical terms this may cause severe central chest pain or serious ventricular arrhythmias (which may prove fatal within a few minutes); low cardiac output accompanied by peripheral vasoconstriction (cardiogenic shock); or chronic cardiac failure. In structural terms, the morphological features of death of the underperfused muscle will develop over the next 24 hours or so. In most instances, if the patient lives, the dead muscle will be replaced by scar tissue. This lacks the contractile properties of muscle and may eventually stretch permanently, leading to the formation of a bulge or **aneurysm** on the wall of the left ventricle. If the patient dies within a few minutes of the cutting off of the arterial blood supply, the structural changes that indicate cell injury or cell death do not occur.

Reducing the concentration of certain lipid classes in the plasma of patients with clinically overt coronary atherosclerosis by changing diet or using drugs does not significantly alter the size of the atherosclerotic lesions but does significantly reduce the risk of both new clinical events and atherosclerosis-related death. The lesion has not been removed but its natural history has been modified.

2 Cell injury and its manifestations

CELL ADAPTATION

Under most circumstances cells try to maintain a **steady state**. If their milieu is altered, they will try to adapt to the change without significant loss of function (cell adaptation). Obvious examples of this are to be found where there is an alteration in the **functional demands** made on cells. An increase in demand usually leads to one or both of the following:

- an increase in **size** of individual cells (**hypertrophy**)
- an increase in **number** of cells (**hyperplasia**).

An example of such adaptation is the hypertrophy of heart muscle fibres that occurs when their work load is increased because of high pressure in the left ventricular outflow tract (e.g. in aortic valve stenosis or systemic hypertension). This hypertrophy leads to a significant increase in left ventricular wall thickness. Conversely, when functional demands decrease, this may be mirrored by a marked **decrease** in cell size (**atrophy**), as in the rapid muscle wasting that may follow immobilization of a limb in plaster following a fracture.

If the environmental changes are so great that cells cannot adjust to a changed milieu, then some loss in the normal range of functions is likely. This may well be accompanied by characteristic structural alterations. These functional and structural changes are the correlates of **cell injury** and may be reversible. Irreversible injury leads to loss of vital cellular functions and thus to **cell death**. *Cell death is not always a pathological event.* It is also the means for maintaining normal numbers of cells and acts in many contexts. Such cell death is a programmed phenomenon known as **apoptosis** (see pp. 39–42).

REQUIREMENTS FOR MAINTENANCE OF THE STEADY STATE

A steady state requires the performance by a cell of a range of basic functions which include:

- Preservation of **normal DNA templates** for the synthesis of nucleic acids and proteins.
- **Normal enzyme content.** Normal amounts and types of enzymes are required for carrying out a variety of intracellular functions.
- **Intact membranes and transmembrane proteins.** The transport of metabolites via energy-dependent transport systems requires intact membranes if osmotic and fluid homeostasis are to be preserved and if signals are to be normally received and acted upon.
- **Adequate supply of substrates and oxygen.** Aerobic energy production is vital for cells and requires adequate oxygenation and normal amounts of suitable substrates. **Hypoxia** (a reduction of the amount of oxygen delivered to cells), often mediated via **ischaemia** (a reduction in the perfusion of a part relative to its needs), is one of the commonest and most important causes of both sub-lethal and lethal cell injury.

These systems are interrelated. Thus it is easier to identify targets of cell injury in terms of anatomy than of function. There are occasional exceptions, however, such as in cyanide poisoning (in which cytochrome oxidase is specifically inactivated, leading to a block in aerobic respiration) and in relation to certain bacterial toxins (see pp. 17–23). It is reasonable, therefore, to consider cell injury either in terms of the part of the cell microanatomy that is primarily affected, or in terms of the type of injury applied. Where possible, these two approaches should be combined.

SITES AND TYPES OF CELL INJURY

TYPES OF INJURY

The reaction patterns to the many types of cell injury are limited and the results of any such injury depend in part on the severity of the injury, and in part on the innate resistance of the cell. *Thus a given degree of injury will have different effects on different cell types.* For example, hypoxia of short duration can cause irreversible injury to neurones but does not damage cells such as cartilage.

Common types of cell-damaging factors in the microenvironment include:

- **Hypoxia** and **anoxia**. These are most often caused by ischaemia, in which perfusion by oxygenated blood is insufficient to meet the metabolic needs of the affected organ or tissue.
- **Reoxygenation**. Reperfusion of acutely ischaemic tissue may considerably increase cell damage. This is believed to be due to the generation of oxygen free radicals (see pp. 11–14).

- Extremes of **heat** or **cold**.
- **Chemical agents** that produce cell damage in many different ways.
- **Immunologically mediated mechanisms** operating through either the humoral or cellular arms of the immune system (see pp. 137–181).
- **Infectious agents**. Bacteria may cause cell injury either by releasing toxic chemicals (see pp. 17–23) or by eliciting cell-damaging immune responses, as in tuberculosis. Viruses too may kill cells directly (e.g. poliovirus) or via immune-mediated mechanisms.
- **Irradiation.**
- **Nutritional deficiencies.**

SITES OF INJURY

The nucleus

The cell nucleus may be altered in a number of ways.

Inherited and congenital abnormalities

Inherited abnormalities may involve **a single gene** only (as in sickle cell disease), in which case there will be no structural abnormality in the nucleus or its constituent chromosomes. In other instances, recognizable chromosomal abnormalities may be present. These may be:

- Alterations of the normal diploid number, as in Down's syndrome or one of the other trisomy syndromes which can lead to multiple congenital abnormalities. These and other chromosomally determined disorders are discussed on pp. 549–553.
- Alterations in the structure of individual chromosomes. Abnormalities may occur in the form of chromosomal breakages, as in syndromes such as **ataxia–telangiectasia** in which there are complex intertwined bundles of abnormally and permanently dilated blood vessels in the eyes and skin. This is associated with a severe immunological deficiency and such extreme radiosensitivity that even diagnostic X-rays can be followed by leukaemia. There appears to be a very close link between chromosomal breakage syndromes and an increased risk of developing leukaemia or other malignant conditions involving the lymphoid system. It is important to avoid exposure of these patients to chemical or physical agents, such as irradiation, that are known to damage DNA.

Other structural chromosomal alterations may also occur in the form of translocations or deletions of portions of chromosomes.

Toxic nuclear damage

This occurs in the treatment of malignant disease with cytotoxic drugs. Several different mechanisms operate depending on the chemotherapeutic agent used. Some, such as the alkylating agents (e.g. cyclophosphamide), combine directly with DNA; some, such as vincristine (the periwinkle

alkaloid), damage the mitotic spindle; others act as analogues of normal metabolites and block some enzyme-controlled steps in nucleic acid synthesis.

Nutritional deficiencies and nuclear damage

Nutritional damage to the nucleus may be seen in folic acid or vitamin B_{12}
deficiency, the latter being associated with pernicious anaemia. Here the
nuclei are larger than normal, but contain less DNA than is optimal for
mitosis. These changes are present in many tissues but are most prominent
among the red cell precursors in the bone marrow.

The cell membranes

Cell membranes mediate many functions. These range from maintenance of
normal osmotic relationships between the intracellular and extracellular
environments, to a variety of receptor and transduction functions. Some
inherited defects of membrane structure and function have been identified;
two examples are given below.

Transport defects

The cells of some individuals are unable to transport **lysine** and **ornithine**
across the luminal membrane of the renal tubular epithelial cell, so that these
dibasic amino acids appear in the urine in significant amounts. A similar
transport defect operates in **Hartnup's disease**, where there is a reduction in
the ability to transport tryptophan from the gut across the small intestinal
epithelium. Because tryptophan is an important source of nicotinic acid, a
deficiency of the latter develops and leads to the appearance of the clinical
signs of **pellagra**.

Receptor defects

Several membrane receptor defects have been described. A paradigm is
familial type IIa hypercholesterolaemia in which cells lack high-affinity
receptors (coded for by a gene on chromosome 19) for the cholesterol-
transporting low density lipoprotein (LDL). Failure to internalize LDL at
receptor sites leads to failure to control cell synthesis of cholesterol via its
rate-limiting enzyme 3-hydroxy-3-methylglutaryl coenzyme A (HMG CoA)
reductase, as well as failure to catabolize circulating LDL. The consequence
is a grossly raised plasma concentration of LDL cholesterol, associated
with abnormally early development of atherosclerosis and ischaemic heart
disease (*Fig. 2.1*).

If only one allele of the receptor gene is mutated, plasma cholesterol
concentrations are about twice the ideal level and there is a markedly
increased risk of coronary heart disease striking in the fifth decade.
Homozygous individuals have much higher cholesterol concentrations and
symptomatic coronary disease in the second decade of life. Transplantation
of a normal liver can normalize the plasma cholesterol concentration in these
homozygotes.

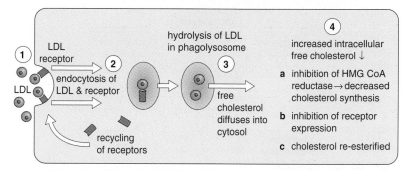

Fig 2.1   Cell biology of familial type IIa hypercholesterolaemia.

The diagram shows the course of events in normal cells that bind low density lipoprotein (LDL) at specific high-affinity receptor sites on the plasma membrane. This LDL is then endocytosed and broken down within phagolysosomes, with the consequent release of free cholesterol in the cytoplasm. The intracellular concentration of free cholesterol controls the level of activity of HMG CoA reductase. As intracellular free cholesterol rises, the enzyme is inhibited and cholesterol synthesis by the cell diminishes. Free cholesterol in the cytoplasm is esterified under the influence of acyl coenzyme A transferase. Patients with type IIa hypercholesterolaemia either lack receptors or have receptors which do not function adequately.

Complement-related membrane injury

Activation of complement (see pp. 66–69), fixed to antigen–antibody complex bound to the cell surface, leads to the generation of a **membrane attack complex** mediated by components 8 and 9 of the complement sequence of proteins. This causes focal lysis of the cell membrane and escape of the cell contents into the extracellular environment. An example of this is the red blood cell lysis that follows incompatible blood transfusions or other immune-mediated forms of haemolysis.

FREE RADICALS AND CELL INJURY

It has become increasingly clear that the formation of free radicals is the common effector pathway for a number of different types of cell injury (*Fig. 2.2*) including:

- reperfusion injury following a period of ischaemia
- certain drug-induced haemolytic anaemias
- paraquat poisoning
- carbon tetrachloride (CCl_4) poisoning
- radiation injury (as in therapeutic irradiation)
- certain cellular correlates of ageing (e.g. accumulation of lipid products within cells – lipofuscins and ceroid)
- oxygen toxicity

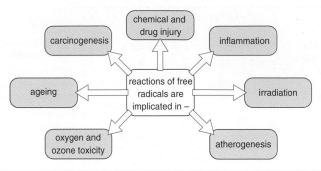

Fig. 2.2   Free radicals and cell injury.

- atherogenesis, where LDL within the arterial wall undergoes oxidative modification.

What is a free radical?

A free radical is an atom or molecule with a single unpaired electron in its outer orbital. Such chemical species are very active; not only do they react with molecules within the cell membrane, but often convert these to free radicals as well, thus forming a **positive amplification system** (*Fig. 2.3*).

Free radicals can arise in a number of ways. One is through the absorption of radiant energy. Thus the cell damage caused by therapeutic irradiation is, to a considerable extent, brought about by the generation of free radicals from cell water.

The reduction of molecular oxygen results in the gain of one rather than two electrons, forming a highly reactive anion O_2^- known as a **superoxide anion**. Superoxide anions in the presence of water undergo what is termed a 'dismutation reaction' to form hydrogen peroxide and molecular oxygen. This is catalysed by the enzyme superoxide dismutase (SOD). The generation of superoxide is an important part of our defences against bacterial infection, and bacterial killing by neutrophil leucocytes and macrophages cannot take place effectively without the formation of oxygen free radicals (see Chapter 5).

Another interesting model of free radical-mediated injury is carbon tetrachloride poisoning. CCl_4 is changed by mixed function oxidases into the free radical $CCl_3^{\cdot}$ in the smooth endoplasmic reticulum of liver cells. This leads to peroxidation of phospholipids in liver cell membranes, first in the smooth endoplasmic reticulum where CCl_4 oxidation has taken place, and later in all the intracellular membranes. If the P450 enzyme system has been induced by previous administration of barbiturates, the amount of free radical formation will be increased and the degree of cell damage will be greater than would be expected for that dose of CCl_4.

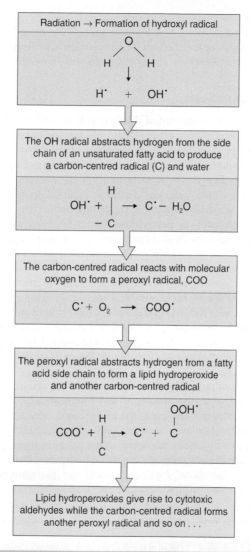

Fig. 2.3 Hydroxyl radicals damage cell membrane via a process of lipid peroxidation.

Both cells and the extracellular environment contain 'scavenging' chemical species. This suggests that generation of free radicals is a regular accompaniment of cell and tissue redox reactions and is not merely an occasional event associated with such abnormal circumstances as irradiation or poisoning. An important scavenger is the group of enzymes, the **superoxide dismutases** (SODs), whose function is the catalytic dismutation of the superoxide anion to hydrogen peroxide and molecular oxygen. SODs are so widely distributed as to suggest that the superoxide anion is an important byproduct of oxidative metabolism. Hydrogen peroxide formed by dismutation is further detoxified to water by catalases and peroxidase.

Effects of free radicals

The **peroxidation of unsaturated lipids** in cell membranes is an important effect of free radical action; other effects are damage to protein (especially thiol-containing proteins) and DNA. Membrane lipid peroxidation is associated with the formation of blebs on the plasma membrane of affected cells. The mechanisms that normally control entry of calcium to the affected cells break down and calcium deposits accumulate in mitochondria. Peroxidation is normally inhibited by hydrophobic scavengers such as **vitamin E** and **glutathione peroxidase**. Chain-breaking anti-oxidants like vitamin E are found in fresh vegetables and fruit, and it is interesting that diets high in these foodstuffs are associated with a reduced risk of atherosclerosis-related diseases and cancer.

Free radicals can also react with molecules in the ionic or water compartments of the cell. Molecules that have scavenging potential in ionic environments include reduced glutathione, ascorbic acid and cysteine. In ex vivo circumstances the importance of these scavengers can be demonstrated by depleting their concentration within isolated cells. This leads to functional and morphological changes of lipid peroxidation even though free radical generation is not increased.

The effect of free radicals depends not only on the activity of the radicals generated, but also on the structural and biochemical environment. For instance, in the extracellular space, the glycosoaminoglycans of connective tissue ground substance may be degraded by free radicals; this can contribute to destructive processes occurring in the joints in rheumatoid arthritis. So far as **plasma membranes** are concerned, uncontrolled activity of free radicals leads to membrane blebbing and failure to maintain the normal fluid and ionic relationships between the intracellular and extracellular compartments.

LYSOSOMES AND CELL INJURY

Lysosomes are involved in disease in three main ways: storage diseases, lysosomal disruption and secretion of enzymes.

Storage diseases

These result from an inherited deficiency of one of the lysosomal enzymes responsible for the normal degradation and turnover of a wide range of molecules. The non-degradable substrates accumulate in lysosomes, mainly within macrophages but also in hepatocytes, neurones, fibroblasts and renal tubular epithelium.

Carbohydrates (e.g. glycogen), complex mucopolysaccharides and a wide variety of sphingolipids are some of the molecules that may accumulate in this way, and many clinical and pathological syndromes are recognized. Cultured cells from affected individuals usually show the same metabolic abnormalities. In some instances (e.g. Hurler's syndrome, one of the mucopolysaccharidoses) the inexorable advance of the disease has been halted by transplanting bone marrow from unaffected and histocompatible donors to the affected children.

Lysosome disruption

The release of intra-lysosomal enzymes into the cell cytoplasm may cause significant damage. Lysosomal membrane rupture, mediated by a single mechanism, occurs in two apparently widely disparate diseases: **gout** and **silicosis**. In the first, neutrophils are affected; in the second, macrophages are the source of the released enzymes. In both diseases, phagocytosis of crystalline material is followed by lysosomal fusion and abnormal hydrogen bond formation between the particle surface and lysosomal membrane. This leads to rupture, and the enzyme content spills out into the cell cytoplasm and the surrounding area (*Fig. 2.4*). A florid inflammatory reaction – acute in the case of gout, chronic in silicosis – results.

Secretion of enzymes from lysosomes

Lysosomes may contribute to disease when lysosomal enzymes are secreted (usually from macrophages) into the immediate environment of these cells. The possibility that such events might be associated with the development of some forms of arthritis was mooted after the observation of Fell and colleagues that, if articular cartilage was incubated with an excess of vitamin A, the glycosaminoglycan of the matrix was destroyed, although the cartilage cells themselves appeared to be viable. In vivo, injections of large doses of vitamin A or papain, both of which render lysosomal membranes unstable, into rabbits led to a loss of the rabbits' ability to prick up their ears; the histological correlate of this was once again a loss of the complex carbohydrate in the cartilage matrix. In humans, joint fluid from patients with rheumatoid arthritis contains lysosomal enzymes. These data have been interpreted as suggesting that inappropriate release of lysosomal enzymes is an effector pathway for articular cartilage damage in the destructive arthritides.

STRESS PROTEINS IN RELATION TO CELL INJURY

Many stresses can cause an increase in the intracellular concentrations of a

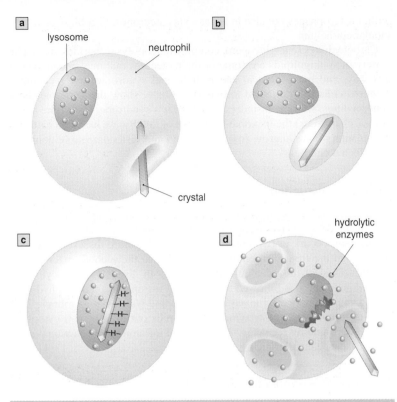

Fig. 2.4 Lysosome disruption.

Tissue injury resulting from intracytoplasmic release of lysosomal enzymes following the formation of abnormal hydrogen bonds between the lysosomal membrane and the surface of an ingested particle, as seen in gout and silicosis. **a** Phagocytosis of crystal. **b** The primary lysosome fuses with the phagosome. **c** Hydrogen bonds form between the crystal surface and the lysosome membrane. **d** As a result of this 'adhesion' between the crystal and part of the lysosomal membrane, the latter ruptures and spills its content of hydrolytic enzymes.

group of highly conserved proteins (stress proteins). A rise in temperature 5–10°C higher than is optimal for the cell type in culture is the model most often used to study stress protein release, and so this group of proteins has been given the name of **heat shock proteins** (hsps). This is a misnomer, however, because many stresses cause increases in the concentration of these proteins, including:

- fever
- ischaemia
- oxidant injury
- infection by certain microorganisms
- cancer

- a wide range of chemical species including transition metals (which cause the generation of free radicals), calcium ionophores, alcohol, metabolic poisons such as azide and various oxidants.

It is believed that this response by cells is essentially protective. These proteins not only help the cell to withstand the original stress but equip them to resist stresses even greater in severity. In the context of cardiac ischaemia, this upregulation of resistance by stress proteins is called **ischaemic preconditioning**.

Stress protein production is an example of inducible gene expression. With regard to the functions of stress proteins, it is believed that they act as **molecular chaperones** by:

- ensuring that other proteins produced by the cell are correctly folded
- taking part in the disassembly of certain oligomeric structures such as those involved in DNA replication.

Classification of stress proteins

The stress proteins are classified into four main groups according to their migratory behaviour during electrophoresis and their molecular weight (*Table 2.1*).

BACTERIAL TOXINS AND CELL INJURY

Many of the striking clinical features associated with certain bacterial infections result from the synthesis and release of highly active chemical species known as **bacterial toxins**. Some of these are the most poisonous molecules ever identified. Two kilograms of the exotoxin of *Clostridium botulinum* would be sufficient to exterminate the world's population.

Table 2.1 Stress proteins

Stress protein	Functions
hsp90	Regulates activity of other proteins by binding to them Prevents aggregation of refolding polypeptides (in vitro)
hsp70	Dissociates some oligomers Binds to extended polypeptides Has ATPase activity
hsp60 (also known as chaperonin)	Weak ATPase activity Binds to partly folded polypeptides and plays a part in their correct folding
hsp15–30	?

Classification of bacterial toxins

There are two principal groups:

- exotoxins
- endotoxin.

Their defining criteria are outlined in *Table 2.2*. The actions of bacterial endotoxin are discussed in the section on shock (pp. 389–391). Exotoxins differ functionally from endotoxin in the precision of their cellular targets. The action of an exotoxin might be likened to that of an arrow which always strikes the target at the same point. Endotoxin resembles, instead, a stone flung into a pool: although the stone makes contact with the surface of the water at one point, from this point ripples fan out in all directions and, in the same way, endotoxin produces a variety of functional perturbations brought about by the generation of many mediators.

EXOTOXINS

Exotoxins exert their effects in the following ways:

- The toxin enters the cell and acts as an intra-cellular enzyme. The commonest type of enzyme action is **irreversible adenosine 5′-diphosphate (ADP) ribosylation** in which ADP ribose is transferred from nicotinamide adenine dinucleotide (NAD) to some intracellular protein, the function of which is thus inhibited. The effects on cell function depend on which protein is ribosylated (e.g. cholera toxin, diphtheria toxin).

Table 2.2 Defining criteria of bacterial exotoxins and endotoxins

Characteristic	Exotoxin	Endotoxin
Secretion product of living microorganism	Yes	No
Part of structure of microorganism; often released from dead organisms	No	Yes
Basic chemical nature	Protein	Combination of lipid and a complex sugar (lipopolysaccharide)
Immunogenic	Yes	Weakly, if at all
Can be 'toxoided' (process by which toxic properties can be removed without impairing immunogenicity)	Yes	No
Heat labile or stable	Usually labile	Stable
Biochemical target	A precise intracellular process, membrane component or neurotransmitter	Several cell types and plasma protein cascade systems associated with inflammation

- The toxin **lyses cell membranes** enzymatically (e.g. α-toxin of *Clostridium perfringens* causing 'gas gangrene').
- The toxin **inhibits neurotransmission** (e.g. acetylcholine at the motor end-plate is blocked by the toxin of *C. botulinum*).

Toxins that ribosylate intracellular proteins

Vibrio cholerae *toxin*

Vibrio cholerae has been responsible in the past for huge numbers of deaths and still causes much disease. Cholera is characterized by the abrupt onset of **profuse, watery diarrhoea** (11–30 litres of stool every 24 hours). This causes severe dehydration and electrolyte disturbance. This devastating effect is accomplished entirely by the bacterial exotoxin; the organism itself fails to invade the tissues and remains within the gut lumen (*Fig. 2.5*).

Cholera toxin has two portions: a single A portion and a pentameric B portion. These operate by perverting a normal cell-signalling system – the adenylate cyclase system.

The adenylate cyclase system consists, functionally, of three parts:

a) The GM_1 receptor.
b) The G_s protein, which is attached by farnesyl bonds to the plasma membrane. This G protein both binds guanosine 5'-triphosphate (GTP) and can act as a GTPase, thus constituting a molecular 'on–off' switch' for signal transduction.
c) Adenylate cyclase which converts adenosine 5'-triphosphate (ATP) to adenosine 3',5'-cyclic monophosphate (cAMP).

Normal operation of the adenylate cyclase system

1) Binding of a ligand to the GM_1 receptor produces a conformational change, which exposes a binding site for the G protein.
2) By diffusion within the membrane, the G protein associates with the ligand–receptor complex and is activated to displace guanosine 5'-diphosphate (GDP) and bind GTP.
3) Binding GTP causes the α portion of the G protein to dissociate from the ligand–receptor complex and exposes a binding site on the G protein for adenylate cyclase.
4) The G protein binds to and activates adenylate cyclase, and cAMP is produced.
5) The G protein now normally hydrolyses the GTP. This returns the G protein to its inactive conformation and it dissociates from adenylate cyclase. The production of cAMP therefore ceases.

In cholera, the **B portion** of the toxin binds irreversibly to and activates the GM_1 ganglioside receptor on the luminal aspect of the small gut epithelial cell. This receptor is functionally coupled to adenylate cyclase via a stimulatory G protein, G_s. The **A portion** of cholera toxin enters the small

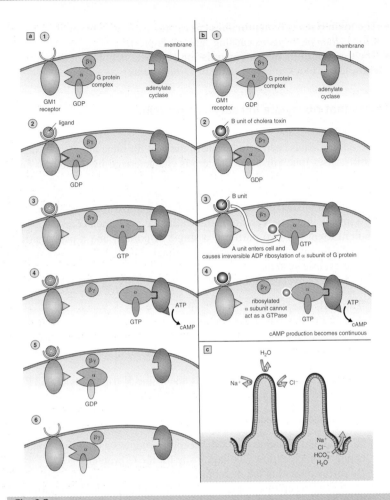

Fig. 2.5

a Activation of the adenylate cyclase system in small intestinal epithelium. (1) The inactive system showing a GM_1 receptor, a G (stimulatory) protein complex which binds GDP and adenylate cyclase. (2) Binding of a ligand to the receptor exposes a binding site for the G protein. (3) Binding of the G protein to the receptor–ligand complex causes the exchange of GDP for GTP and leads to dissociation of the α subunit of the G protein, thus exposing a binding site for adenylate cyclase. (4) The α subunit of the G protein binds to adenylate cyclase, causing activation and the production of cAMP. (5) The α subunit of the G protein now acts as a GTPase and the GTP is exchanged for GDP, leading to dissociation of the α subunit from adenylate cyclase and cessation of cAMP production. This cycle of events is repeated as long as the ligand remains bound to the receptor. It ends (6) when the ligand dissociates from the receptor and the receptor returns to its inactive configuration. **b** The irreversible ADP ribosylation of the α subunit of the G protein leads to the latter being unable to function as a GTPase. As a result, activation of adenylate cyclase continues with continuing production of cAMP. **c** Cholera toxin causes sustained production of cAMP by small gut epithelium leading to blocking of water, sodium and chloride absorption by villous cells and increased transport of water, sodium, chloride and bicarbonate into the gut lumen by crypt cells.

gut epithelial cell and irreversibly ribosylates the G protein. This inactivates its GTPase function and cAMP production thus continues in an uncontrolled manner. Such unregulated cAMP production has effects on both **villous** and **crypt** epithelial cells:

- at the villus, cAMP **inhibits entry** of water, sodium and chloride
- in the crypt, cAMP **promotes the pumping out** into the gut lumen of water, sodium, chloride and bicarbonate.

The combination of these effects causes the water and electrolyte depletion that is seen in cholera and which also occurs in the diarrhoeal illnesses caused by the heat-labile toxin of *Escherichia coli* and, interestingly, by a protein of *Rotavirus*. The latter causes millions of cases of diarrhoea annually and is responsible for 800 000–900 000 deaths per annum, mainly in young children.

Patients can be rescued from this dire state only by adequate replacement of lost water and electrolytes. As both cholera and severe infantile gastro-enteritis usually occur in populations that are both economically and socially deprived, it is important that such treatment be simple and cheap. Cholera toxin does not block the passage of glucose from the gut lumen into the gut wall, and both water and electrolyte can gain access to the gut wall in association with the glucose. The discovery of this glucose transport mechanism has formed the basis for successful oral rehydration in severe diarrhoeal illnesses.

Diphtheria toxin

Diphtheria toxin is significant in establishing infection within the pharynx because it is lethal for defending phagocytes and is the single factor responsible for severe disease in corynebacterial infections. It is extremely toxic for the cells of susceptible species: a **single molecule** is sufficient to kill that cell.

Unlike cholera toxin, which exerts its effect locally on gut epithelium, diphtheria toxin spreads within the bloodstream and affects many organs and tissues, most notably the heart, kidneys and nervous system, while the organisms themselves remain confined to the epithelium of the pharynx.

If the disease is established, treatment with neutralizing antibody (antitoxin) is mandatory. Of even greater importance is prevention of disease by actively immunizing infants with diphtheria toxoid. The toxoid retains its immunogenicity but its toxicity is removed. These preventive measures have made diphtheria rare in the West but this rarity depends on persisting with active immunization programmes. In some of the republics of the former Soviet Union, which have undergone considerable disturbance, diphtheria has once again become a common disease.

Only toxin-producing strains of *Corynebacterium diphtheriae* (toxigenic strains) cause diphtheria; non-toxigenic strains cause a mild sore throat only. Toxigenicity is conferred by a bacterial virus (bacteriophage), which possesses the gene encoding the toxin, being incorporated into the genome of the corynebacterium. This situation, where an inserted phage codes for toxin production by a bacterium, also occurs in the case of the toxin of *Clostridium botulinum* types C and D, the toxin of *C. novyi* and the erythrogenic toxin of β-haemolytic streptococci.

tox gene expression is normally regulated by a corynebacterial repressor protein which binds to the tox gene in the presence of ferrous iron. If intra-bacterial iron concentrations fall, production of the toxin commences. In mutant strains of *C. diphtheriae* that cannot produce the repressor protein, toxin production proceeds uninfluenced by the intra-cellular iron concentration.

Like the toxin of *V. cholerae*, diphtheria toxin consists of two portions: one binds to a receptor on the plasma membranes of target cells; the other enters the cells and irreversibly ribosylates a protein known as elongation factor 2 (EF-2). EF-2 plays a vital part in translation of messenger RNA within the ribosomes. Once ribosylated it cannot perform its normal function, and protein synthesis within the affected cell ceases.

Toxins that damage cell membranes

Several toxins cause cell injury in this way. They include:

- the α-toxin of *C. perfringens* which causes gas gangrene (see pp. 44–45)
- haemolysins produced by *Staphylococcus aureus*
- haemolysins produced by *Streptococcus pyogenes*.

The tissue damage occurring in gas gangrene is an archetype of this variety of toxin-mediated injury. It is caused by the α-toxin of *C. perfringens*; this molecule acts as a lecithinase and cleaves the phospholipids in the plasma membrane of affected cells.

Clostridia are strictly anaerobic, Gram-positive, spore-forming bacilli. They multiply in deep wounds where there is abundant devitalized tissue and resulting low oxygen tension. Thus, gas gangrene has been most commonly seen in military practice where deep wounds, associated with much tissue destruction, become contaminated by soil driven into the tissues. In civilian practice, gas gangrene is most likely to occur where above-knee amputation has been carried out because of severe lower limb ischaemia (see p. 45). Stumps in which the flaps are at the margin of viability because of poor arterial perfusion may become contaminated by *Clostridia* derived from the patient's own large gut (auto-infection).

The presence of the toxin in material derived from wounds can be demonstrated by its lecithin-splitting properties. If cultures are set up using agar plates that incorporate egg yolk, toxin causes the appearance of an opaque zone of diglyceride in relation to the organisms (Nagler's reaction).

Toxins that interfere with neuro-transmission

Only two organisms produce toxins that act in this way: *C. botulinum* and *C. tetani*.

Botulinum toxin

The toxin of *C. botulinum* is one of the most toxic substances known: a dose of 1 μg is lethal to humans. The toxin is preformed in contaminated foods and then ingested by the victims. Unlike all the other forms of toxin-related injury discussed here, it is *not* necessary for an affected individual to be infected by the organism: a very small amount of the toxin suffices.

Botulinum toxin exists in eight antigenic forms (A, B, C1, C2, D, E, F and G), each produced by a different strain of *Clostridia*. Botulism in humans is caused by toxins A, B, E and F; toxin type A accounts for about 60% of cases. Toxin A may occur in preserved fruits, vegetables and meat; B is usually found in meat and E in uncooked sea-food.

The toxin is carried in the bloodstream to peripheral neuromuscular junctions where it blocks transmission of acetylcholine (ACh) by inhibiting its release from nerve terminals. The inevitable result is flaccid paralysis of the affected muscles, which may be widespread and is particularly lethal if muscles used in breathing are affected. This action of the botulinum neurotoxin in blocking ACh transmission has led to use of the toxin as a therapeutic agent in certain dystonic disorders such as vocal cord spasm, eyelid spasm and spasmodic torticollis. Local injection of toxin at affected sites causes paralysis which lasts for about 3 months.

Tetanus toxin

C. tetani produces two toxins; the one responsible for the muscle spasms and contracture characteristic of tetanus is known as **tetanospasmin**.

The organisms most often enter the tissues as a result of deep penetrating wounds. In some parts of Africa neonatal tetanus occurs when the umbilical stumps of neonates are anointed with cow dung (a rich source of *Clostridia*). If the organisms can multiply within the tissues, the toxin they release enters the motor nerve fibres by binding to ganglioside receptors and then travels in a cephalad direction up the axons until the anterior horn cells of the spinal cord are reached. The toxin acts by blocking transmission of **glycine** from inhibitory interneurones. This leads to over-excitability of the motor neurones, expressed in the form of spasms, rigidity and trismus (lockjaw).

RADIATION AND CELL INJURY

All forms of radiation may be harmful to living cells. This fact underlies the use of irradiation in the treatment of certain malignant neoplasms. All of us are exposed to a certain amount of background radiation due to:

- **cosmic radiation** derived from the sun and outer space; the higher the altitude, the greater the exposure
- **radioactive elements** in the earth's crust (radium is the best-known example)
- certain naturally occurring **radionuclides** present within the body.

About 80% of the annual dose of ionizing radiation that we receive comes from these sources. The remainder comes from:

- radiation in **medical diagnosis and treatment**
- radioactive **minerals** in fertilizers and certain building materials
- **nuclear fall-out**
- **domestic products** such as television sets and smoke detectors.

THE NATURE OF RADIATION

Basically, radiation is of two types: electromagnetic and particulate.

Electromagnetic radiation

This represents energy that is propagated by wave motion. Forms of electromagnetic radiation that are relevant from the biological viewpoint include γ- and X-rays. γ-Rays are emitted spontaneously from radioactive materials; X-rays are produced artificially. These forms have a short wavelength and are of high frequency. These attributes are associated with sufficient energy to ionize the materials through which they pass.

Particulate radiation

This is brought about by the movement of sub-atomic particles. It occurs either because of the decay of radioactive substances or as a result of the acceleration of sub-atomic particles to very high speeds (e.g. in a cyclotron).

The radiation dose is measured in rads – 1 rad results in the absorption of 100 ergs of energy per gram of absorbing substance; 100 rads = 1 Gray (Gy)

THE BIOLOGICAL RESPONSE TO RADIATION

The biological response of cells and tissue to radiation depends on the interaction of:

- physical factors
- chemical factors
- biological factors.

Physical factors.   These include the total dose of radiation, the character of the radiation and the time over which administration occurs.

Chemical factors.   These may serve either to protect cells against radiation damage or to potentiate that damage. The most active potentiating agent is molecular oxygen, which serves as a substrate for the generation of tissue-damaging oxygen free radicals (see pp. 11–14). Thus, in the treatment of certain malignant tumours, attempts are made to increase oxygen tension within tumours by hyperbaric oxygen therapy before irradiation. Chemical species, such as sulphydryl groups, that act as free radical scavengers tend to protect cells against radiation damage.

Biological factors. These are complex and incompletely understood. An important consideration is the point during the cell cycle when exposure to radiation occurs. Cells are most sensitive during the G2 phase (between DNA synthesis and mitosis) and during mitosis, and least sensitive during the S phase (when DNA is being synthesized). Thus cells that are undergoing rapid division are likely to be more radiosensitive than those in which turnover is slow. Sublethal radiation injury can be repaired and the differing ability of cells to accomplish this is clearly related to their degree of radiosensitivity.

The relative sensitivity of normal organs and tissues to radiation is shown in *Table 2.3*.

Acute, potentially lethal, damage occurs after a single dose of whole body irradiation of sufficient strength

A single dose of irradiation about 10 000 times the average daily background exposure (0.001 rad) is required before any functional or morphological changes occur. At this point (10 rad) specific functional and morphological abnormalities are noted in certain lymphocyte sub-populations.

- **100 rad.** This causes radiation sickness of mild degree associated with nausea and vomiting. The rate of division in haemopoietic cells decreases and there is a short-lived lymphopenia.

Table 2.3   Relative radiosensitivity of various organs and tissues

Very high	High	Intermediate	Low
Bone marrow	Kidney	Adult bone	Uterus
Testis	Liver	Adult cartilage	Vagina
Ovary	Lung	Mucosa of mouth	Pancreas
Breast (in childhood)	Heart	Oesophagus	Adrenal
Growing cartilage	Growing bone	Bladder	
Lens	Small bowel		
	Colon		
	Thyroid		
	Cornea		
	Pituitary		
	Spinal cord		
	Growing muscle		
	Salivary gland		
	Brain		
	Skin		
	Rectum		

- **1000 rad.** This causes severe necrosis in the haemopoietic stem cell compartment with resulting pancytopenia. There is extensive loss of gut epithelium. This is severe radiation sickness, death occurring usually within 2 weeks.
- **10 000 rad.** This causes severe disturbances in central nervous system function. Death occurs within hours.
- **100 000 rad.** This dose kills most cells; death within minutes is likely.

Radiation effects in specific tissues

Blood vessels

Blood vessel damage is a common and important component of both acute and delayed irradiation damage. Acutely, there is dilatation and increased permeability of both arterioles and capillaries, this is manifest as skin reddening (erythema) and oedema. At a slightly later stage endothelial cells undergo necrosis and there may be patchy necrosis of the smooth muscle cells of arterioles.

Months or years after exposure small blood vessels may still show damage. Depending on the part of the vascular bed affected, various secondary effects may occur:

- atrophic changes in the skin, often associated with scarring of the sub-epidermal tissue
- interstitial scarring in the myocardium
- ulcer formation in the gut
- renal cortical atrophy associated with interstitial tissue scarring
- necrosis of white matter in the brain associated with increase in glial fibres; spinal cord damage.

Skin

In the early stages (up to 4 weeks after exposure) there is likely to be erythema, loss of hair and dryness (due to death of hair follicle cells and sebaceous glands). Delayed injury is characterized by some degree of atrophy, dilatation of blood vessels, hyperkeratosis and a marked degree of homogenization of the dermal collagen.

Haemopoietic and lymphoid systems

These are very sensitive to radiation. Large doses of radiation cause severe lymphopenia, and a decrease in the size of spleen and lymph nodes. In sublethal irradiation, recovery takes place. In the long term, severe irradiation may cause leukaemia as demonstrated by the increased risk seen in survivors of the nuclear attacks on Japanese cities in 1945 and in nuclear accidents.

Heart

Radiation affects the heart of 2–9% of patients who receive treatment to the mediastinum for lymphoma and about 3% of those irradiated because of breast carcinoma. The most common expression of cardiac damage is peri-carditis, which often goes on to scarring, thus producing constriction of the underlying myocardium. Interstitial fibrosis may also occur, and is attributed to vascular damage (see above).

Lung

A dose of 35–40 Gy administered in 3 to 40 fractions produces radiation pneumonitis in 10–15% of patients receiving irradiation to the chest area, usually about 8–15 weeks after exposure.

Alveolar capillary damage leads to oedema of the inter-alveolar septa. At a slightly later stage the epithelial cells lining the air spaces (alveolar pneumo-cytes types 1 and 2) are affected. Necrosis and desquamation of the type 1 cells occurs and type 2 cells tend to proliferate. The damaged air spaces often show an eosinophilic membrane plastered down on their walls (hyaline membrane). This is a non-specific sign of respiratory distress syndrome. Later (after 16 weeks) interstitial scarring develops, which causes restrictive lung disease.

All forms of radiation-induced lung damage carry an increased risk for the subsequent development of malignancy within the lung.

Gastro-intestinal tract

The mouth shows evidence of radiation damage very early after therapeutic irradiation of the head and neck. Changes in the oral mucosa are similar to those described in the skin. Damage to the salivary glands leading to scarring and loss of secretory acini may cause permanent dryness of the mouth.

The principal change encountered in the rest of the gastro-intestinal tract is denudation of surface epithelium. This occurs because radiation decreases the regenerative ability of the stem cell precursors of intestinal epithelial cells. The normal rate of loss of mature epithelial lining cells is not com-pensated for by the generation of new cells, and large areas of shallow ulceration result.

In the long term, strictures, chronic ulcers, fistulae and neoplasms may complicate irradiation of the gut. The small gut, colon and rectum are most commonly affected and it is believed that the most potent mechanism involved in long-term damage is radiation-mediated injury to small gut wall blood vessels.

Liver

Doses of 40 Gy or more are required before clinically obvious liver damage occurs. This usually manifests about 3 months after exposure. The principal anatomical target is the venous drainage of the liver. The endothelial cells of these vessels swell and in some cases die. This is associated with fibrin deposition within the vessel lumina. If the fibrin is not lysed, collagen strands grow into the vessels and obstruct their lumina. This situation (veno-occlusive disease) is not specific for radiation injury and also occurs in association with liver damage caused by certain chemical poisons. The end-result is congestion and, ultimately, necrosis, in the central part of the liver lobule (acinus zone 3).

Radiation-induced liver tumours have also been reported, particularly following the use of thorium dioxide, an α particle-emitting imaging material. This collects in the fixed macrophages in the liver (Küpffer cells) and can cause significant local changes including malignant neoplasms of the liver cells, bile ductules and blood vessels.

Endocrine system
Tumours have been reported following radiation in all endocrine glands. The thyroid is by far the most commonly affected, thyroid carcinomas having been reported in survivors of nuclear fall-out and in individuals who received therapeutic irradiation during childhood.

The skeleton
The risk of radiation damage occurring in the skeleton depends largely on the age of the individual at the time of exposure. Growing cartilage and bone are radiosensitive; adult bone and cartilage are relatively resistant. Many cases of malignant neoplasm of bone following radium exposure have been reported.

Testis and ovary
The germinal epithelium in both sexes is very sensitive to irradiation. Acute radiation damage is expressed in the form of suppression of meiosis in both ovary and testis. This is followed by necrosis of germinal epithelium, the spermatogonia being most severely affected. Recovery tends to be slow.

Urinary tract
The urinary **bladder** is very susceptible to radiation injury. Acute damage is expressed as suppression of regenerative activity of epithelial stem cells, and this leads inevitably to ulceration. Scarring in the deeper portions of the bladder wall is an important and clinically most disadvantageous complication because the bladder's capacity may be greatly reduced. This leads to a crippling degree of increased frequency of micturition.

In the **kidney**, radiation may cause vasodilatation, oedema of the interstitium and some degree of loss of the normal molecular sieving functions of the glomeruli, leading to proteinuria. Functional recovery from this phase is the rule, but after a long latent period progressive scarring of glomeruli and consequent loss of tubules may occur.

Breast
Irradiation of the breast is associated with an increased risk of breast cancer, the peak incidence occurring 15–20 years after exposure.

Nervous system
The mature nervous system is moderately resistant to acute radiation-

mediated injury. Both the brain and spinal cord show necrosis associated with a degree of myelin loss. These changes are believed to be secondary to small blood vessel damage. In the spinal cord, severe post-irradiation damage may be expressed clinically in the form of paraplegia.

As in many other tissues, radiation increases the risk of subsequent malignancy.

Eye

The principal target for radiation damage to the eye is the lens. Opacities develop in the substance of the lens and may progress to full-blown cataracts.

SOME MORPHOLOGICAL EXPRESSIONS OF CELL INJURY

Injury can often be correlated with morphological changes within the affected cells. The pathological literature of the nineteenth and early twentieth centuries abounds with graphic, but rather meaningless, descriptive terms for cell injury such as cloudy swelling or hyaline (glassy) degeneration.

Sub-lethal cell injury is usually manifested by:

- alterations in cell volume (**acute cellular oedema**)
- accumulation of excess triglyceride (**fatty change**).

CHANGES IN CELL VOLUME

The control of volume within fairly narrow limits is characteristic of mammalian cells. This control is exerted largely by energy-dependent sodium and potassium transport mechanisms, linked with membrane-bound enzymes.

If these mechanisms break down, large amounts of isotonic fluid collect within the cell and increase its volume. The mitochondria swell; it is for this reason that, on light microscopic examination, the cytoplasm appears granular. This increase in intracellular fluid content, or **acute cellular oedema**, occurs particularly if the cells become **hypoxic**, but also in the course of fever or cell injury by certain bacterial toxins and chemical poisons.

Normal cells have a higher potassium and a lower sodium content than extracellular fluid. These differentials in respect of sodium and potassium are maintained by the ATP energy-dependent membrane transport system called the **sodium pump**; part of this system is the ouabain-sensitive ATPase within the plasma membrane of the cell.

Hypoxia and the other forms of cell injury mentioned above cause a decrease in ATP production, and the ratio of ATP to ADP thus falls significantly. This leads to partial failure of the sodium pump. Potassium ions diffuse out of the cell into the extracellular fluid, and the reverse applies to sodium ions, which enter the cell in large amounts. Because the hydration shell of sodium is greater than that of potassium, water enters the cells from the extracellular fluid as well. This will, of course, lead to an increase in cell volume.

The effects of hypoxia on the cell involve the following sequence of events (*Fig. 2.6*).

1) As the oxygen tension falls, mitochondrial phosphorylation decreases rapidly with a consequent fall in ATP.
2) This drop in ATP stimulates the activity of the enzyme **phospho-fructokinase**.
3) This leads to an increase in the rate of anaerobic glycolysis.
4) This, in turn, causes an accumulation of lactate which, together with the increase in inorganic phosphate concentration, decreases the intracellular pH. Morphologically this is believed to be reflected in the appearance of clumping of the nuclear chromatin.

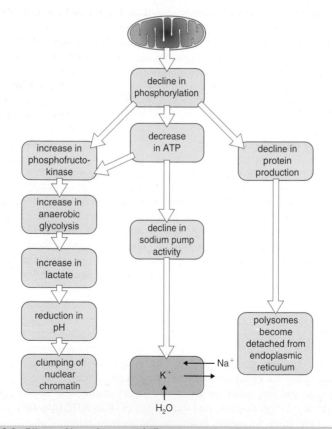

Fig. 2.6   Effects of hypoxia on metabolic events within cells.

5) At this point the decline in ATP will have produced its effect on the sodium pump, and the accumulation of sodium and water mentioned above takes place.
6) Protein production is also adversely affected at this stage, expressed in morphological terms by **detachment of polysomes** from the membranes of the endoplasmic reticulum and scattering of both free and bound polysomes into monomeric ribosomes.

At this stage the process is still reversible: both function and structure of the protein-secreting apparatus can be brought back to normal if the cell's oxygen supply is restored. By now the cytoskeleton also appears to be affected and the plasma membrane of the cells may show blebs or the appearance of microvilli. If hypoxia continues, the degree of cell damage may reach a point at which restoration of normal structure and function cannot occur and the cell will die.

1) The mitochondria become markedly swollen and accumulate dense flocculent material (probably calcium and lipid), and the intracellular membranes become fragmented.
2) Nuclear chromatin starts to undergo attack by enzymes (presumably of lysosomal origin) and as this proceeds the nucleus becomes digested away (this is known as **karyolysis**; see p. 38).
3) At this stage not only is there equilibration between extracellular and intracellular ionic concentrations, but other molecules begin to move freely across the plasma membrane so that dyes in the extracellular fraction can move into the cell, while the cell's own enzymes leak out (*Fig. 2.7*). This alteration in plasma membrane permeability can constitute a valuable marker of cell injury in the patient. For example, **death of cardiac muscle cells** is associated with the release into extracellular fluid, and then into plasma, of intracellular enzymes such as **creatine kinase** and **β-hydroxybutyric acid dehydrogenase**. The plasma concentrations of these enzymes can be monitored in patients with a suspected diagnosis of ischaemic damage to the myocardium and can provide an additional method for assessing whether the degree of ischaemic damage is increasing. Raised plasma concentrations of **aspartate** and **alanine amino-transferases** similarly provide a valuable marker for **liver cell injury**.

PARENCHYMAL CELL FATTY CHANGE: ACCUMULATION OF EXCESS TRIGLYCERIDE

Fatty change is the term applied when parenchymal cells, notably those of the **liver**, **heart** and **kidney**, contain stainable triglyceride. On microscopic examination the fat may be seen either as small droplets or, if these coalesce, as large single drops which occupy most of the cell area and push the remaining cytoplasmic contents and nucleus to the cell edge. In conventionally prepared tissue sections, which must be dehydrated in alcohol and

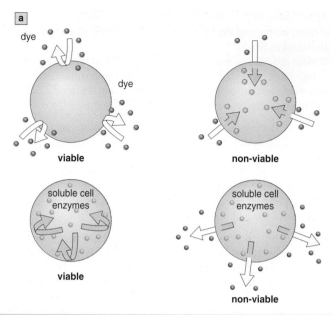

Fig. 2.7   Lethal cell injury.

Lethal damage to cells is associated with change in permeability of the cell plasma membrane. The viable cell normally excludes dye molecules in the incubating medium. Lethal injury is associated with staining of the cells. Similarly, water-soluble intracellular enzymes do not leak out of a viable cell, but lethal cell damage is associated with escape of such enzymes into the intracellular fluid. The concentration of these enzymes can be monitored in samples of plasma.

'cleared' in various organic solvents before being embedded in paraffin wax, the fat droplets are dissolved away to leave intracytoplasmic spaces. Therefore, the presence of triglyceride cannot be confirmed by staining. The fat can, however, be demonstrated by cutting sections from blocks of tissue that have been frozen rapidly. Dyes that dissolve preferentially in triglyceride, such as mixtures of Sudan III and IV or Oil-Red O, will then stain the fat-containing droplets a bright orange-red.

Macroscopic features

Organs affected by severe fatty change are a pale yellowish-brown and may feel greasy.

In the **liver**, the degree of fat accumulation may be so great that blocks of tissue float in water or fixative solutions. The distribution of fat is usually diffuse in the organ as a whole, although not necessarily in individual liver acini.

In the **kidney**, fatty change shows up as a series of yellowish streaks in the cortex, as the accumulation of fat is non-uniform and tends to be confined to epithelial cells lining the convoluted tubules.

In the **heart**, severe fatty change is commonly seen as a pale and rather flabby myocardium. However, the fatty change sometimes seen in patients suffering from chronic anaemia produces a curious striped appearance, which is most obvious in the subendocardial layer of the inter-ventricular septum in the papillary muscles. In a rare departure from the well-known tendency of morbid anatomists to characterize morphological alterations in terms of food, this appearance has been called 'tabby cat' or 'thrush-breast' striation.

Origin of the excess intracellular triglyceride

The fat accumulating in affected cells is derived largely from adipose tissue stores; it does not appear as a result of some 'unmasking' of fat already present within the cell. A variety of experimental models show this. For example, if an animal is poisoned with phosphorus it develops acute liver damage associated with severe fatty change. Starving the animal before administration of the phosphorus, with resulting depletion of adipose tissue fat stores, prevents development of the fatty change, even though the liver cell damage occurs as before. Similarly cells grown in culture can accumulate triglyceride only if triglyceride is present in the culture medium.

The causes of triglyceride accumulation within liver cells

The liver occupies a central place in fat metabolism; disorders (including various types of poisoning) that result in hepatic fatty change can be understood most easily in terms of disturbance of the various processes related to fat metabolism.

The liver cell normally receives fat in two forms and from two sources:

1) non-esterified **free fatty acid** (FFA), released from adipose tissue stores by lipolysis
2) the **chylomicron**, a large molecule synthesized within the small intestinal epithelium and consisting of triglyceride (90%), phospholipid and apoproteins B, C and E.

If apoprotein B cannot be synthesized, then chylomicrons cannot be assembled and triglyceride derived from the diet accumulates within the intestinal epithelium (abetalipoproteinaemia). In the blood vessels draining the intestine, chylomicrons are acted on by a lipoprotein lipase, which removes some of the triglyceride. This is then either used to provide energy in muscle or stored in adipose tissue. The remaining portion of the chylomicron (remnant particle) binds to a receptor on the liver cells (the ligand being apoprotein E) and is internalized by the liver cell.

Within the liver cell, hydrolysis of the chylomicron remnants takes place, liberating FFAs and glycerol. Acetate, from which additional FFAs can be synthesized, is also present within the liver cell. Irrespective of their origin, most of the FFAs are esterified to form triglyceride, some are incorporated into phospholipid, and others into cholesterol esters. The triglyceride within the liver cell, which is kept in the form of a micelle by phospholipid, is then coupled to a lipid-acceptor protein or apoprotein and secreted from the liver in the form of very low density lipoprotein (VLDL).

KEY POINTS

Accumulation of triglyceride in the liver
It should therefore be clear that accumulation of excess triglyceride may reflect either one or both of the following:

- an increase in the amount of lipid being brought to the liver, particularly in the form of non-esterified fatty acids (NEFAs)
- an inability of the liver cell to carry out the functions outlined above if a normal amount of lipid is delivered to it.

High NEFA levels in the presence of normal liver cells

High plasma concentrations of NEFAs in the presence of normal liver cells occur when there is a decrease in the energy normally supplied by carbohydrates. Increased fat catabolism is needed to make up for the energy shortfall, leading to lipolysis of adipose tissue fat and a rise in the plasma concentration of FFAs. This occurs:

- in **starvation**
- where there is a block in normal carbohydrate metabolism, such as in **uncontrolled diabetes mellitus**, **galactosaemia** and some forms of **glycogen storage disease**.

Normal plasma NEFA levels in the presence of injury or abnormality of liver cells

Because of the many functions carried out by liver cells in respect of the FFAs delivered to the liver, the number of ways in which liver cell injury causes fatty change is correspondingly great. Relevant modes of injury include:

- anoxia due to severe congestive cardiac failure
- severe protein and calorie undernutrition
- chronic alcholism
- other chemical and bacterial toxins.

Anoxia due to severe congestive cardiac failure.   The cells first affected are those in the centrilobular zone. This gives the affected organ a mottled red and yellow appearance known as '**nutmeg liver**'.

Severe protein and calorie undernutrition (known as **kwashiorkor** when seen in children).   In this condition, the liver cell (because of a shortage of the necessary amino acid substrates) is not able to synthesize the lipid-acceptor proteins needed for the export of triglyceride in the form of VLDL. Triglyceride accumulation may be so great that post mortem samples of liver float in water or aqueous fixatives. Sequential liver biopsy shows that fatty change of this type is completely reversible by a diet containing adequate amounts of protein.

Chronic alcoholism.   This is one of the commonest causes of significant hepatic fatty change in over-privileged Western communities. The metabolic effects on the liver cell of ingestion of excess amounts of alcohol are complex. The substitution of large amounts of alcohol for part of the diet in healthy non-alcoholic volunteers quickly produces hepatic fatty change. Interference with **oxidation of fatty acids** is likely to be the most important cause of intracellular triglyceride accumulation in alcoholics, but there may also be an associated **hyperlipidaemia** (Frederickson type V) characterized by a rise in plasma triglyceride concentrations.

Other chemical and bacterial toxins.   Many chemicals are capable of inducing hepatic fatty change both in humans and experimental animals. These include CCl_4, puromycin, ethionine and phosphorus, to name only a few. The fact that CCl_4 can damage liver cells through the generation of free radicals has been mentioned earlier. There is some evidence that the metabolic events associated with this, which lead to the death of liver cells, are different from those that result in the accumulation of fat within the liver cell. CCl_4 reduces protein synthesis by the liver, and it is suggested that fat accumulates because of lack of synthesis of enough lipid-acceptor protein. However, work with other models such as **orotic acid** poisoning has shown that inhibition of protein secretion is not a prerequisite for intracellular fat accumulation; the fault may be, at least in the early stages, a **failure of coupling** between triglyceride and lipid-acceptor protein.

Decline in protein synthesis

The decline in protein synthesis associated with some examples of both toxic and non-toxic hepatic fatty change may be brought about in various ways. For example, **puromycin**, an antibiotic with a structure resembling the terminal portion of transfer RNA, is a powerful inhibitor of protein synthesis in the rat. Inhibition is accomplished by a decrease in the rate of transcription of ribosomal RNA, this being associated with a later effect on RNA maturation.

Ethionine, on the other hand, decreases protein secretion by acting as a drain on hepatic ATP. This is because ethionine, which is the ethyl analogue of the amino acid methionine, competes successfully with the latter for ATP and combines with the ATP to form *S*-adenosyl-ethionine plus inorganic orthophosphate. *S*-adenosyl-ethionine is inactive with respect to the transfer of methyl groups and simply acts as an adenosyl trap. Hepatic ATP is thus drained and there is a consequent reduction in messenger RNA synthesis, a break-up of polyribosomes and a decline in protein synthesis.

CELL INJURY AND ITS MANIFESTATIONS

- Cells unable to adapt to environmental change show structural and functional changes (**injury**).
- **Cell death** results if these changes are irreversible.
- In sub-lethal injury common structural changes includes increases in cell volume (cellular oedema) and accumulation of fat.
- There are many **causes** of cell injury:
  — trauma
  — extremes of temperature
  — radiation
  — bacterial toxins
  — chemical poisons
  — enzymes released from lysosomes
  — immune-mediated mechanisms
  — hypoxia
  — anoxia and re-oxygenation
  — nutritional deficiencies.
- A common **mechanism** is free radical-mediated damage. Free radicals are highly reactive chemical species with unpaired electrons in the outer orbital. They damage DNA, proteins and cell membranes (via peroxidation of lipids), and react with intracellular water. Free radicals operate in the context of drug and radiation injury, ageing, atherogenesis and oxygen toxicity.

3 Cell and tissue death

If micro-environmental changes are such that cells cannot achieve a new steady state, the integrated functions break down and these cells die. We must remember that cell death can be a normal phenomenon and some cell populations have a high turnover. Nevertheless, in many diseases, cell death causes the characteristic clinical picture, and the extent of such cell death may determine the outcome.

The character of a disease is often determined by the **type of cell** that dies. In poliomyelitis the anterior horn cells of the spinal cord are the targets for destruction by the poliovirus. The patient thus develops a lower motor neurone type of paralysis in muscles whose motor nerve supply is related to the affected neurones. Many other such examples could be given.

The **extent of cell death** has a significant effect on the natural history of disease. In **myocardial infarction**, if more than 35% of the muscle cells die, pump failure occurs with a sudden and severe fall in cardiac output.

MORPHOLOGICAL CHANGES IN CELL DEATH

Cell death may be defined, in physiological terms, as the *irreversible breakdown of the energy-dependent functions of the cell*. For the histopathologist, cell death means the series of morphological changes occurring in a cell or group of cells following lethal injury. The differences between functional and structural cell death are the expression of:

- elapsed **time** since the injury
- the unfettered action of **enzymatic degradation** and/or **protein denaturation**.

Thus the cells of a piece of tissue removed at operation or biopsy and placed immediately in fixative are dead but show no structural abnormalities indicating cell death. The appearances of dead cells vary depending on which of the two processes – enzymatic digestion or protein denaturation – is dominant. Some degree of enzymatic degradation is nearly always present, and is manifested by various nuclear and cytoplasmic changes.

AUTOLYSIS

If enzymatic degradation dominates, then dead cells are likely to be removed completely. This process is accomplished by activation of enzymes normally present within affected cells. The process of **self-digestion** is known as autolysis.

Microscopic features

The **cytoplasm** shows decreased basophilia (indicating loss of RNA and protein) and an increased affinity for acid dyes like eosin (eosinophilia). This increased eosinophilia is due to denaturation of some of the cytoplasmic proteins with exposure of basic groups that bind the eosin.

Irreversible damage to the **nucleus** shows itself in one of three patterns:

1) **pyknosis**: the nucleus shrinks and becomes intensely basophilic
2) **karyorrhexis**: the nucleus undergoes fragmentation
3) **karyolysis**: there is a gradual fading away of the basophilic nuclear material, presumably as a result of the activity of DNases.

The immediate result of these changes (as seen in haematoxylin and eosin stained sections) is a highly eosinophilic cell that has lost its nucleus. Its survival in this form depends on whether further enzymatic digestion takes place. The enzymes are derived largely from lysosomes. The factors that lead to activation and release of lysosomal enzymes are not known, but it is likely that decreased intracellular pH is important. Release of lysosomal enzymes can be inferred from the following:

- ultracentrifugal fractionation of dead cells shows that lysosomal enzymes are no longer particle-bound but present in the supernatant
- there is evidence of enzymatic digestion of cell components in the form of loss of DNA and RNA protein and glycogen.

HETEROLYSIS

If enzymatic digestion is accomplished 'from outside', the process is termed heterolysis. Here the enzymes are derived from the lysosomes of cells such as neutrophils or macrophages. Heterolysis may occur as a result of **endocytosis**, in which phagocytes ingest portions of dead or dying cells and segregate them into phagocytic vacuoles (**phagosomes**). The phagocyte lysosomes then fuse with the phagosomes to form secondary lysosomes in which digestion of the ingested cell occurs. However, phagocytosis is not an absolute prerequisite for heterolysis, which can occur because of local release of lysosomal enzymes by phagocytes.

APOPTOSIS (PROGRAMMED CELL DEATH)

Cell turnover implies that all the fully differentiated cells populating a given tissue must die and be replaced in a controlled and 'programmed' manner. The term apoptosis (literally a 'dropping off', as in relation to petals and leaves) has been suggested for this controlled type of cell deletion. Apoptosis plays a role opposing that of mitosis in regulating the size of cell populations.

Apoptosis differs from necrosis

In contrast with necrosis there is *no*:

- breakdown in the mechanisms supplying cellular energy
- failure in the maintenance of normal cell volume
- rupture of plasma membranes
- acute inflammatory reaction elicited by the death.

The process:

- is energy dependent
- involves protein synthesis.

MORPHOLOGICAL CHANGES IN APOPTOSIS (*Fig. 3.1*)

In structural terms apoptosis appears to take place in clearly defined stages:

- The affected cell separates from its neighbours.
- Characteristically the nuclear chromatin becomes condensed, and well-defined masses of chromatin form under the nuclear membrane.
- The cell then breaks up into a number of membrane-bound, ultra-structurally well-preserved, fragments (**apoptotic bodies**).
- These fragments are then either shed from epithelium-lined surfaces or are phagocytosed by other cells, where they undergo a series of changes resembling *in vitro* autolysis within phagosomes. This phagocytosis must involve a ligand–receptor interaction between the apoptotic bodies and the cells that engulf them; this is discussed in the section on effector mechanisms (pp. 41–42).

Microscopically, apoptosis is usually inconspicuous. This is because of the short duration of the process as it affects a single cell (1–2 hours or less). Accurate assessment of the extent of apoptosis in tissue sections requires several thousand normal cells to be inspected, as the proportion of recognizable apoptotic cells is less than 1%. Because they are recognizable for so short a time, even a small proportion of recognizable apoptotic cells may indicate major reductions in cell population.

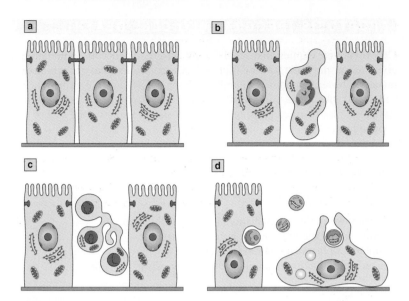

Fig. 3.1   Programmed cell death (apoptosis).

a Normal. **b** The middle cell shrinks away from its neighbours. The nuclear chromatin is condensed along the nuclear membrane, forming well-defined masses. The organelles, however, show no evidence of damage. **c** The affected cell now breaks up into several membrane-bound, ultrastructurally well-preserved, fragments (apoptotic bodies). **d** These are then engulfed either by neighbouring parenchymal cells or macrophages. Some apoptotic bodies are shed from epithelial surfaces in large numbers (e.g. in the small gut lining).

APOPTOSIS IS INVOLVED IN BOTH PHYSIOLOGICAL AND PATHOLOGICAL PROCESSES AFFECTING THE CONTROL OF CELL POPULATIONS

Apoptosis is involved not only in cell turnover in many healthy adult tissues but also in the focal elimination of certain cells during normal embryonic development. It occurs spontaneously in some untreated malignant neoplasms and also in some types of therapeutically induced regression of malignant tumours. It is implicated in both physiological involution and atrophy of various tissues and organs:

- **organogenesis during embryonic life** (e.g. in the separation of digits during limb development)
- **elimination of effete cells** in cell populations with a high turnover, such as small gut epithelium
- **cell death following the removal of hormonal stimuli** (e.g. in the endometrial shedding phase of the menstrual cycle)
- **clonal elimination of lymphocytes that might otherwise react with 'self' antigens** and thus lead to autoimmune disease

- **atrophy of hormone-dependent tissues** after removal of the stimulating hormone (e.g. the prostate after orchidectomy)
- **atrophy of the secretory epithelial component** in exocrine glands after **prolonged duct obstruction** (e.g. the salivary and lacrimal glands and pancreas)
- **spontaneous elimination of part of the cell population in certain tumours**
- **viral damage to cells** – this is seen in certain types of viral hepatitis
- **cytotoxic T lymphocyte-mediated cell death**, as in graft rejection
- **preventing genome instability** from developing in cells in which there has been some damage to the genome (p. 507).
- **cell death associated with low doses of certain injurious stimuli** including therapeutic irradiation, cytotoxic drugs used to treat cancer, and heat.

EFFECTOR MECHANISMS IN APOPTOSIS

These mechanisms include:

- chromatin condensation
- insoluble proteins
- proteases
- ligand–receptor interactions.

Chromatin condensation is associated with chromatin cleavage, first to fragments corresponding to the loop and rosette domains in which the chromatin is organized. Later these fragments are further broken down to mononucleosome and oligonucleosome size. This process is mirrored by the appearances seen when DNA from apoptotic cells is electrophoresed; such DNA shows a characteristic 'laddered' pattern on electrophoresis, whereas that of necrotic cells is seen as an unstructured 'smear'. These features suggest that the DNA is broken down by **endonucleases**; indeed, some endonucleases have been identified in apoptotic cells.

Apoptotic bodies contain proteins that are insoluble in ionic detergents. This results from **cross-linking** brought about by a **transglutaminase**.

Apoptosis may be blocked in several cell types by protease inhibitors. Specific proteases are necessary for cell death to be brought about by cytotoxic T cells. The same is true in relation to the programmed cell death occurring in the hermaphrodite worm *Caenorhabditis elegans*, in which 131 of the 1090 cells normally undergo apoptosis. In *C. elegans* two gene products are necessary for apoptosis to occur, one of which (the product of *ced-3*) is a cysteine protease. Cysteine protease activation via many different stimuli is a common effector pathway for apoptosis. These proteases, known as **caspases**, cleave their substrates preferentially at aspartate residues.

Engulfment of apoptotic bodies results from ligand–receptor interactions. When macrophages engulf apoptotic neutrophils, two receptors on the macrophage surface become occupied. These are the vitronectin receptor (an integrin) and CD36, a thrombospondin receptor. These receptors bind thrombospondin which, in turn, acts as an intercellular bridge between the macrophage and the apoptotic body.

GENETIC REGULATION OF APOPTOSIS

Because apoptosis involves protein synthesis, it is likely that the process is regulated by the genome. This hypothesis finds support from studies with *C. elegans*, which contains:

- two genes that appear to **promote cell death** (*ced-3* and *ced-4*)
- one gene that **protects** the worm cells against apoptosis (*ced-9*).

The gene product of *ced-3* resembles the mammalian protein interleukin 1β-converting enzyme (ICE), while that of *ced-9* resembles the product of the mammalian proto-oncogene *bcl-2* with which it also shares functional similarities.

Genetic survival factors

The activity of certain genes protects cells in a high-turnover state from programmed cell death. The products of such genes should be regarded as **survival factors** rather than as factors promoting cell division (**mitogens**). Examples include:

- the *bcl-2* gene; this was first discovered from molecular analysis of a chromosome translocation (14:18) which is present in most cases of a human B cell follicle-centre lymphoma.
- the proto-oncogene *c-abl*, which produces a tyrosine kinase; translocation of the *abl* gene occurs in chronic myeloid leukaemia and in certain acute lymphoblastic leukaemias of childhood.
- the *LMP-1* gene of the Epstein–Barr virus; this has the ability to induce neoplastic transformation, which may result indirectly via induction of *bcl-2*.
- the adenovirus early region gene *E1b*.

Presence of gene *p53*

The presence of normal ('wild-type') tumour-suppressor gene p53 *is responsible for the initiation of apoptosis, especially in cell injury characterized by DNA double-strand breaks* (p. 507). In human cancer treatment, this is extremely important, because tumour cells which lack wild-type *p53* do not undergo apoptosis when exposed to ionizing radiation. In addition, lack of *p53* is likely to result in the survival of cells with DNA mutations and thus to increase the chances of cancer development (p. 506).

NECROSIS

Necrosis is the term applied when cell death occurs in part of an organ or tissue in continuity with neighbouring viable tissue. Various morphological forms exist and may, as in the case of caseation necrosis, provide a clue to the cause of tissue injury.

COAGULATIVE NECROSIS

Here **denaturation of intracytoplasmic protein** is the dominant process. The dead tissue becomes firm and slightly swollen. Protein molecules within the cytoplasm become unfolded, making the tissue more opaque than normal and more reactive with certain dyes such as eosin. Microscopically, the cells show the signs of nuclear death described previously, but the most noteworthy feature is the **retention of the general architectural pattern** of the tissue, despite the death of its constituent elements.

Coagulative necrosis occurs typically in ischaemic injury, such as may occur in the heart or kidney. However, for reasons that are not clear, ischaemic injury in the central nervous system leads to necrosis dominated by enzymatic digestion and liquefaction of the dead tissue.

Caseation necrosis

Caseation necrosis occurs characteristically in **tuberculosis**. It is a form of coagulative necrosis in which no liquefaction is present. On microscopic examination the affected tissue appears completely **structureless** and exhibits a greater than usual affinity for dyes such as eosin. Caseation necrosis owes its somewhat unfortunate name (caseous = cheese-like) to its macroscopic appearance, as large areas of caseous necrosis somewhat resemble white crumbly goat's cheese. On chemical analysis, large amounts of **lipid** are found to be present in these necrotic areas in addition to the coagulated protein.

LIQUEFACTIVE (COLLIQUATIVE) NECROSIS

In liquefaction necrosis the effect of hydrolytic lysosomal enzymes is dominant. The end-result is a local accumulation of protein-rich, semi-fluid material. It is not particularly common as a primary event except, as mentioned above, in the brain. However, secondary infection of necrotic tissue by pus-forming organisms commonly leads to liquefaction.

TRAUMATIC FAT NECROSIS

This occurs almost exclusively in the female breast, especially if the breast is heavy and pendulous. It results from rupture of adipocytes with release of their contents. The released fat undergoes lipolysis and is converted to fatty acids and glycerol. Clinically the lesion appears as a hard lump in the breast, and may be mistaken for a malignancy. Excised lesions may show a small, central cystic area in which some oily droplets are present. At the periphery the adipose tissue is much firmer and also more opaque than usual.

Microscopy shows numerous granular macrophages containing phago-cytosed lipid. Fatty acid crystals are also often present and excite a foreign-body giant cell reaction (multinucleate cells formed by fusion of macrophages).

ENZYME-MEDIATED FAT NECROSIS

Another type of fat necrosis occurs in the peritoneal cavity in **acute haemorrhagic pancreatitis**. Here the pancreatic enzymes are released from acini and ducts, and thus reach the interstitial tissues. The proteolytic and lipolytic enzymes damage cell membranes and convert intracellular tri-glyceride into glycerol and fatty acids. These combine with calcium in inter-stitial fluid to form **soaps**, which appear as small, intensely white and opaque patches on the adipose tissue of the pancreas, omentum and other areas of the peritoneum.

GANGRENE

Strictly speaking, the term gangrene should be limited to necrosis of tissues associated with a superadded infection by putrefactive microorganisms. The responsible organisms include:

- *Clostridia* species (anaerobic, Gram-positive, spore-forming bacilli) derived from the gut or soil
- anaerobic streptococci
- members of the family Bacteroidaceae.

Clinically, the term gangrene is often used for any black foul-smelling area in continuity with living tissues. This can result primarily from the actions of bacterial toxins, or secondarily from a combination of ischaemia and superadded infection. True gangrene may occur, for example, in the gastrointestinal tract. This is most commonly due to the blood supply being cut off, leading to extensive necrosis. Resident potentially putrefactive organisms provide an ideal source for superadded infection.

Another example of true gangrene is so-called **gas gangrene**. This is a rapidly spreading form of tissue necrosis, often involving muscle. It results from infection by saccharolytic and proteolytic *Clostridia* which secrete a wide range of toxins that destroy cell membranes and the macromolecules of interstitial ground substance. These toxins constitute the basis for the spread-ing that is so menacing a feature of gas gangrene. *Clostridia* infection of this type not infrequently complicates deep penetrating injuries sustained in battle. It may also occur as a rare complication of acute suppurative appen-dicitis, in strangulation of the gut, in the puerperium and in the stumps of mid-thigh amputations carried out for ischaemia of the lower limbs (p. 45).

The presence of dead tissue as a result of injury, and a poor oxygen supply favour the multiplication of these anaerobic organisms. The affected muscles and adjacent soft tissues are oedematous and often very painful. They may feel **crepitant** (crackly) on palpation because of the formation of gas bubbles (carbon dioxide) in the tissue as a result of fermentation of sugars by bacterial toxins. The infection may remain localized or may become generalized (**septicaemia**). Evidence of such spread may be seen at post-mortem examination in the form of:

- bubbles in some of the solid viscera (most notably the liver)
- signs of haemolysis such as haemoglobin staining of the aortic intima.

Gangrene brought about by ischaemia may occur, as already stated, in the gut. It is also not uncommon in the lower limb. The background to this is usually severe atherosclerosis (pp. 323–341) of the large and medium-sized arteries of the limb. The stenosing lesions are composed partly of pro-liferated fibromuscular tissue and partly of lipid accumulations derived mainly from the plasma. These then become complicated by superimposed thrombosis. Diabetic patients and cigarette smokers are particularly at risk. In younger patients ischaemic necrosis of the lower limbs may occur as a result of **thromboangiitis obliterans** (**Buerger's disease**). In this condition an inflammatory process involves the whole vascular bundle (veins as well as arteries) and leads to arterial occlusion.

If the limb is oedematous and a fairly thick layer of adipose tissue is present, the ischaemic necrosis may be associated with infection by putre-factive organisms. The typical appearances of **wet gangrene**, with large blebs on the skin surface, occasionally accompanied by gas production, may then be seen.

Where these conditions do not occur, and where the arterial narrowing has progressed slowly over a long period, so-called **dry gangrene** is seen. Starting at the most distal extremities the tissues become desiccated and black. The affected areas are very cold; there is no unpleasant smell and no bleb or gas formation. The black discolouration of the skin is due to staining by haemoglobin, which diffuses from the small vessels into the extravascular compartment. Not infrequently a line of demarcation forms at the junction between the living and dead tissues, and the latter may actually separate off (so-called **spontaneous amputation**).

CELL AND TISSUE DEATH

- Cells that are unable to achieve a new 'steady state' in the face of injurious factors **die**. This cell death may determine the clinical features of a disease, e.g. death of anterior horn cells in the spinal cord causes paralysis.
- The structural changes of cell death reflect the effects of time and either enzymatic digestion or protein denaturation.
- Cell death may occur as a 'programmed phenomenon' (**apoptosis**) involving protein synthesis and use of energy. It is important and operates in many contexts:
  — normal tissue turnover
  — organ development in fetal life
  — viral injury
  — atrophy.
- Death of cells in continuity with living tissue is termed **necrosis**. This occurs basically in two forms – coagulative and liquefactive. Some variants, e.g. **caseation necrosis**, seen in tuberculosis, have diagnostic value.
- Necrosis associated with super-added infections by certain bacterial species is termed **gangrene**. Affected tissues are black and foul smelling.

4 Acute inflammation I: introduction

Injury to living tissue results in a process in which **phagocytic cells and elements of circulating plasma enter the damaged area**. This process is acute inflammation, and it usually continues as long as the tissue injury persists.

Acute inflammation is, in evolutionary terms, very ancient: many of the processes involved in inflammation, such as chemotaxis and phagocytosis, are present in simple unicellular and multicellular organisms. The acquisition of a complicated circulatory system adds significantly to the complexities of the inflammatory response: it is the changes that occur in the **calibre** and **permeability** of arterioles, capillaries and venules (the **microcirculation**) that dictate the most prominent of the symptoms and signs of acute inflammation.

The acute inflammatory response is mediated via two pathways, one involving the microcirculation and the other, leucocytes. Understanding is aided if each of these pathways is viewed as a set of distinct operations (*Fig. 4.1*).

Changes in the microcirculation

The changes that occur in the microcirculation are:

- An **increase in the calibre** of arterioles, capillaries and venules. This results in an increase in the amount and speed of blood flow in the injured area, leading to **redness** and **heat**.
- An **increase in the permeability** of the affected blood vessels. This causes the escape of larger than normal amounts of water and also of high molecular weight proteins such as fibrinogen, not normally found in extravascular interstitial fluid. This process, termed **exudation**, leads to **swelling** (inflammatory oedema).

Leucocyte activity

The activities of phagocytic cells in inflammation are complex and involve several distinct steps, discussed in detail on pp. 58–65 and 81–90. They include:

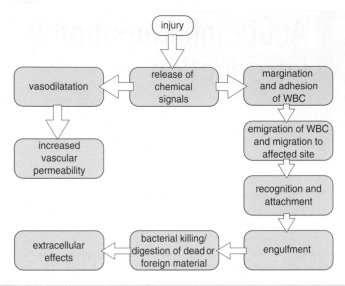

Fig. 4.1 Vascular and cellular pathways in acute inflammation.
WBC, white blood cells.

- **adhesion** of neutrophils and monocytes to the endothelial cells of microvessels in the affected area of tissue
- **migration** of these leucocytes between endothelial cells and through the basement membranes of microvessels to reach the extravascular fluid compartment.
- **attachment** to infecting microorganisms, or to dead or injured cells and tissue elements
- **engulfment** (phagocytosis) of the organisms, cell or tissue debris, etc.
- **killing** of the phagocytosed organisms and digestion of cell or tissue debris
- effects on surrounding tissue of **chemical mediators** secreted or otherwise released from phagocytes.

Is the inflammatory process helpful or harmful?

John Hunter, the famous London surgeon, stated in 1794 that 'inflammation in itself is not to be regarded as a disease but as a salutary operation consequent upon some violence or disease'. This is not the whole truth. Inflammation is, indeed, a defence mechanism, but some inflammatory reactions can have crippling or life-threatening consequences, for example the filling up of airspaces in the lung and the resulting blockage of gas exchange that occurs in pneumonia.

CAUSES OF ACUTE INFLAMMATION

In general terms, any process that injures cells may cause an inflammatory reaction. Such processes include **mechanical trauma**, such as cutting or crushing, and **chemical injuries**, such as those produced by acids, alkalis and phenols. An important cause of chemical injury of tissues is the presence of physiological substances in inappropriate locations. For example, gastric juice is harmless in the stomach, its natural milieu, but causes severe inflammation in the peritoneal cavity after perforation of a peptic ulcer.

Injury may also be caused by:

- ultraviolet or X-irradiation
- extremes of cold or heat (burns and frostbite)
- reduction in the arterial blood supply sufficient to cause death of the underperfused tissue (**ischaemic necrosis**)
- living organisms such as bacteria, viruses, parasites, worms and fungi
- inappropriate or excessive operation of immune mechanisms.

CLINICAL CHARACTERISTICS OF ACUTE INFLAMMATION

Anyone who has suffered from, say, a boil can give an excellent account of the clinical features of acute inflammation. The affected area is **hot**, **red**, **swollen** and **painful**. These are the so-called **cardinal signs** of inflammation, described by the Roman physician Celsus in the first century of the Christian era as **calor**, **rubor**, **tumor** and **dolor** respectively.

The translation of these clinical observations into pathophysiological terms had to wait for the microscopic studies of Julius Cohnheim, who first observed that injury was followed by changes in small blood vessels, adhesion of white blood cells to the inner lining of these vessels and finally, by migration of these cells into the extravascular space. We can now correlate the cardinal signs of acute inflammation with a distinct series of events in the microcirculation (*Fig. 4.2*).

REDNESS AND HEAT

The only logical explanation for redness and heat is **persistent dilatation of small vessels** and an **increased blood flow** in the affected area leading to increased capillary and venular filling. Normally, only part of the microcirculation is filled with circulating blood at any one time. As capillaries have no smooth muscle cells in their wall, they constitute a set of passive channels whose blood content depends largely on flow in feeding arterioles. Thus redness and heat, so striking in acute inflammation, must depend on an increase in the calibre of the arterioles feeding the injured area; this, in turn, must represent the result of **arteriolar smooth muscle relaxation**.

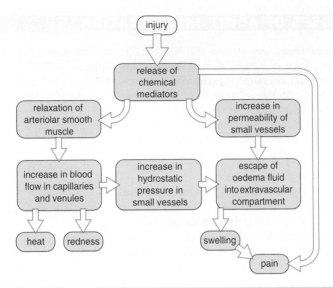

Fig. 4.2 Vascular events that underlie the cardinal signs of inflammation.

The tone of arterioles, acting as precapillary sphincters, is controlled in two ways:

1) Under normal circumstances the circular smooth muscle coat of the arteriole is controlled by the autonomic nervous system, in particular the sympathetic vasoconstrictor nerves. These nerves are largely responsible for controlling the blood pressure, cardiac output and distribution of blood flow among the different organs and tissues. Blushing in response to some embarrassing circumstance constitutes an easily observed example of this control system in operation.

2) However, arteriolar smooth muscle cells also react to local chemical mediators. The accumulation of such compounds at and around the site of injury plays a dominant role in the arteriolar dilatation of acute inflammation. This is demonstrated by the fact that acute inflammation in tissue that has long been denervated shows no essential differences from that occurring in normally innervated areas.

SWELLING

In simple terms, local tissue swelling must mean that something has been added to the bulk of the formed tissue elements or to the gel-like ground substance in that area. Chemical analysis of such a swollen area shows that the increase in bulk is due to the local **accumulation of excess interstitial fluid**, containing solutes and proteins derived from the plasma. This extravascular fluid accumulation is called **oedema**.

In inflammatory oedema the fact that there has been a net transfer from the intravascular to the extravascular compartment can be shown by injecting the dye 'Evans' blue' intravenously into a small animal. If a mild thermal injury is produced at some site, the skin at the site of injury shows blue staining. Evans' blue circulates in the plasma bound to albumin, and the staining therefore indicates that albumin has passed from the small vessels into the extravascular compartment.

Exudation of protein-rich fluid in inflammation

Inflammatory exudation is synonymous with the escape of high molecular weight proteins from small vessels. To understand this, we need to know something of the normal routes of transport across endothelial barriers and the forces that determine the rates of such transport. Endothelium of all types is permeable to a wide range of molecules. Most of the available data suggest the existence, in a functional sense, of a 'two-pore' system.

The **large-pore component** has a diameter of about 50 nm. Using the appropriate ultrastructural tracers, the structural equivalent of the large-pore system is shown to be the plasmalemmal vesicles. These vesicles are present in large numbers in endothelial cells and are concentrated along the luminal and abluminal membranes. They have a diameter of about 70 nm. Once the vesicles have incorporated a large molecule by pinocytosis, they bud off from the luminal plasma membrane and travel across the endothelial cytoplasm towards the abluminal aspect of the cell. Here they fuse with the abluminal plasma membrane and discharge their contents.

The structural equivalent of the '**small-pore**' system is more equivocal, but the available evidence suggests that it may correspond to the junctions between adjacent endothelial cells. It has a diameter of 9 nm.

The mechanisms underlying the escape from the microcirculation of water and solutes on the one hand and plasma proteins on the other may well be different, and merit separate consideration.

Ultrafiltration

Transport of water and solute across the endothelial cell barrier shows many of the features of ultrafiltration, in which the movement of fluid and electrolytes is controlled largely by physical forces. There are two sets of such forces acting in opposition to each other:

1) Hydrostatic forces within the microcirculation tend to push fluid out into the extravascular compartment.
2) Intravascular osmotic pressure is exerted by the plasma proteins. The hydrostatic pressure of the extravascular tissues combines with plasma osmotic forces to push fluid back into the vessels.

Normally the result of these opposing sets of forces is a small net outflow of fluid from the microcirculation, which then drains from the extravascular compartment via the lymphatic channels. An increase in the intravascular hydrostatic pressure in the vessels of the microcirculation, such as occurs in acute inflammation, increases the amount of water and solute driven out of the vessels, although the oedema fluid produced in this way still has a relatively low protein content. Obviously loss of protein from the intravascular compartment potentiates this process, because the intravascular osmotic pressure falls and there is a corresponding rise in the osmotic pressure of the extravascular tissue fluid.

Protein leakage

Chemical analysis of the exudate invariably shows a protein concentration that is simply not attainable by the processes of ultrafiltration or **transudation** discussed above. Some other explanation for this high concentration of plasma-derived protein must exist.

The technique of vascular labelling in small animals elegantly shows that very large molecules escape from the microcirculation in the course of the formation of inflammatory oedema. It also serves the purpose of identifying the vessels from which leakage has occurred. A few drops of indian ink are injected intravenously into a small animal such as a rat. Except in the liver and spleen where the endothelium is normally 'leaky', the tissues do not blacken and the vessels of the microcirculation are not outlined by the ink particles, which instead are taken up by phagocytic cells in the sinusoids of the liver and spleen. However, if a mild injury is produced *after* the injection of the ink, some of the vessels in the injured area become outlined by the ink particles.

On microscopic examination, these particles are seen to have crossed the endothelial cells and to be lying piled up against the basement membrane, which they do not cross. Careful examination shows that the vessels so labelled are small **venules** measuring up to about 80 or 100 μm in diameter; capillaries, larger venules and arterioles are not labelled when the injury has been mild.

It is not clear on light microscopy what cellular events underlie the passage of such large molecules as indian ink or ferritin across the normal endothelium. This question was answered by the electron microscopic studies of Guido Majno, who showed that, when small doses of histamine or other vasoactive substances were injected into the cremaster muscle of rats, the endothelial cells in venules contracted, creating gaps through which the particles could pass. In due time the endothelial cells presumably relax and the gaps disappear, as particles can be found lying deep to apparently intact interendothelial junctions. A combination of ultrastructural and immunocytochemical studies has shown that endothelial cells contain contractile filaments.

It should be emphasized that the change in microvascular permeability described above is what is seen when the injury is **mild**. In reality the alterations in vascular permeability following injury are more varied, both in nature and timing. The major factor affecting these changes appears to be the **degree of severity of the injury**, which is reflected in the magnitude of the functional and structural change in the endothelial cells (*Fig. 4.3*).

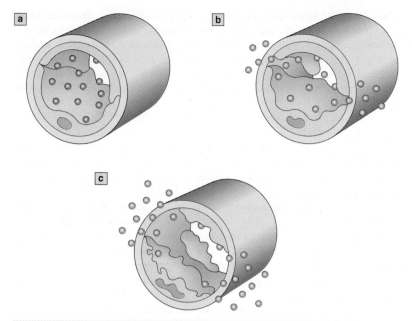

Fig. 4.3   Endothelial cell damage in relation to the escape of large molecules from the microvasculature.

a Normal vessel. **b** If injury is mild, the endothelial cells contract and create gaps through which particles can pass. **c** In severe injury, the endothelial cells may be damaged or even killed, and the amount and duration of the escape of large molecules from the vascular compartment is greatly increased.

Patterns of increased vascular permeability

Most of our knowledge here is derived from studies carried out in small animals, where the experimental conditions, in particular the type and severity of injury, are clearly defined. It is likely that in human inflammation the processes are much more complex. The patterns of increased vascular permeability following injury are characterized in terms of two variables:

- the **time** between infliction of the injury and recordable changes in microvascular permeability.
- the **duration** of the change in vascular permeability.

On this basis, three patterns can be observed: the immediate transient response, the delayed persistent response and the immediate persistent response.

Immediate transient response.   As its name implies, the immediate transient response follows almost immediately on mild injury. The alteration in vascular permeability reaches a peak within 5 minutes or so and returns to normal within 15 minutes. Carbon labelling shows that the **escape of fluid is confined to small venules**. The development of leaky venules extends more widely than the immediate area of injury, suggesting that a chemical signal is involved. Because the increase in vascular permeability can be blocked by predosing animals with antihistamine compounds, it is reasonable to suppose that this signal is histamine. The short duration of the change strongly suggests that the increase in venule permeability is brought about by **endothelial cell contraction** and that the endothelial cells are not seriously damaged.

Delayed persistent response.   The delayed persistent response takes longer to develop. In some instances the peak effect occurs about 4 hours after injury, while in others there may be an interval of up to 24 hours before increased vascular permeability becomes greatest. Such increased permeability is not blocked by the prior administration of antihistamines. In cases where the peak effect is noted after 4 hours, labelling with carbon shows that **fluid and macromolecules escape from the capillaries**. When the reaction peaks later (e.g. 24 hours after injury), both **venules and capillaries** are labelled. Some affected capillaries contain small aggregates of platelets, and damaged and broken endothelial cells are also seen. While interendothelial cell gaps are found in affected venules, it is believed that these result from direct endothelial injury rather than from the operation of a chemical mediator such as histamine.

A good example of the delayed type of response is to be found in **sunburn**, which is mediated by **ultraviolet radiation**. Exposure to sunlight on the first day of the holidays, while enjoyable, may be followed some hours after exposure has ceased by the onset of an uncomfortable inflammatory reaction.

Immediate persistent response.   The immediate persistent response is associated, experimentally, with the application of relatively powerful agents. The affected vessels begin to leak within a few minutes and permeability becomes maximal 15–60 minutes after injury. Labelling studies show that **small vessels of all types** leak, and electron microscopy reveals **severe damage to endothelial cells** and pericytes, with the former sloughing away from their basement membranes. Exudation continues until the endothelial cells have been replaced by ingrowth of new cells, derived from the uninjured part of the vessel lining, along the basement membrane. It may therefore last for many days and be of impressive proportions. This type of response is seen in patients who have been badly burned or suffered severe mechanical trauma.

Blood flow patterns

Understanding how the fluid exudate forms in acute inflammation leads naturally to an understanding of why the flow of blood slows in some parts of the microcirculation in injured areas. This change in flow is associated with packing and sludging of red cells. Loss of water from the leaking venules and capillaries leads to increased concentrations of blood cells in these vessels. Although plasma proteins also escape from the vessels, the loss of fluid may be so great as to increase the plasma protein concentration within these vessels; this will add further to the tendency for an increase in blood viscosity. Rouleaux formation by the red cells is enhanced. The tendency of white cells to adhere to the endothelial surface of the postcapillary venules and to each other may also impair flow through the injured vessels.

PAIN

Pain is less well understood than the other cardinal clinical features of the acute inflammatory reaction and, indeed, may not always be present. The **local increase in tissue tension** is clearly one factor; the denser the tissue affected, the greater the degree of pain. Palpating or squeezing an acutely inflamed area will either increase existing pain or produce pain where none existed; it seems reasonable to ascribe this also to an increase in local tissue pressure. However, some of the endogenous chemical compounds released in the course of the acute inflammatory reaction can cause pain in their own right when injected subcutaneously or intradermally. These may also contribute to the pain experienced in many inflammatory reactions.

ACUTE INFLAMMATION I: INTRODUCTION

- Acute inflammation is the series of microvascular and cellular events that occur after tissue injury.
- Affected tissues become *red, hot, swollen and painful*, due to **dilatation** of arterioles, capillaries and venules, and an **increase in the permeability** of the affected vessels.
- Cellular events involve **migration of phagocytes** from small blood vessels to the site of injury where they engulf and kill microorganisms or engulf and break down tissue debris. This process involves:
  - **adhesion** of phagocytes (neutrophils and monocytes) to the inner lining of small blood vessels
  - **migration** between adjacent endothelial cells
  - **movement** through extravascular tissues
  - **attachment** to infecting organisms or to tissue debris
  - **engulfment**
  - **killing** or digestion.
- In evolutionary terms, inflammation is a protective system but inflammatory reactions can have serious, even fatal consequences, as, for example, in pneumonia.
- The **causes** of inflammation include:
  - trauma
  - chemical injury
  - ultraviolet or X-irradiation
  - extremes of heat or cold
  - ischaemia
  - infection
  - inappropriate or excessive operation of immune mechanisms.

5 Acute inflammation II: cellular events and chemical mediators

In evolutionary terms, one of the first defences to develop against the presence of 'foreign' material, whether living or dead, was **phagocytosis** or engulfment by specialized cells. Migration of phagocytic cells to a site of injury remains one of the most fundamental components of the host's response. It is vital for a successful defence against infection by living microorganisms. *Its central role is demonstrated by the increased susceptibility to infection shown by persons who either have insufficient phagocytic cells or whose cells cannot seek out, engulf or destroy pathogenic microorganisms.*

NEUTROPHILS

In the early stages of acute inflammation most of the cells migrating to the injured area are neutrophils, although a small number of eosinophils and basophils may also be present. Neutrophils:

- are present in relatively large numbers in the blood
- can be replaced rapidly from precursors in the bone marrow
- move more quickly than other leucocytes.

The number of neutrophils present at sites of tissue damage depends on the severity of such damage and the nature of the injury. Physical injury rarely evokes a significant neutrophil response, whereas infection by certain organisms such as *Escherichia coli* or staphylococci elicits a striking response.

Neutrophils make up 40–75% of circulating white cells. They have a diameter of about 15 μm, characteristically segmented nuclei and granular cytoplasm containing two types of granule:

1) larger granules staining densely with Romanowsky-type dyes and containing lysozyme (accounting for about one-third of their

content), lysosomal enzymes, peroxidase and certain cationic proteins, the last of which may be important signals for the recruitment of further neutrophils.

2) smaller granules, also lysosomal in nature, also containing lysozyme (about two-thirds of their content), alkaline phosphatase and lactoferrin, an iron-binding protein, which inhibits bacterial multiplication.

The energy source of the neutrophil is glucose, normally stored as glycogen. The cell can produce energy by glycolysis under anaerobic conditions, which is useful because oxygen tension may fall to a very low level in areas of tissue damage.

In general, the early peak of neutrophil migration to an inflammatory focus is followed some hours later by a further wave of cell migration, this time by mononuclear phagocytes (**macrophages**). This biphasic pattern of cell accumulation is found in most inflammatory reactions, but the precise timing may vary with the nature of the injury.

NEUTROPHIL OPERATIONS IN ACUTE INFLAMMATION

Adhesion of neutrophils to endothelium and their subsequent emigration

The mechanisms of emigration are not completely understood. With the change in blood flow, the white cells, which are heavier than red cells, come to lie at the periphery of the column of flowing blood cells. Some **adhere** to the endothelium, a process known as '**margination**'. Adhesion of the leucocyte to the endothelium is clearly a pivotal step in emigration of the neutrophil. The importance of adhesion is made plain by the existence of a rare inherited defect known as the **leucocyte adhesion deficiency syndrome**, in which adhesion of leucocytes to the microvascular endothelium cannot occur. Patients suffering from this disorder have repeated episodes of life-threatening bacterial infection because their neutrophils cannot emigrate from the vascular compartment.

Until recently adhesion was difficult to understand, because the negative charges associated with carboxyl groups of the sialic acid residues on the plasma membranes of the endothelial cells and the neutrophil should repel each other.

It is now known that there is a wide range of molecules causing cell–cell adhesion as a result of a receptor–ligand interaction. Many of these have transmembrane domains and almost certainly mediate not only cell adhesion but transmembrane signalling as well. Some are normally expressed on cell surfaces; others appear only after the cells that can produce them have been 'instructed' to do so. Divalent cations, especially calcium and magnesium, appear also to play a part in adhesion; the pretreatment of experimental animals with chelating agents that remove these cations inhibits the margination and adhesion of white cells. It is also known that exposure of neutrophils to chemotactic factors decreases their negative surface charge and increases their adherence to endothelial cells. It has recently been suggested that exocytosis of lactoferrin from the specific granules of the neutrophil may also be a factor in neutrophil–endothelial adhesion. There has been a case report in which neutrophils deficient in lactoferrin would not stick to endothelium when stimulated by chemotactic factors.

Adhesion molecules on endothelial cells and circulating leucocytes

Adhesion molecules expressed on the **endothelial cell surface** are of two basic types (*Figs 5.1* and *5.2*):

1) **Selectins** derive their name from the resemblance of part of their structure to lectins, a series of proteins, widely distributed in nature, that bind with high affinity to sugars and that have a remarkable ability to distinguish between different sugars.
2) Members of the **immunoglobulin gene superfamily**. This includes heavy and light chains of immunoglobulin, T-cell receptor α and β chains, major histocompatibility complex (MHC) class I and II peptides, β_2-microglobulin, CD4 and CD8 molecules on T lymphocytes, and certain adhesion molecules expressed on endothelium.

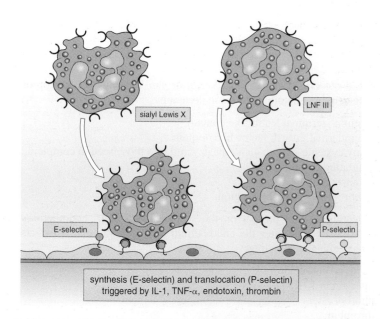

sialyl Lewis X

LNF III

E-selectin

P-selectin

synthesis (E-selectin) and translocation (P-selectin)
triggered by IL-1, TNF-α, endotoxin, thrombin

Fig. 5.1   The 'rolling' phase of leucocyte adhesion to vascular endothelium.

Adhesion is mediated by interaction between sugars on the leucocyte plasma membrane and selectins expressed on the surface membranes of endothelial cells.

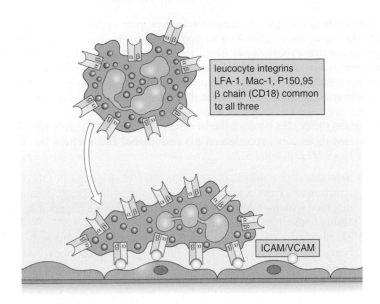

leucocyte integrins
LFA-1, Mac-1, P150,95
β chain (CD18) common
to all three

ICAM/VCAM

Fig. 5.2   Flattening of leucocytes on the endothelium before emigration.

Interaction occurs between β₂ integrins on the leucocyte surface and adhesion molecules of
the immunoglobulin gene superfamily on the endothelium.

The endothelial selectins. The selectins are a family of glycoproteins
having certain structural features in common:

- an amino terminal lectin-like domain
- an epidermal growth factor-like domain
- many cysteine-rich tandem repeats similar to those seen in complement-regulating proteins
- a transmembrane region
- a short intracytoplasmic region.

Selectins are *not* present on the surface of 'resting' endothelium but
are expressed only after the endothelium has been stimulated by various
chemical signals, including:

- bacterial endotoxin
- interleukin 1 (IL-1)
- phorbol esters
- thrombin
- tumour necrosis factor α (TNF-α).

Two endothelial selectins have so far been identified. These are E-selectin
and P-selectin.

E-selectin is also known as **endothelial leucocyte adhesion molecule 1 (ELAM-1)**. The ligand for E-selectin is believed to be a complex carbo-hydrate called **sialylLewisX**, present on the surface of the white cells (neutrophils and monocytes) that bind to E-selectin. The selectin itself is expressed on the endothelium within 30 minutes of stimulation, reaches its peak concentration somewhere between 2 and 4 hours after stimulation, and is expressed for about 24 hours.

P-selectin was originally cursed with the name **platelet activation-dependent granule to external membrane protein (PADGEM)**. This molecule is also present within the α granules of platelets. In the endo-thelium, P-selectin is synthesized constitutively and is stored in rod-shaped cytoplasmic organelles known as Weibel–Palade bodies, from which it is transported to the luminal membrane when endothelial cells are stimulated. The ligand for P-selectin has been identified as a sugar, **lacto-*n*-fuco-pentaose III (LNF-III)**, which contains the sialylLewisX structure within its core. P-selectin binds neutrophils and monocytes and is maximally expressed on the endothelial surface membrane within 10–30 minutes.

Adhesion of neutrophils and monocytes to the endothelial selectins appears to be important in the early stages of the inflammatory reaction and is responsible for the phenomenon of the **leucocytes rolling along the surface of the endothelium** in the affected area.

Immunoglobulin gene superfamily of adhesion molecules. These receptors are so named because each contains several domains resembling the structure of immunoglobulin. Three such molecules have so far been identified and cloned. They are known as:

- **vascular cell adhesion molecule 1 (VCAM-1)**
- **intercellular cell adhesion molecule 1 (ICAM-1) (CD 54)**
- **intercellular cell adhesion molecule 2 (ICAM-2).**

All three are glycoproteins: it is the two ICAM molecules that are thought to be especially involved in the acute inflammatory reaction. Both are expressed constitutively by endothelial cells but ICAM-1 is expressed at very low levels, being increased in acute inflammation by stimulants such as **IL-1** or **TNF-α**. Induction of high levels of ICAM-1 on endothelium takes 4–6 hours; levels reach a maximum by 24 hours, at which point they plateau. Leucocytes bind to the ICAMs with high affinity; they then flatten and spread over the endothelium before migrating between adjacent endothelial cells.

The ligands on the surface of the neutrophils and monocytes that bind to the adhesion molecules of the immunoglobulin gene superfamily belong to a group known as the **integrins**. Integrins are a family of cell surface proteins that mediate the adhesion of cells to:

- **extracellular matrices** such as fibronectin and vitronectin
- **fibrillar proteins** such as collagen and laminin, both of which are present in basement membranes
- **endothelial cells** during inflammation.

All integrins have two subunits, termed α and β. Eleven α subunits and six β subunits have been described, and these, in different combinations, form at least 16 integrins. Many cells express integrins, some of which are clearly cell type-specific. These include the **gpIIb/IIIa** molecule, which is expressed only by **megakaryocytes and platelets** and which mediates **platelet aggregation**. Three others, **LFA-1**, **Mac-1** and **p150,95** are expressed only on leucocytes and it is these that adhere to the endothelial ICAMs in acute inflammation. They are known as the β_2-integrins; all three have the same β chain (CD18), although their (subunits are different.

Emigration

Once the neutrophils lie in close contact with the plasma membranes of the endothelial cells, they put out pseudopodia. These enter the gap between two adjacent endothelial cells, forcing it open. Neutrophils then move into the basement membrane substance, through which they soon pass, within 2–9 minutes (*Fig. 5.3*).

For unknown reasons, leucocytes from neonates and myeloblasts from leukaemic patients cannot attenuate their cytoplasm sufficiently to squeeze through the interendothelial cell gaps. The chemoattractants responsible for this movement are believed to belong to a family of low molecular weight proteins known as the **C-X-C chemokines** (see pp. 74–75, 78). IL-8 is probably the most important in this context.

Emigration involves movement, and the mechanisms responsible for leucocyte movement are also responsible for phagocytosis and for movement of the leucocyte's intracellular granules. They involve both the plasma membrane and the cytoplasm.

Neutrophils move by crawling forward; this is accomplished by the protrusion of clear pseudopodia from the aspect of the neutrophil facing the direction of travel. Pseudopodia become transiently attached to underlying substrates and, during this phase, the rest of the cell body is pulled forwards.

The movement of macrophages appears less polarized than that of the neutrophil: macrophages extend a thin layer of plasma membrane and cytoplasm round their whole circumference. This is known as 'ruffling'. At the same time, the macrophage cell surface not attached to underlying substrates becomes covered with spiky projections, giving the plasma membrane a very 'restless' appearance.

Observations of moving leucocytes suggest a dominant role for the **peripheral part of the cytoplasm**, where pseudopodia are formed. Heating activated leucocytes to 40°C leads to loss of pseudopodia. The pseudopodia retain the capacity to move and even to respond to chemotactic signals, however, suggesting that the 'motor' that drives leucocyte movement resides in this periphery of the cytoplasm.

The fact that the peripheral cytoplasmic zone of an activated leucocyte always excludes cell organelles suggests that it is in a **gelled state**. This is supported by studies in which aspiration of the plasma membrane of

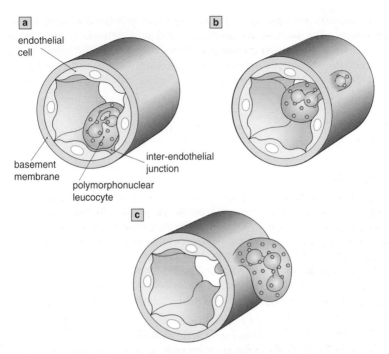

Fig. 5.3   Emigration of leucocytes from small blood vessels in acute inflammation.

a Margination of white cells within the flowing blood occurs and granulocytes adhere to the endothelial cells. **b** The granulocyte inserts a cytoplasmic pseudopodium between adjacent endothelial cells. **c** The granulocyte has almost completely passed through the interendothelial gap and the underlying basement membrane, and will soon be seen free in the perivascular space.

activated white cells shows that the peripheral zone of the cytoplasm exhibits **viscoelastic behaviour**. This means that initially there is resistance to the aspiration, which is followed by a free flow of peripheral cytoplasm into the pipette. This behaviour is characteristic of a gel.

The mechanical properties of this zone of cytoplasm are believed to depend on its principal component: **actin filaments**. The fungal metabolite **cytochalasin**, which inhibits actin filament assembly from their monomeric subunits, powerfully inhibits leucocyte movement, phagocytosis and granule movement. Support for a primary role for actin in the mechanical responses of white cells comes from a number of different sources:

- proteins that can gel actin in vitro are present in leucocytes (α-actinin and actin-binding protein)
- actin gel contracts in the presence of adenosine 5′-triphosphate (ATP)
- purified leucocyte myosin causes contraction of actin gels in vitro.

The architectural arrangement of actin filaments in activated leucocytes favours movement. The actin filaments are arranged in a network attached to the inner side of the plasma membrane of the leucocyte on the aspect that is attached to an underlying substrate. Three-dimensional study of these organized actin networks shows:

- features adapted for maximal extension of pseudopodia
- exclusion of cell organelles
- a pore size that allows water, solutes and small molecules to penetrate through the meshwork.

This arrangement is promoted by two proteins: **actin-binding protein** and α-**actinin**. Another compound promoting actin filament assembly is the phosphoinositide, PIP$_2$.

Actin filaments assemble in response to chemotactic signals. In resting leucocytes, about half the actin is in the form of filaments while the rest can be extracted easily from the cell by treatment with detergents. In leucocytes stimulated by chemotactic signals, the fraction of actin that resists solubilization by detergents rises. What is of some interest is how the 50% of non-polymerized actin is kept in this state in the resting leucocyte, preventing inappropriate activation of the leucocyte. Two mechanisms have been suggested:

1) A molecule identified as **profilin**, a basic protein present in many cell types, **sequesters monomeric actin molecules**.
2) **A molecule binds to the growing ends of actin filaments**, preventing the addition of monomers to these ends. In addition some of the previously assembled filaments are severed. The responsible molecule appears to be **gelsolin**, a protein that can be purified from leucocytes.

Myosin powers the contraction of the leucocyte cytoplasm. There is abundant evidence that contraction of the peripheral zone of the cytoplasm in leucocytes is mediated by **myosin**. This includes the facts that:

- when extracted leucocyte gels contract, myosin concentrates in the contracted areas
- addition of myosin to actin gels causes them to contract
- anti-myosin antibodies inhibit the contraction of leucocyte cytoplasm extracts.

Chemotaxis

Chemotaxis is the directional, purposive movement of phagocytic cells towards areas of tissue injury or death or the sites of bacterial invasion. It is mediated by a series of chemical messengers. Chemotaxis must be distinguished from chemokinesis, a chemically induced increase in activity of phagocytic cells with no vectorial component. Clearly a process of this sort must have two aspects:

1) **signals that attract the phagocyte** towards the appropriate area

2) **the ability of the phagocyte to respond to the signal** by moving towards the point from which the signal has been generated (**reception** and **transduction**).

That phagocytic cells are capable of responding in a directed way to a variety of stimuli has been shown in several ways. In my view the most elegant of these is the system devised by Harris in which neutrophils are incorporated into clotted plasma between a coverslip and a slide. When such preparations are examined by dark-field microscopy, the cells show up as white spots against a black background, and movement in any direction can be recorded as white tracks by long exposure of a single photographic frame. Harris found that various bacteria were chemotactic under these circumstances.

CHEMICAL MEDIATORS

GENERATION AND RECEPTION OF SIGNALS

Many substances are now known to be chemotactic for neutrophils in vitro, although, of course, their significance in vivo is less clear. These substances include **low molecular weight compounds** which are products of protein synthesis by invading microorganisms, and **endogenous compounds**.

Formylated peptides

These are low molecular weight compounds produced by microorganisms. They have methionine as the N-terminal residue. It is not certain whether such compounds as f-Met-Leu-Phe (formylated methionine-leucine-phenyl-alanine) have any role to play in mammalian inflammation. However, it is interesting that, in prokaryotes, ribosomal synthesis of new proteins starts with formyl-methionine, which may later be cleaved. Eukaryotic protein synthesis does not proceed in this way (except, interestingly enough, in mitochondria), and this therefore provides a recognition system by which prokaryotic bacterial invaders can be distinguished from eukaryotic cells. Neutrophils possess receptors for f-Met-Leu-Phe, and the latter can also cause endothelial cells to express some adhesion molecules.

Endogenous mediators

These are classified in *Table 5.1*. In this section we shall seek briefly to characterize them and to see how some of the systems interact with one another.

In theory, no substance should be labelled a chemical mediator of acute inflammation unless, when given in a concentration likely to be found in human disease, it can reproduce the features of inflammation, and unless it

Table 5.1   Broad groupings of inflammatory mediators

Source	Mediators
Activated plasma protein cascades	Complement system Kinin system Intrinsic blood clotting pathway Fibrinolytic system
Stored within cells and released on demand	Histamine 5-Hydroxytryptamine Lysosomal components
Newly synthesized in and released from cells on demand	Prostaglandins Leukotrienes Platelet-activating factor Cytokines such as IL-1 and TNF-α

Table 5.2   Plasma-derived mediators in acute inflammation

System	Mediator in acute inflammation
Complement	C3a C5a C567 trimolecular complex
Kinin	Kallikrein Bradykinin and other short peptides
Clotting	Fibrinopeptides
Fibrinolytic	Plasmin

can always be identified at sites of inflammatory reactions. However, it is not always possible to operate with such a degree of certainty and some compounds discussed here retain for the present a putative rather than a proven role.

As outlined in *Table 5.1*, the main sources for endogenous mediators are the **plasma** and the **tissues**; these will be considered separately (*Fig. 5.4*).

Endogenous mediators derived from plasma include those shown in *Table 5.2*. All these plasma systems are interconnected (see *Fig. 5.6*), the interconnections serving the purpose of **positive amplification loops**.

THE COMPLEMENT SYSTEM

The complement system consists of about 20 different proteins that are functionally interlinked to play an important role in immune responses and inflammation. Activation of complement is discussed more fully in the section dealing with the immune system (see pp. 137–181).

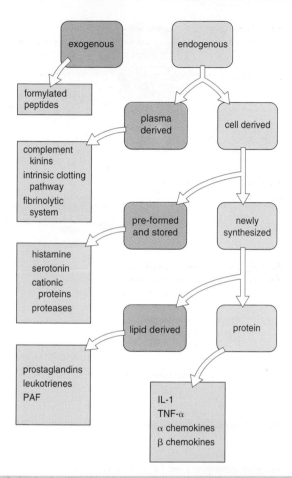

Fig. 5.4   A simple classification of the mediators of acute inflammation.

Activated complement (*Fig. 5.5*):

- yields particles that coat, for example, microorganisms and function as adhesion molecules for neutrophils and macrophages (**opsonins**)
- leads to **lysis of bacterial cell membranes** via the membrane attack complex
- yields biologically active fragments influencing the **vascular and cellular pathways of acute inflammation**.

One of the most important chemotactic factors for neutrophils is the 5a component of the **complement cascade**, although a trimolecular complex of C567 also operates as an attractant for phagocytes, and some workers maintain that C3a also does.

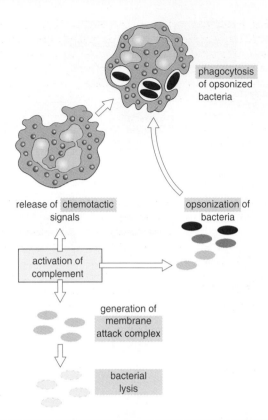

Fig. 5.5   Actions of complement in defence against infection.

The complement cascade can be activated in at least two ways. The first of these, known as the **classical pathway**, is through the **formation of antigen–antibody complexes**, to which C1q then binds. The second, known as the **alternate pathway**, operates via the **direct cleavage of C3** with consequent activation of the rest of the sequence. The alternate pathway can be activated by certain lipopolysaccharides derived from Gram-negative bacteria (endotoxins), by cobra venom and by polysaccharides derived from the cell walls of certain yeasts (zymosan). A number of aggregated immuno-globulins, notably immunoglobulin (Ig)A and IgE, also act in this way. **Plasmin**, a product of the fibrinolytic cascade, acts via both the classical and alternate pathways.

The part played by the complement system extends beyond the bounds of chemotaxis to involve the vascular component of acute inflammation as well. The increased vascular permeability produced by activation of the comple-ment cascade is attributed to the formation of '**anaphylatoxins**', the cleav-age products of C3 and C5 – **C3a** and **C5a**. If C3a and C5a are injected into human skin they cause local reddening and leakage from the microvascula-ture; C5a is 1000 times more active than C3a in this respect. Thus both C3a and C5a are mediators of the vascular and cellular components of the inflam-matory reaction, C5a being the more active. The C567 complex exerts its effect solely in respect of chemotaxis. In addition C3 fragments can induce the release of neutrophils from bone marrow reserves, and C5a may induce the release of lysosomal enzymes. The effects of C5a on the microvessels probably result from its effect on mast cells, which are stimulated to produce large amounts of leukotriene B_4.

THE KININ SYSTEM

The kinin system consists of a series of enzymes leading to the conversion of plasma precursors into active polypeptides. The latter share an ability to **induce change in the tone of vascular smooth muscle**. Some kinins, notably bradykinin, are powerful vasodilators and are also able to cause pain when injected intradermally.

The kinin-generating cascade starts with the activation of **Hageman factor (clotting factor XII)**. Hageman factor can be cleaved by a number of different substances including:

- glass
- kaolin
- collagen
- basement membrane
- cartilage
- trypsin
- sodium urate crystals
- kallikrein (a later member of the kinin-forming cascade)
- clotting factor XI
- bacterial endotoxins
- plasmin.

This wide range of activators signifies its central and important biological position. Once Hageman factor is activated, it acts on three **plasma pro-enzymes** to convert them to their active form (*Fig. 5.6*):

1) **Clotting factor XI** is activated to initiate the intrinsic clotting cascade.
2) **Plasminogen proactivator** is activated to **plasminogen activator** ultimately to form plasmin, the fibrinolytic enzyme.
3) **Prekallikrein** is cleaved to **kallikrein**, thus leading to kinin generation.

Plasma kallikrein (which is itself chemotactic for neutrophils) cleaves a plasma substrate, kininogen, releasing the active nonapeptide **bradykinin**. Bradykinin is a powerful hypotensive agent that produces vascular dilatation and increases vascular permeability in extremely small doses. Bradykinin is destroyed by two peptidases, and the other enzymes of the kinin-generating

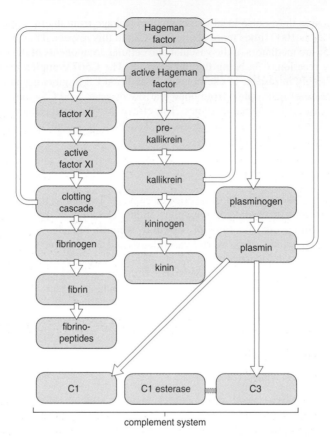

Fig. 5.6   Interrelationships between the plasma cascade systems and acute inflammation.

system can be interrupted at various points along the cascade. The precise role of the kinin system in inflammation has yet to be determined. Clearly it is not the only system involved, as patients with no Hageman factor can still mount a normal inflammatory response. It may be that the kinin system is important because of its interrelationships with other inflammation-mediating plasma cascades.

THE CLOTTING SYSTEM

Hageman factor cleavage also activates clotting factor XI. This active form of factor XI feeds back to cleave more Hageman factor, thus providing the third positive amplification loop. Of the three enzymes that act in this way – factor XI, plasmin and kallikrein – the last is by far the most active on a molar basis. The fibrinopeptides released from fibrinogen by the action of thrombin may both induce vascular leakage and be chemotactic for neutrophils.

THE FIBRINOLYTIC SYSTEM

Activated Hageman factor also triggers the fibrinolytic system, leading to the production of **plasmin**. Apart from its fibrinolytic powers, plasmin is well fitted to play an important part in the generation and maintenance of the inflammatory reaction. It feeds back to activate more Hageman factor and also digests the Hageman factor into particles that tend to activate prekallikrein rather than clotting factor XI. Thus plasmin forms the second positive amplification loop in the kinin-generating system (kallikrein itself constituting the first). In some species, when fibrin is cleaved by plasmin, fibrin degradation products are formed which are chemotactic for neutrophils; these also have the ability to enhance vascular permeability. Plasmin also activates C1 to trigger the classical pathway of complement activation and can cleave C3 directly; thus it also initiates the alternate pathway of complement activation.

TISSUE-DERIVED MEDIATORS

PREFORMED COMPOUNDS

Vasoactive amines

The first vasoactive amine to be linked with the acute inflammatory reaction was **histamine**. Histamine, formed by the decarboxylation of histidine, is found in mast cell granules and in the parietal cells of the stomach mucosa.

Mast cells are distributed throughout the body and can usually be found in relation to small vessels in the connective tissue. They are recognized by their metachromatic reaction with blue-violet dyes such as toluidine blue: their intracytoplasmic granules stain red. This reaction is caused by sulphated mucopolysaccharides within these granules. In addition to histamine, the granules contain heparin, 5-hydroxytryptamine (in rats and mice) and a variety of other enzymes. The name 'mast' cell is curious; it is derived from the German (*mästen*, to stuff or fatten), presumably because of the many cytoplasmic granules. Mast cells have considerable pharmacological potential and play a significant part in early acute inflammation and in type I hypersensitivity reactions (**anaphylaxis**) (see pp. 196–199).

A wide range of non-cell-killing stimuli may release mediators from the mast cell granules (*Fig. 5.7*). These include:

- physical injury such as heat, mechanical trauma and irradiation
- chemical agents such as immunoglobulins, snake venoms, bee venom, dextrans, chymotrypsin and trypsin, certain surfactants and cationic proteins released from the lysosomes of neutrophils, C3a and C5a; and,

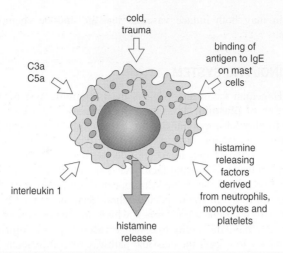

Fig. 5.7   Mechanisms leading to degranulation of mast cells and the release of histamine.

in connection with type I hypersensitivity reactions, an antigenic challenge to IgE-coated cells.

The mechanism of release of granule contents depends on an increase in intracellular guanosine 3′,5′-cyclic monophosphate (cGMP) and a corresponding inhibition of adenosine 3′,5′-cyclic monophosphate (cAMP). Any treatment that increases the concentration of cAMP in the mast cell will inhibit the release not only of histamine but of certain other active substances which are synthesized and released following a rise in cGMP concentration.

Histamine (and, in small rodents, 5-hydroxytryptamine) causes vascular dilatation and increased vascular permeability. However antihistamines only inhibit the immediate phase of the vascular response to injury, suggesting that vasoactive amines are of significance only during this phase.

Compounds released from lysosomes

The cell population of an acutely inflamed area can contribute potential mediators derived from lysosomes. This applies not only to the neutrophils, but also to other cell types, notably platelets. Candidate mediators include:

- cationic proteins
- acid proteases
- neutral proteases.

Cationic proteins.   Some of these attract mononuclear phagocytes in in vitro systems, whereas others induce the release of histamine from mast cells and so affect vascular permeability.

Acid proteases. The lysosomes of neutrophils contain many proteases, most active at approximately pH 3.0. In many areas of acute inflammation, the pH tends to fall because of the increased production of lactic acid due to neutrophil glycolysis. However, the pH does not usually fall so low as to provide the optimal condition for these enzymes.

Neutral proteases. Although acid proteases play only a limited role, the same is not true of the lysosomal enzymes active at neutral pH. We believe these are of considerable importance in causing tissue breakdown in a number of pathological situations. The range of targets for such proteolysis is wide, because neutrophil lysosomes contain collagenases, elastases and enzymes that degrade cartilage and basement membranes. It may be that tissue damage caused by release of lysosomal contents and the generation of oxygen free radicals occurs much more frequently and is of much greater significance than has hitherto been appreciated. Apart from the direct tissue damage caused by release of lysosomal enzymes, some of these can also generate chemotactic fragments from C5 and produce kinins from plasma precursors. In addition, damaged or activated neutrophils release substances that attract other neutrophils by a mechanism independent of complement.

Acidic lipids: the products of arachidonic acid peroxidation

In 1970 it was discovered that certain 20-carbon-chain fatty acids are released in experimentally induced inflammatory states and in type I hypersensitivity reactions. These are known as **prostaglandins** (so named because they were first identified in seminal fluid). This was followed by a series of studies showing that:

- peroxidation of arachidonic acid, a major constituent of the lipid in cell membranes, occurs in many inflammatory conditions in a wide variety of species (including humans)
- injection of prostaglandins produces the vascular changes of acute inflammation.

Some potent anti-inflammatory drugs, most notably aspirin and indomethacin, selectively inhibit prostaglandin synthesis. Corticosteroids, the other major group of anti-inflammatory agents, do not inhibit prostaglandin synthesis. They stabilize membranes and in so doing may block the release of fatty acids from membrane phospholipids. Thus the supply of starting material for the synthesis of prostaglandins is cut off.

Arachidonic acid can be metabolized in two ways. First, the stable prostaglandins, such as prostaglandin (PG) E_2, the potent vasoconstrictor and platelet aggregator thromboxane A_2, and the dilator and anti-aggregatory compound PGI_2 are all produced via two unstable endoperoxides. These are produced from arachidonic acid via an enzyme pathway known as the **cyclo-oxygenase pathway**. This cyclo-oxygenase system is blocked by aspirin and indomethacin. Both PGE_2 and PGI_2 have a strong vasodilator effect and also produce some increase in vascular permeability. Prostaglandins of the E series are hyperalgesic and also act synergistically with other pain-producing mediators of inflammation such as bradykinin.

Another pathway of arachidonic acid peroxidation exists, known as the **lipo-oxygenase pathway**. This can occur in platelets, neutrophils and mast cells, and the initial step is the formation from arachidonic acid of an intermediate, 5-hydroperoxyeicosotetraenoic acid (HPETE). From this intermediate, a family of compounds known as the **leukotrienes** is produced. Much less is known about the inflammatory activity of these compounds than of the prostaglandins, but some are certainly chemotactic (most notably LT B_4) and others are chemokinetic.

Leukotrienes C_4, D_4 and E_4 are now known to be identical to a compound discovered over 40 years ago known as **slow-reacting substance A**, remarkable for its ability to produce **slow and sustained contraction of smooth muscle**, in contrast to the more rapid and short-lived effect of histamine. This substance can be found in the lungs of sensitized guinea-pigs challenged with the appropriate antigen, and is believed to be the effector substance that causes contraction of bronchiolar smooth muscle, leading to narrowing and obstruction of small airways in type I hypersensitivity reactions. Eosinophils tend to accumulate in the tissues of patients with type I hypersensitivity reactions, and it is now known that eosinophils contain large amounts of **aryl sulphatase**, which can destroy slow-reacting substance A. Thus the eosinophil reaction in tissues, for so long regarded simply as a useful marker of allergic injury, can now be seen to be the expression of a protective mechanism against excess leukotriene.

Platelet activating factor

The term 'platelet activating factor' (PAF) is an example of scientific terminology telling the truth but not the whole truth. This compound, derived from membrane phospholipid, does activate platelets but it also has a wide range of other activities, acting in the context of inflammation as a general upregulator of the processes so far described (*Fig. 5.8*).

PAF (1-*O*-alkyl-2-acetyl-sn-glycerol-3-phosphocholine) is generated after activation of phospholipase A_2 and is released at the same time as other membrane lipid-derived mediators.

PROTEIN MEDIATORS: THE CYTOKINES

Many low molecular weight proteins are synthesized and released from cells active in inflammation and in determining immune responses. These are shown in *Tables 5.3–5.7*; some, active in the acute inflammatory process, are discussed here.

IL-8 and other chemokines

Chemokines are low molecular weight proteins (8–11 kD) that are important

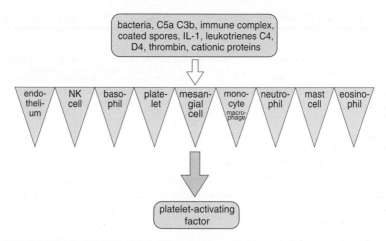

Fig. 5.8   Mechanisms leading to, and cell sources of, PAF release.
NK, natural killer.

in initiating and sustaining inflammatory reactions. Some preferentially attract neutrophils; others attract monocytes.

Chemokines are classified into two subfamilies: α and β.

The α family is coded for by genes located on chromosome 4. These chemokines are characterized by an amino acid sequence in which two terminal cysteines are separated by some other amino acid, thus giving the sequence Cys–X–Cys. Included in this group are IL-8, β-thromboglobulin *gro*-α, β and γ, and platelet factor 4.

α Chemokines are mostly produced by monocytes, although some are also produced by T lymphocytes, endothelial cells and platelets. **IL-8** mediates the rapid accumulation of neutrophils in inflamed tissues by inducing the formation of **neutrophil-binding ligands on the endothelial cells of microvessels** in the injured area. The chemokine *gro* (MIP-2α or 2β) also acts as a neutrophil chemoattractant as well as promoting the release of pro-inflammatory lysosomal enzymes. **β-thromboglobulin** and **platelet factor 4**, which are released from activated platelets, stimulate the fibroblasts that take part in the organization of thrombi and haematomas.

β Chemokines are encoded by genes located on chromosome 17. These mediators have a cysteine–cysteine amino acid arrangement (Cys–Cys). They include:

- RANTES (Regulated on Activation, Normal T cell Expressed and Secreted): RANTES is a potent attractant for 'memory' T cells but not for naive T cells, and also attracts monocytes
- macrophage-activating factor (MAF)
- MIP-1α
- MIP-1βα.

Table 5.3   Peptide cytokines – interleukins

Cytokine	Source	Functions
IL-1	Chiefly monocytes/ macrophages but many other cells including epithelial and endothelial cells	A multifunctional protein; many of its activities are similar to those of TNF-α. Acts as an **endogenous pyrogen**. Induces macrophages to produce **additional IL-1** and **IL-6**. Also induces glucocorticoid, prostaglandin and collagenase synthesis and release. Induces expression of adhesion molecules on vascular endothelium, thus stimulating leucocyte adhesion. Stimulates the production by macrophages of chemokines such as IL-8 which activate neutrophils
IL-2	T cells after stimulation by antigen or mitogen	Major growth factor for both helper and cytotoxic T cells and lymphokine-activated killer cells. Also involved in B-cell development
IL-4	Chiefly T_H2 cells	Pivotal in development of T_H2 subset; involved in B-cell help; causes switching of antibody production to IgE; growth factor for mast cells and stimulates production of VCAM
IL-5	T_H2 cells and activated mast cells	Stimulates growth and differentiation of eosinophils and thus promotes killing of helminths; promotes growth and differentiation of B cells and, together with other cytokines, induces synthesis of IgA and IgM in mature B cells
IL-6	Macrophages, fibroblasts, stromal cells in bone marrow, vascular endothelium and some T cells	Causes terminal differentiation of immunoglobulin-producing B cells; inhibits macrophage production of IL-1 and interferon-γ (IFN-γ); stimulates liver cells to produce acute-phase proteins such as fibrinogen, serum amyloid protein A, α_2-macroglobulin; promotes formation of osteoclasts
IL-7	Stromal cells in bone marrow and thymus	Stimulates proliferation of B-cell progenitors which show no rearrangement of heavy and light chain genes in germ cell line, and pre-B cells in which rearrangement of these genes has occurred but which have no surface immunoglobulin as yet. Stimulates mature T cells and enhances cytotoxicity
IL-9	T lymphocytes	Promotes proliferation of T cells
IL-10	T and B lymphocytes, activated mast cells and epidermal cells	Downregulates production of cytokines including IL-1, macrophages, IFN-γ and TNF-α by macrophages; inhibits nitric oxide (NO) production; stimulates B-cell proliferation, differentiation and activity
IL-11	Stromal cells	Promotes both lymphopoiesis and growth of haemopoietic cells
IL-12	Has two subunits: one produced by T, B, natural killer (NK) cells and macrophages; the other by activated macrophages and B cells	Strong stimulator of NK cells, growth factor for activated T cells and maturation factor for cytotoxic T cells; induces formation of IFN-γ and thus enhances formation of T_H1 cells
IL-13	Activated helper and cytotoxic T cells	Suppresses proinflammatory cytokine, chemokine and growth factor production by macrophages and also downregulates the production of NO; enhances expression of MHC class II proteins and thus antigen presentation; causes human B cells to switch antibody production to IgE and IgG4. Shares some features with IL-4
IL-14	T cells and malignant B cells	Induces proliferation of activated but not of resting B cells, and inhibits immunoglobulin production
IL-15	Epithelial cells	Stimulates T-cell proliferation by binding to IL-2 receptor

Table 5.4 Peptide cytokines – interferons

Cytokine	Source	Functions
IFN-α and IFN-β	Leucocytes and fibroblasts	Antiviral; activates phagocytes
IFN-γ	T and NK cells	Antiviral; pivotal for development of T_H1 from T_H0 cells and inhibits development of T_H2 cells; it is the most powerful macrophage-activating factor (MAF) and is therefore important in cell-mediated immunity; increases expression of MHC class I and II proteins, thus enhancing antigen presentation; causes the expression of adhesion molecules on the surface of vascular endothelium (as does TNF-α); causes differentiation of cytotoxic T cells; antagonizes several IL-4 actions; promotes synthesis of IgG_{2a} by activated B cells

Table 5.5 Peptide cytokines – cytotoxins

Cytokine	Source	Functions
TNF-α	Macrophages, mast cells and T cells. Macrophages stimulated to produce TNF by IFN-γ and migration inhibition factor (MIF). MIF production by T cells is stimulated by endotoxin	Derives its name because serum of animals given endotoxin produces haemorrhagic necrosis in tumours. At **high concentrations** (as may be induced by endotoxin), TNF acts systemically. It functions as a **pyrogen**, activates the **clotting system**, stimulates production of **acute-phase proteins** by the liver, inhibits myocardial contractility by stimulating production of NO, and over long periods causes cachexia. At **low concentrations** TNF-α upregulates the inflammatory response; it induces expression of the adhesion molecules ICAM-1, VCAM-1 and E-selectin, which promote adhesion and migration of leucocytes from the microvessels to the extravascular compartment. It enhances the killing of intracellular organisms such as *Leishmania*, and *Mycobacterium tuberculosis*. It activates several leucocyte types leading to the production by macrophages of various cytokines including IL-6, chemokines and TNF-α itself
TNF-β	Activated T cells	Shares many of the actions of TNF-α. Lyses tumour cells but not normal cells; activates neutrophils; increases adhesion of leucocytes to vascular endothelium and promotes their migration

Table 5.6   Peptide cytokines – colony-stimulating factors

Cytokine	Source	Functions
Granulocyte–macrophage colony-stimulating factor (GM-CSF)	T cells, macrophages, mast cells, endothelium, fibroblasts	Stimulates growth of granulocyte and macrophage colonies; activates macrophages, neutrophils and eosinophils
G-CSF	Fibroblasts, endothelium	Stimulates proliferation of mature granulocytes
M-CSF	Fibroblasts, endothelium, epithelium	Stimulates growth of macrophage colonies
IL-3	T cells and mast cells	Stimulates growth and differentiation of haemopoietic precursors
Steel factor	Stromal cells in bone marrow	Causes mitotic division of haemopoietic stem cells (binds to the c-*kit* ligand)
Transforming growth factor β (TGF-β). This is a family of five closely related proteins. TGF-β is secreted in an inactive form and must be cleaved before it can bind to its receptor	Monocytes, T lymphocytes and platelets	Has an autocrine effect on monocyte–macrophages and regulates its own production by these cells. It also upregulates the production of IL-1, fibroblast growth factor (FGF), platelet-derived growth factor (PDGF) and TNF-α. It increases production of connective tissue matrix proteins and is a potent angiogenic factor. It has an immunosuppressive effect by inhibiting the proliferation of T lymphocytes

Table 5.7   Peptide cytokines – chemokines

Cytokine	Source	Functions
α Chemokines All have Cys–X–Cys amino acid sequence Includes IL-8 and gro-α, β, γ	Principally by monocytes, some also by T cells, endothelial cells and platelets	Induce rapid accumulation of neutrophils by mediating formation of neutrophil-binding ligands on endothelium
β Chemokines All have Cys–Cys amino acid sequence Includes RANTES and MAF	T lymphocytes and monocytes	Potent attractants for memory T cells and monocytes

These chemokines are produced by T lymphocytes and monocytes. MAF acts exclusively on monocytes, attracting them to sites of injury, activating them and regulating the expression of integrins on their surfaces.

IL-1 and TNF-α

IL-1 and TNF-α are peptides that have many activities in common.

The principal sources of **IL-1** are monocytes and macrophages, but other cells such as endothelial cells and some epithelial cells may also produce this cytokine. IL-1 has a molecular weight of 17–18 kD and is a potent regulator both of local inflammatory events and of many systemic ones (*Fig. 5.9*). Its synthesis is stimulated by various microbial products, most notably

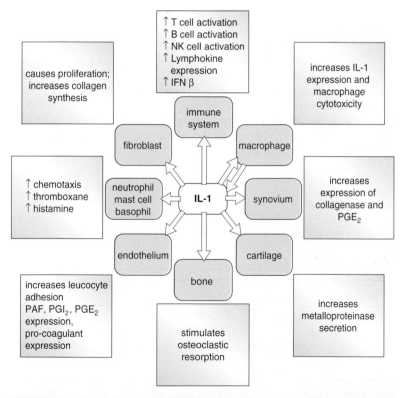

Fig. 5.9 Targets and effects of interleukin 1.

NK, natural killer; IFN, interferon; PG, prostaglandin.

bacterial endotoxin, and other cytokines. Locally, it upregulates adhesion molecule expression on endothelial cells, leading to adhesion of both leucocytes and platelets and to stimulation of macrophage production of chemokines (such as IL-8) that activate neutrophils. Systemically, IL-1 acts as an endogenous pyrogen (inducer of fever) and induces glucocorticoid synthesis and the release of prostaglandins, collagenase and acute-phase proteins. It lacks the ability of TNF-α to produce necrosis of tumour cells and tissue injury, to increase the expression of MHC-coded proteins or to mediate the Schwartzmann reaction.

TNF-α belongs to a family of ligands (currently with ten known members). Among many other functions mentioned below, all of these ligands bind to receptors on target cells that initiate signals either for cell proliferation or for apoptosis. TNF exists almost entirely as a secreted protein, but the others are transmembrane proteins acting chiefly through cell–cell contact.

TNF-α binds to two receptors, one a 55 kD and the other a 75 kD transmembrane protein (*Table 5.8*). It is one of the cytokines produced in the greatest amounts by stimulated macrophages, especially if the stimulatory signal has been bacterial endotoxin.

TNF-α plays an important part in host defence against infections by Gram-negative bacteria, its production being greatly modulated by endotoxin. When endotoxin is present at low doses TNF-α mediates a protective response by enhancing macrophage killing and cytokine production, activation of B lymphocytes and induction of fever. TNF upregulates the expression of MHC class I proteins and the cytotoxic potential of CD8 T lymphocytes, thus increasing host defence against intracellular parasites. At high concentrations it is one of the potent mediators concerned in the pathogenesis of endotoxin-related shock.

Table 5.8   TNF-α and its receptors

Receptor occupied	Effects
55 kD	Apoptosis Tumour cell lysis in vitro
75 kD	T-lymphocyte proliferation Skin necrosis Insulin resistance
Both	Bone resorption Haemorrhagic necrosis in tumours Fever

PHAGOCYTE RESPONSE TO CHEMOTACTIC SIGNALS

RECEPTION AND TRANSDUCTION OF THE SIGNAL

Chemotactic substances can be likened to hormones in that they are soluble molecules acting on cells distant from the point at which the chemical signal is generated (*Table 5.9*). As with hormones, it is likely that the first site of interaction between the chemotactic molecule and the phagocyte is a **specific receptor** or series of receptors on the plasma membrane of the phagocyte. We know this is correct for at least two of the chemotactic signals mentioned above: the formylated peptides and the 5a component of the complement system.

Formylated peptides bind saturably and with high affinity to the surface of both human and rabbit neutrophils, and there appear to be definable populations of these peptide receptors on the neutrophil surface. It is unlikely that a single receptor on the plasma membrane of the phagocyte binds all the chemotactic substances mentioned, because exposing cells to excessive

Table 5.9   Effects of inflammatory mediators

Inflammatory event	Responsible mediator(s)
Dilatation of microvessels	Histamine Bradykinin Prostaglandins
Increase in microvessel permeability with production of oedema	Complement fractions C3a and C5a Histamine Bradykinin PAF Leukotrienes C_4, D_4, E_4
Chemotaxis	f-Met-Leu-Phe C5a, ?C3a Cationic proteins derived from neutrophils TNF-α, IL-8
Tissue damage	Lysosomal enzymes Oxygen free radicals generated by acute inflammatory cells
Pain	Bradykinin PGE_2
Fever	TNF-α IL-1 Both act in this way by mediating production of prostaglandins

amounts of the chemotactic peptides does not appear to block their ability to respond to C5a; the reverse is also true.

Signal transduction (*Fig. 5.10*) has been studied by exposing neutrophils to chemotactic peptides. This is followed by release of arachidonic acid, suggesting activation of a membrane phospholipase. This increase in arachidonic acid may induce changes in membrane ion permeability (especially for calcium). Ion fluxes are now believed to play an important role in chemotactic signal transduction: changes in both sodium and calcium flux are involved.

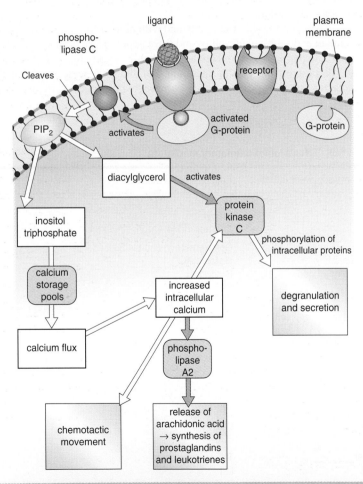

Fig. 5.10 Transduction of chemotactic signals within leucocytes after ligand binding to the appropriate receptor on the leucocyte plasma membrane.

Cyclic nucleotides also play an important part in the initiation of movement of phagocytes. The balance between release of cAMP and cGMP may well constitute a control system for the activation and blocking of both chemotaxis and certain other events (such as the release of active compounds from the granules of mast cells) in the acute inflammatory reaction. **cGMP** enhances:

- chemotactic movement
- the release of histamine and leukotrienes from mast cells
- the release of lysosomal enzymes and lymphokines from neutrophils and T lymphocytes respectively.

cAMP produces the *opposite* effect in each of these instances. The main effect of the cyclic nucleotides within the neutrophil is probably exerted on the cytoskeleton, the principal target being the microtubule system. **Microtubules** are hollow fibres with a diameter of 24 nm; they appear to be inserted at the periphery of the cell in the region where the contractile microfilaments are concentrated. The microtubules are in equilibrium with the protein from which they are formed, known as **tubulin**. This is a dimeric protein which, when assembled into tubules, plays an important role not only in chemotaxis and cell secretion but also, in other cells, in mitosis.

A rise in the intracellular concentration of cGMP promotes assembly of the microtubules, and a rise in cAMP levels inhibits tubule assembly. Anything that inhibits microtubule assembly will also inhibit migration of neutrophils in response to chemotactic signals. This is the basis of an old treatment for acute gouty arthritis – **colchicine**. The acute local inflammation in gout results from a perversion of normal neutrophil function. Sodium biurate crystals are deposited in the synovium because of abnormal uric acid metabolism. These 'foreign' bodies attract neutrophils, which engulf them. However, abnormal hydrogen bonds form between the surface of the urate crystals and the phagolysosomal membrane, with resulting rupture of the membrane and spillage of the lysosomal enzymes into the extracellular space. It is this that causes the intense pain of acute gouty arthritis. Colchicine, through its interference with microtubule assembly, prevents phagocyte migration and interrupts this cycle of events. Vinca alkaloids, used in treating certain malignancies, act in the same way.

In contrast, drugs that *raise* the intracellular content of cGMP enhance the movement of phagocytes towards attractants. One such drug is **levamisole**, which can be shown to reverse chemotactic deactivation in vitro. More interestingly, levamisole has been shown to reverse the depression in movement of human neutrophils and monocytes induced by a number of viruses, including herpes simplex.

PHAGOCYTOSIS

Phagocytes arriving at the site of tissue damage and/or bacterial invasion must recognize which structures to attack and become attached to them.

In vivo, phagocytes demonstrate remarkable selectivity as to what they will ingest, presumably by recognizing certain specific features on cell surfaces. For example, mononuclear phagocytes (macrophages) ingest old or damaged red cells but disregard normal ones.

Opsonization

It has been known for a long time that bacterial cells coated with immunoglobulin or damaged cells that have interacted with fresh serum are phagocytosed more readily than those that have not. This coating of particles with proteins is called **opsonization** (preparation for eating, from the Greek *opsonein* meaning a 'relish') (*Fig. 5.11*).

Opsonins are either:

- **specific antibodies of the IgG class:** for opsonization to occur, the Fc fragment of the immunoglobulin must be intact
- the **C3b component of complement:** this is a non-specific activity of great biological value to the host, as invading microorganisms can be opsonized even on the first occasion that the host is infected with a particular organism.

The apparent restriction of opsonization to these two protein classes indicates that the plasma membrane of the phagocytic cell possesses specific receptor sites for the C3b subunit (one of the β_2 family of integrins) and for the Fc fragment of IgG.

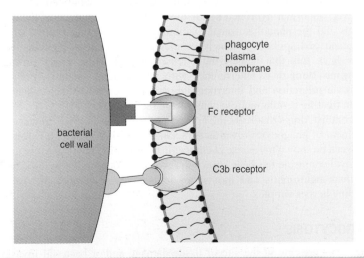

Fig. 5.11   Opsonization through the medium of immunoglobulin and C3b.

Engulfment

Engulfment of a bacterium or foreign object occurs through fusion of pseudopodia projecting from the phagocyte plasma membrane in the form of long finger-like projections. The pseudopodia fuse on the far side of the object to be phagocytosed, thus locking it within a membrane-bound vesicle or **phagosome**. The phagosome then buds off from the plasma membrane of the phagocyte and comes to lie within the neutrophil or macrophage cytoplasm. The phagosome membrane is obviously composed of part of the phagocyte plasma membrane which has become inverted; the inner layer of the phagosome membrane is therefore identical with the outer layer of the plasma membrane. Engulfment is an active, energy-dependent process which is inhibited by substances interfering with ATP production. This suggests that a mechanism such as actin–myosin contraction 'drives' engulfment as well as cell movement. Support for this view comes from the fact that colchicine inhibits engulfment as well as phagocyte migration.

Lysosomal fusion and degranulation

Once the phagosome has formed, lysosomal granules move towards it and apposition of their membranes, followed by membrane fusion, occurs. The lysosomal granules disappear as this happens (hence the expression 'degranulation of polymorphonuclear cells'). These events take place with great speed; fusion of lysosomes with phagosomes occurs more or less in concert with ingestion and ends when the process of ingestion is over. Compounds known to inhibit migration and phagocytosis also inhibit degranulation.

METABOLIC EVENTS ASSOCIATED WITH BACTERIAL KILLING

As well as triggering ingestion and fusion of phagosomes and lysosomes, recognition of an invading microorganism and attachment to it by the phagocyte is associated with a burst of oxidative activity (the **respiratory burst**). This results essentially in the step-wise **reduction of molecular oxygen to hydrogen peroxide**:

- This respiratory burst is associated with a 2–20-fold increase in oxygen consumption compared with a resting cell, and there is a considerable increase in glucose metabolism via the **hexose monophosphate shunt**.
- Reduction of molecular oxygen is catalysed by a non-haem protein oxidase believed to be localized on the external surface of the phagocyte plasma membrane.
- The hydrogen donor for the reduction is either reduced nicotinamide adenine dinucleotide (NADH) or reduced nicotinamide adenine dinucleotide phosphate (NADPH). The presence of one or other of these pyridine nucleotides is an essential link in the chain because, if regeneration from NAD to NADP cannot take place, hydrogen peroxide will not be formed. Hence adequate amounts of glucose-6-phosphate

dehydrogenase (G6PD) are required within the cell if bacterial killing is to proceed in the normal way.

- In reduction, oxygen gains only one electron and is converted into an **oxygen free radical**, the superoxide anion (O_2^-). About 90% of the oxygen consumed in the respiratory burst is converted into superoxide anion.
- When two molecules of this anion react with each other, one is oxidized and the other reduced, forming **hydrogen peroxide** and oxygen in a **dismutation** reaction, catalysed by the enzyme **superoxide dismutase**. Other highly reactive oxygen-derived metabolites have been identified or have been predicted to exist as a result of activation of phagocytic cells. These include an active hydroxyl radical ($OH^\bullet$), singlet oxygen and hypochlorous acid.

Phagocytes cannot kill ingested organisms in the absence of the respiratory burst and without production of the superoxide anion. Both superoxide dismutase and catalase can inhibit phagocyte-mediated bacterial killing. However, superoxide appears to have little bactericidal effect on its own, and it is now widely believed that the most important bactericidal activity within phagocytes resides in hydrogen peroxide. Hydrogen peroxide by itself has significant bactericidal activity, but this is potentiated 50-fold when the hydrogen peroxide reacts with the myeloperoxidase (one of the phagocyte's lysosomal enzymes) and halide ions. The most likely product, in chemical terms, of the hydrogen peroxide–myeloperoxidase–halide complex is hypochlorous acid (HOCl).

The bactericidal mechanism appears to involve halogenation or oxidation of the bacterial surface. It is also likely that decarboxylation of cell walls and/or cell membrane proteins occurs, with local generation of toxic aldehydes. In addition to the activity of the hydrogen peroxide–myeloperoxidase–halide complex, evidence suggests that hydroxyl radicals formed by the interaction between hydrogen peroxide and the superoxide anion are also important in bacterial killing; mannitol, a scavenger of hydroxy radicals, inhibits the bactericidal activity of an acetaldehyde–xanthine oxidase system which can trap and reduce molecular oxygen, generating active oxygen free radicals.

DETOXIFICATION OF HYDROGEN PEROXIDE

As hydrogen peroxide can diffuse out of phagosomes, it is important that mechanisms should exist to prevent lipid peroxidation of the cell's own membranes. The scavenger systems involved are catalase and, perhaps even more importantly, glutathione peroxidase. The activity of the latter implies a need for a constantly replenished supply of reduced glutathione. This, once again, emphasizes the importance of G6PD, as reduced glutathione must be regenerated through coupling mechanisms linked to the hexose monophosphate shunt. Thus G6PD is involved in both the production and detoxification of bactericidal peroxides.

OTHER MECHANISMS OF BACTERIAL KILLING

While the oxygen-dependent bactericidal mechanisms in phagocytes are fundamental, there are other systems that injure ingested microorganisms. These are related to various aspects of lysosomal function and include:

- **Low pH within the phagolysosome**. The pH inside the vacuole is 3.5–4; this in itself may be bactericidal or bacteriostatic (preventing multiplication without killing organisms). In addition, the low pH promotes the production of hydrogen peroxide from superoxide.
- **Lysozyme (muramidase)**. This is a low molecular weight cationic enzyme which attacks the mucopeptide cell walls of some bacterial species.
- **Lactoferrin**. This iron-binding protein inhibits the growth of a number of microorganisms.
- **Cationic proteins** with antibacterial activity also enter the phagosome in the course of fusion and degranulation.
- **Lysosomal hydrolases** entering the phagosome in the course of phagosome–lysosome fusion may have some antibacterial activity, but are probably more important in digesting the remains of organisms killed by other means.

DEFECTS OF NEUTROPHIL FUNCTION

NEUTROPENIA

Even if the operations discussed above occur normally, this is of no avail in protecting the host if there are **insufficient cells** to cope with the number of invading microorganisms. This situation occurs in various forms of bone marrow failure:

- drug or poison induced (e.g. chloramphenicol, benzene)
- infiltration of the marrow by large numbers of tumour cells
- bone marrow fibrosis
- other forms of marrow failure.

DISORDERS OF MIGRATION AND CHEMOTAXIS

These may occur as a result of an intrinsic defect in the cell, from inhibition of locomotion or because of deficiencies in the generation of chemotactic signals.

Intrinsic cell defects

The 'lazy leucocyte' syndrome. The nature of this defect has not been identified.

Job's syndrome. This typically affects fair-skinned, red-haired females and is characterized by recurrent 'cold' staphylococcal abscesses.

Diabetes mellitus.   Leucocytes from diabetic patients with poorly con-trolled diabetes show impairment of locomotion. This is at least partially reversed by adding insulin and glucose to the leucocytes.

Chediak–Higashi syndrome.   This rare congenital autosomal recessive disorder occurs in humans, cattle, mink and certain strains of mouse. In all species it is characterized by partial albinism, the presence of giant lyso-somal granules in neutrophils, and increased susceptibility to bacterial in-fection. In humans, death usually occurs in childhood and is often preceded by the development of a malignant process involving lymphoid cells. Two major defects have been documented in the neutrophils of patients suffering from this syndrome:

1) failure to show directed movement in response to chemotactic stimuli both in vivo and in vitro
2) a delay in intracellular bacterial killing which appears to result from a reduced rate of phagosome–lysosome fusion.

It has been proposed that this combination of defects results from a failure in microtubule assembly from tubulin; the addition of cGMP or agents that increase intracellular cGMP generation to the neutrophils might reverse the situation. The lysosomes in Chediak–Higashi leucocytes lack elastase and cathepsin G.

Leucocyte adhesion deficiency syndrome.   This is due to absence of the CD18 β subunit of the β_2 integrins expressed on the surface of leucocytes. It affects neutrophils only; monocytes, lymphocytes and eosinophils can make use of the β_1 integrin system, which involves binding of very late activation antigen 4 (VLA-4) on the leucocytes with VCAM on endothelium.

Inhibition of locomotion

The serum of certain patients inhibits neutrophil chemotaxis; certain drugs such as corticosteroids and phenylbutazone also do this.

Deficiencies in the generation of chemotactic signals

The most important of these are deficiencies in the complement system.

DISORDERS OF PHAGOCYTOSIS
Opsonin deficiencies

These include deficiencies of complement or IgG. Some patients with sickle cell disease have opsonin deficiencies, apparently associated with failure of alternate pathway activation of the complement system.

DEFECTS OF ENGULFMENT

These can be brought about by drugs, such as morphine analogues. They also occur under hyperosmolar conditions, such as may be seen in diabetic keto-acidosis.

DISORDERS OF LYSOSOMAL FUSION

This may occur with drugs, such as corticosteroids, colchicine and certain antimalarials. Failure of lysosomal fusion in the neutrophils of patients with Chediak–Higashi syndrome is mentioned above.

DISORDERS OF BACTERIAL KILLING

The most important disorder of bacterial killing is **chronic granulomatous disease of childhood**. This is a rare childhood disorder, sometimes X-linked, which is characterized by recurrent bacterial infections involving skin, lung, bones and lymph nodes. Affected children show increased susceptibility to infection by a rather mixed bag of organisms including *Staphylococcus aureus*, *Aerobacter aerogenes* and certain fungi such as *Aspergillus* species. Draining lymph nodes are often enlarged and show proliferation of mononuclear phagocytes lining the sinuses or aggregations of mononuclear cells tightly packed together to form granulomatous foci.

The neutrophils in this condition respond normally to chemotactic signals and phagocytose normally. However, the burst of respiratory activity that normally follows engulfment does not take place and there is no superoxide or hydrogen peroxide production. Failure to produce reactive oxygen intermediates is due to a defect in the cytochrome b-245 oxidase system. This cytochrome has two subunits, large (92 kD) and small (22 kD).

The **X-linked form** of the disease is due to a mutation in the gene coding for the larger subunit. In most cases this results in failure to produce **any** gene product but in some cases a low level of gene product is present; these patients can be treated with interferon γ with some success.

About one-third of children with chronic granulomatous disease inherit the disease in an **autosomal recessive** pattern. The defect results either from a mutation in the gene encoding the smaller 22 kD subunit or in the cytosolic components of the NADPH oxidase system.

Interestingly, neutrophils from patients with chronic granulomatous disease can kill certain pathogenic microorganisms such as streptococci and pneumococci. These organisms produce a certain amount of hydrogen peroxide themselves but *do not produce catalase*. Within the phagosome the concentration of hydrogen peroxide produced by the microorganism rises gradually until, in a sense, the organisms 'commit suicide'. However, bacteria that also produce catalase are safe from the effects of their own hydrogen peroxide.

The role of G6PD in the production and detoxification of hydrogen peroxide has been mentioned above. If the degree of deficiency of this enzyme is very severe, a clinical picture resembling that encountered in chronic granulomatous disease of childhood may be seen. Absence of myeloperoxidase brings about some reduction in the efficiency of intracellular, oxygen-dependent bactericidal mechanisms, but the functional defect is usually not very severe.

KEY POINTS: NEUTROPHIL FUNCTION AS A MEANS OF HOST DEFENCE

- As part of the host's system of defence against infection by pathogenic microorganisms, the role of the neutrophil is to **seek out, ingest and kill a wide range of these organisms**. These processes can be looked at most easily as a set of distinct operations, any of which can go wrong and thus render the neutrophil ineffective as a bacterial 'hunter–killer'.
- As with any instruction, that given to the neutrophil to emigrate from the local microvasculature and to proceed towards the invading microorganisms or the injured or dead tissue elements must involve the **giving** and **receiving** of an appropriate **signal**. **Transduction** of this signal must then take place, so that **migration** of the phagocytic cell can occur towards the point from which the signal emanated. The generation and reception of the signal and the vectorial movement by the neutrophil which follows is known as **chemotaxis**.
- Once the neutrophil has reached the invading microorganism or the dead or effete cells from which the chemotactic signal has been generated, a process of **attachment** occurs between the neutrophil and the object to be phagocytosed. This is facilitated by the latter being coated by either immunoglobulin or one of the components of complement C3b. *Phagocytic cells possess receptors for the Fc portion of immunoglobulin and for C3b.*
- In some instances, one of the acute-phase proteins – C-reactive protein – binds to carbohydrates on certain bacteria and activates complement via the classical pathway, thus leading to coating of the organism by C3b. These coating molecules, which provide binding sites for the phagocytes, are called **opsonins** and the coating process is termed **opsonization**. The foreign material or organism is then engulfed by the plasma membrane of the phagocyte and comes to lie within a membrane-bound vesicle called the **phagosome**. These two steps together constitute the process of **phagocytosis**.
- *Fusion then takes place between the membranes of the phagosome and a lysosome, resulting in the formation of a secondary lysosome or phagolysosome.* In this way the contents of the lysosome are released into the lumen of the phagosome. The morphological correlate of this operation is loss of granules in the cytoplasm of the neutrophil. If the occupant of the phagolysosome is a living organism, killing and digestion of that organism occurs. This is accomplished largely by **oxygen-dependent mechanisms**.

MONONUCLEAR PHAGOCYTES IN ACUTE INFLAMMATION

The cellular component of inflammation includes another type of phago-cytic cell, the mononuclear phagocyte, which exists in two forms. An inter-mediate form, known as the **monocyte**, circulates in the blood; following migration into tissues it either matures or differentiates into the tissue **macrophage**.

The monocyte has a half-life of about 22 hours, approximately three times as long as that of the neutrophil. Despite the fact that it can be regarded as an intermediate cell form, it possesses a range of functional activities shared with the mature tissue macrophage.

Monocytes and macrophages are derived from bone marrow. Bone marrow destruction by X-rays leads to failure of injury to elicit any mono-nuclear cell response, whereas after thymectomy a normal response is pro-duced. The transition from monocyte to macrophage within the tissue is accompanied by a considerable structural and functional increase in the phagocytic, lysosomal and secretory apparatus in that:

- the cell becomes larger
- the plasma membrane becomes more convoluted
- lysosomes increase in number
- both the Golgi apparatus and the endoplasmic reticulum become more prominent.

There is considerable overlap in the phagocytic functions of the macrophage and the neutrophil, so it is not a surprise to find that the plasma membrane of the macrophage has surface receptors for the Fc fragment of immunoglobulin as well as for complement components.

Like the neutrophil, the macrophage depends on glycolysis for its energy needs during phagocytosis and also exhibits a respiratory burst following bacterial engulfment. However, because it has a well-developed protein secretory apparatus, the macrophage can synthesize and replace depleted enzymes, and this allows it to act for a much longer time than the neutrophil.

Many pathogenic microorganisms are phagocytosed by the macrophage. A large number of them are destroyed within the phagosomes as effectively as in the neutrophil. However, some organisms parasitize macrophages and multiply within the phagosomes. Such organisms include *Listeria*, *Brucella*, *Salmonella*, *Mycobacterium*, *Chlamydia*, *Rickettsia*, *Leishmania*, *Toxoplasma*, *Trypanosoma* and *Legionella*. This symbiotic relationship is destroyed by **activation of the macrophage**, which then becomes highly dangerous to its previous symbiotes.

CHEMICAL INFLUENCES ON MACROPHAGE FUNCTION

Macrophage chemotactic factors include those already described for the neutrophil, such as complement cleavage products, microbial products, *N*-formyl methionyl peptides and fibrin degradation products. In addition, however, there is an important group of chemical activators that trigger a wide range of macrophage functions apart from chemotaxis. These are called **lymphokines** and are secreted by **activated T lymphocytes**. It is now will accepted that sensitized T lymphocytes reacting with specific antigen can release products that activate macrophages, both *in vivo* and *in vitro*. The lymphokines include:

- a **macrophage chemotactic factor**, which can recruit macrophages into sites of infection, contact-type hypersensitivity or inflammation

- a **migration inhibition factor**, which can immobilize macrophages in certain lesions
- factors that stimulate the secretion of hydrolytic enzymes by macrophages, rendering them capable of killing neoplastic cells and of limiting the ability of intracellular organisms to reproduce themselves.

Other types of macrophage activation, for example via the action of complement cleavage products, lead to other forms of activity. This topic is discussed further in Chapter 14.

ACUTE INFLAMMATION II: CELLULAR EVENTS AND CHEMICAL MEDIATORS

- **Phagocytes** (neutrophils and macrophages) are pivotal in **defence against infection**. Low cell numbers or defective function increase susceptibility to infection.
- Phagocyte migration requires **adhesion to vascular endothelium**, a two stage process medicated by binding between phagocyte and endothelial molecules.
- The migration is mediated by chemical signals (chemokines), of which IL-8 is the most important in this context; cells move in response to chemical signals (**chemotaxis**).
- **Chemotaxis** involves the reception and transduction of chemical signals.
- Most of the chemical signals are endogenous and are derived from plasma protein cascade systems (the **complement system**, **Hageman factor** – clotting factor XII, the **kinin system** and the **fibrinolytic system**) and cells (**vasoactive amines**, **modified fatty acids** and **low-molecular weight proteins**).
- **Bacterial killing** by phagocytes is largely oxygen-dependent. It involves a burst of oxidative activity leading to the formation of bactericidal metabolites.
- Defects in phagocyte function arise in many ways including:
  — low cell number (neutropenia)
  — failures in chemotactic signal generation/transduction
  — defects in cell movement and/or engulfment
  — failures in bacterial killing.

6 Factors that modify the inflammatory reaction

The processes described in Chapters 4 and 5 are common to some degree to all acute inflammatory responses. However, there are considerable differences between inflammatory reactions, and these differences involve a number of variables. The outcome of an injury is the result of interaction between the **injurious agent** and the **host**; variations in either of these may exert a considerable effect.

FACTORS RELATED TO THE INJURIOUS AGENT

These include:

- the amount or dose of the agent
- its strength (or, in the case of a pathogenic microorganism, its virulence)
- the duration of exposure in the case of physical or chemical agents
- the intrinsic nature of the agent.

The severity of injury produced by any noxious agent, living or not, is a function of its inherent toxicity and the time for which it exerts its effect. Duration of exposure is of particular importance in injury produced by physical and certain chemical agents such as heat, cold, actinic rays, acids and alkalis. In injury produced by pathogenic microorganisms, the inherent power of the organisms to produce tissue damage is of great importance, but here too the **dose** of the agent may determine the outcome of the infection.

MORPHOLOGICAL FEATURES

The intrinsic nature of the agent may correlate with a distinctive morphological reaction in the tissues. Thus, the structural pattern may help the histopathologist to make an aetiological diagnosis.

Suppurative inflammation

Certain organisms, such as *Staphylococcus aureus*, tend to elicit inflammation that is characterized by massive neutrophil accumulation. Many of these neutrophils die after phagocytosis of the microorganisms and release lysosomal enzymes into the damaged area. Because the organisms also produce substances (exotoxins) that damage tissues directly, the end-result is a central area of liquefaction necrosis containing tissue debris and dead and dying neutrophils. This forms a thick, opaque, yellowish-green fluid, known as **pus**. Organisms eliciting this reaction are termed **pyogenic** (i.e. pus forming). The process of pus formation is termed **suppuration**, and a localized suppurative lesion is called an **abscess**.

Membranous inflammation

Corynebacterium diphtheriae and *Clostridium difficile* produce powerful exotoxins that kill surface epithelia. The fluid that exudes from the small subepithelial blood vessels is rich in fibrinogen, which is converted to fibrin, and then becomes densely infiltrated by neutrophils. The end-result is an opaque greyish-white membrane, consisting of a mixture of dead epithelial cells, fibrin and neutrophils. This type of reaction is described as **membranous** or **pseudomembranous**. In the case of diphtheria, the target area is the pharynx and larynx. The clostridium causes pseudomembranous enterocolitis, particularly in patients whose bowel bacterial flora has been altered by previous antibiotic treatment.

Predominantly macrophage cellular reactions

Salmonella typhi, the organism responsible for typhoid fever, does not elicit a neutrophil response. The lesions of typhoid – occurring in the gut, lymph nodes, liver and less often at other sites – are therefore characterized by a predominantly macrophage infiltrate.

Haemorrhagic inflammation

Some organisms attack small blood vessels, producing lesions in which bleeding is prominent. This occurs in certain rickettsial diseases such as typhus, in anthrax, and in some cases of pneumonia caused by the influenza virus.

Fibrinoid necrosis

Inflammatory reactions caused by impaction or formation of antigen–antibody complexes in small blood vessels or by irradiation are characterized by a reaction in which both blood vessels and intercellular collagen show a curious form of necrosis. In sections conventionally stained with haematoxylin and eosin, the affected vessels or collagen fibres appear smudgy and deeply eosinophilic. Appropriate special stains show fibrin to be present in these areas, and this type of tissue damage is accordingly known as **fibrinoid necrosis** (see p. 203).

Extension of inflammatory processes

Where inflammation is due to infection by a pathogenic microorganism, the ability of the organism to spread through the tissues is an important modifying factor. The natural history of the disease depends on whether the tissue reaction keeps the infection localized or whether spread to surrounding tissues or distant sites occurs. Factors influencing this include:

- release of spreading factors by the microorganism
- lymphatic blockage
- the susceptibility of the microorganism to phagocytosis.

Release of spreading factors by infective agents.   Many such agents exist, including exotoxins that can hydrolyse the mucopolysaccharide ground substance in the extracellular space, such as the hyaluronidase produced by both *Streptococcus pyogenes* and *Clostridium perfringens*: both characteristically cause spreading inflammation. Streptococci also produce streptokinase, which lyses polymerized fibrin laid down in the course of inflammatory exudate formation; this too may inhibit localization of infection. The clostridia causing **gas gangrene** (*C. perfringens*, *C. oedematiens* and *C. septicum*), not only produce exotoxins such as hyaluronidase and collagenase which facilitate spreading of infection, but also modify the local reaction by the release of powerful necrotizing toxins which break down muscle (see p. 45). The muscle carbohydrate is then fermented by appropriate enzymes also produced by these organisms, forming bubbles of gas which make the affected tissues feel crepitant (crackly).

Lymphatic blockage.   This may assist in localization of infection, presumably being mediated by coagulation of lymph: this process is inhibited if the invading pathogen (such as *S. pyogenes*) is able to elaborate lytic enzymes.

The susceptibility of infecting microorganisms to the normal defensive process of phagocytosis is obviously an important variable. Some organisms have surface material (capsules) which makes phagocytosis difficult. This material may be carbohydrate in nature, such as the capsular polysaccharide of the *Pneumococcus*, or a protein. *S. aureus* has a protein (protein A) in its wall which combines with the Fc fragment of antibody attached to the organism and thus blocks attachment of this fragment to the Fc receptor on the phagocyte.

S. pyogenes and *S. aureus* produce toxins that can kill the threatening phagocytes. These few examples serve to indicate the range of defensive options evolved by prokaryotes against phagocytosis and killing.

FACTORS RELATED TO THE HOST

Factors related to the host operate predominantly, but not exclusively, in relation to the injuries produced by microorganisms. Some of these factors may be inferred from material presented in earlier sections, especially in relation to chemotaxis, phagocytosis and bacterial killing (see Chapter 5).

The general health of the host is important; infections that, under normal circumstances are fairly trivial, may become life threatening if the host is debilitated, undernourished or severely anaemic. For example, measles, which occurs principally in childhood, is usually a mildly unpleasant and inconvenient disorder in developed countries. In malnourished populations, however, measles is a major cause of death in infants and children (the ninth commonest cause of death).

Just as defects in phagocytes render the host more susceptible to infection, so do defects in the B- and T-cell elements of the immune system. These may occur as part of a congenital syndrome or may be acquired either through some disease associated with immunosuppression (such as acquired immune deficiency syndrome or Hodgkin's disease). Immunodeficiency may also result from treatment in which immunosuppression is induced either deliberately (as in patients receiving allogeneic transplants) or as a side-effect (as in patients receiving cytotoxic therapy for malignant neoplastic processes, particularly those involving the lymphoreticular system).

CLASSIFICATION OF INFLAMMATORY REACTIONS

We can use simple **set theory** to classify inflammation. Sets that can usefully be considered are:

- **duration** of the inflammatory reaction
- **type of exudate** associated with the particular type of injury; this may be:
  a) serous
  b) fibrinous
  c) haemorrhagic
  d) catarrhal
  e) purulent (suppurative)
  f) membranous or pseudomembranous
  g) a combination of the above
- the influence on lesion morphology and natural history of the **anatomical location** of the injury; this can be considered under the following simple headings:
  a) **solid tissue**
  b) **epithelium-lined surfaces**
  c) **serosal surfaces**.

Examples of the use of a common set as an expression of a particular inflammatory reaction are shown in *Fig. 6.1*.

DURATION

Inflammation of short duration (days) is termed **acute**. A reaction lasting for some weeks is termed **subacute**, and long-lasting inflammatory reactions (months or even years) are described as **chronic**.

TYPES OF EXUDATE

Serous exudate

A serous exudate is low in protein, particularly fibrinogen, so that there is little formation of polymerized fibrin. This type of reaction is frequently seen in relation to surfaces lined by mesothelial cells, such as the joint spaces

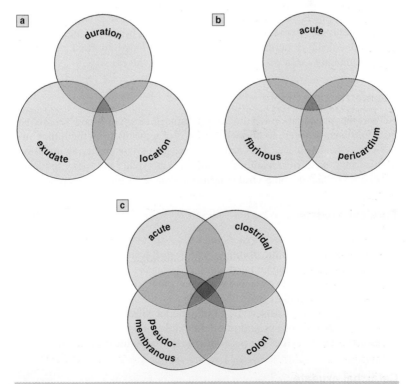

Fig. 6.1 Use of set theory to categorize inflammatory reactions.

a Chosen sets; **b** fibrinous pericarditis; **c** pseudomembranous colitis.

or pleural cavities. A typical example of serous exudation is the fluid that accumulates in a common blister, such as that seen after mild repetitive trauma (e.g. chopping wood, or rowing by those not used to the exercise). Similar serous effusions are not uncommonly seen in tuberculous pleurisy, particularly in young adults.

Fibrinous exudate

Fibrinous exudate is lower in volume than the serous type and has a high protein content, with a large amount of fibrinogen that is converted to fibrin. It occurs particularly in relation to serosa-lined cavities such as pleura, pericardium and peritoneum. The mesothelial linings involved characteristically lose their moist, shiny-looking surface. This becomes dull, granular and opaque as the linings become covered by polymerized fibrin. Clinically, fibrinous serosal exudates are associated with pain elicited by movement of the underlying viscera. Thus, in patients with fibrinous pleurisy, inhalation causes a 'catch' in the breath due to pain. On clinical examination, auscultation reveals a creaking sound known as a 'friction rub'.

Two contiguous surfaces covered in fibrin tend to stick together; if the fibrin is not lysed later in the inflammatory process, bridges of scar tissue are formed and result in permanent loss of function. One important example is postinflammatory stenosis of the aortic or mitral valves.

Haemorrhagic exudate

Haemorrhagic exudation occurs where damage to small blood vessels has been sufficiently severe to allow the escape of red cells from the lumen into the extravascular space. This may be seen in certain bacterial infections such as anthrax, in rickettsial infections such as typhus and rocky mountain spotted fever, and in some viral conditions such as influenzal pneumonia.

Purulent exudate

Certain pathogenic microorganisms cause an inflammation reaction in which the neutrophil is the dominant element. Because of the large number of cells present, the exudate is opaque. The organisms concerned often also liberate toxins producing tissue necrosis, and the lysosomal enzymes liberated from dying neutrophils cause liquefaction of the dead tissue, so that the centre of the lesion consists of the fluid material called pus. Not infrequently a combination of fibrinous and purulent exudation is seen, often in relation to serous surfaces such as the peritoneum (fibrinopurulent exudate).

Catarrhal exudate

Catarrhal exudate usually occurs where mucous membranes are inflamed. The exudate is initially serous in character, but this phase is followed by a profuse discharge of mucus from the glands of the mucosa which converts the exudate into sticky, viscous material. An upper respiratory tract viral infection, such as a common 'cold', is a good example of this.

Membranous and **pseudomembranous exudates** are considered on p. 94.

ANATOMICAL LOCATION AND THE INFLAMMATORY REACTION

The type of tissue in which injury and inflammation occur affects the course of events and hence the structural changes that occur.

Abscess formation

If the injury occurs in a **solid block** of tissue such as the dermis, liver, kidney or brain, and the causal agent is a pyogenic organism, suppuration is likely to occur. The process takes two forms:

1) If the process is localized, the lesion with its necrotic pus-filled centre is termed an **abscess**.
2) If the inflammatory reaction is a spreading one, it is termed **cellulitis**.

An abscess has clearly defined **zones** that mirror the ongoing processes:

- The centre of the roughly spherical mass forming the abscess is made up of partly or completely liquefied dead tissue mixed with the remains of dead and dying neutrophils.
- This is surrounded by a layer in which fibrin and living neutrophils are present.
- At the periphery of this is a membrane consisting largely of proliferating fibroblasts, new capillaries and young collagen fibres.

This last layer represents the **repair process**, which is a possible path of development in the natural history of acute inflammation. This zone of fibroblastic proliferation serves as a barrier to further spread of the inflammatory process, but also prevents discharge of the abscess contents, without which healing cannot occur. It is often necessary, therefore, to lay the abscess open so that it can discharge adequately. In some cases, such as the lung or brain, the lesion must be removed completely with a rim of surrounding tissue.

Ulcers

In epithelium-lined tissue, such as skin, gut, pharynx, larynx or trachea, several different reactions may occur. One, previously discussed, is the pseudomembranous reaction, in which surface epithelium becomes necrotic and, together with fibrin and inflammatory cells, forms a membrane which can be detached to show the raw, subepithelial tissue beneath. A more common type of inflammatory lesion in epithelial surfaces is the ulcer. An ulcer is a **local defect in an epithelial surface**, the defect being produced by the shedding of dead epithelial cells.

Inflammation on serosal surfaces

On serosal surfaces such as the pleura or peritoneum, the exudate is usually serous, fibrinous or fibrinopurulent. Because of the arrangement of the tissue in what are basically flat mesothelium-lined sheets, there is little or no tendency for the process to become localized other than by the 'glueing' together of contiguous affected membranes.

BIOLOGICAL EFFECTS OF THE INFLAMMATORY REACTION

ROLE OF THE EXUDATE

The outpouring of fluid exudate can be protective in a number of ways.

Dilution. The fluid exudate might dilute the toxin if the injurious agent is a chemical poison or if, in the course of infection, tissue-damaging exotoxins are released by the pathogen.

Bacterial killing by antibody and complement. Exudation implies that proteins as well as fluid and solute escape from the microcirculation, so antibodies and complement are likely to form part of the exudate and will contribute to the killing of microorganisms and/or the neutralization of their toxins.

Localization. The transformation of fibrinogen to fibrin and the polymerization of the latter into tough strands may serve some localizing function. The presence of fibrin also assists the phagocytosis of non-opsonized organisms; this process is known as **surface phagocytosis**.

ROLE OF PHAGOCYTIC CELLS

The benefit to the host of the action of phagocytic cells is obvious. These cells play a protective role as a primary means of defence against the consequences of infection. This is made clear by the greatly enhanced risk of serious infections in patients in whom either the number of circulating neutrophils is significantly reduced or one of the functions of these cells is seriously compromised.

HARMFUL EFFECTS OF INFLAMMATION

Inflammation, in the broadest sense, is not purely protective. It may also cause a series of potentially life-threatening or functionally crippling situations. It is worth examining some of the ways in which inflammation can operate to the disadvantage of the patient.

Oedema

Inflammatory oedema may have serious consequences. For example, if the larynx is involved in a patient with a parainfluenza virus infection of the upper respiratory tract, laryngeal oedema may develop and obstruct normal airflow. The patient will experience great difficulty in breathing, the inspiratory and expiratory efforts will be accompanied by a loud noise (**stridor**) and the patient may become cyanotic through lack of oxygen. This event, which is like being strangled, is a medical emergency. The patient may well require tracheostomy to restore normal airflow until the oedema has subsided.

Cerebral oedema, which can occur as a consequence of inflammation as well as in certain other situations, may also have disastrous consequences. Swelling of the brain within its rigid box, the cranium, means that any increase in pressure must be transmitted downwards and backwards through the only available potential avenue of escape, the foramen magnum. This imposes severe shearing stresses on the small perforating blood vessels at the base of the mid-brain and may cut off the blood supply to important areas. At post mortem examination the presence of such displacement due to cerebral oedema may be recognized by deep grooves (formed by the pressure of the tentorium) on the mid-brain or in the cerebellar tonsils if the latter have herniated through the foramen magnum.

Failure to control mediator release

Very rarely, unpleasant consequences may arise from failure to control the generation of chemical mediators of inflammation. One such example is a condition known as **hereditary angioneurotic oedema**, in which patients develop localized areas of oedema in a wide range of anatomical locations; the oedematous areas are often painful. This is believed to be due to the unrestrained activity of a kinin-like particle liberated in the course of activation of the C2 component of complement. Normally this is inactivated by an esterase, but in affected individuals the inactivator substance is not synthesized.

Malfunction caused by exudates

Apart from their association with oedema, exudates can cause malfunctions in particular locations. In lobar pneumonia caused by *Streptococcus pneumoniae*, an exudate rich in fibrin is formed; this spreads through the pores of Kohn to involve large areas of lung tissue. The exudate causes difficulty in oxygen diffusion and in gas exchange across alveolar septa. Fortunately, in most cases blood oxygen levels are not significantly reduced, but considerable disturbance in blood gases may occur if sufficient lung tissue is involved. In underprivileged communities this condition is still an important cause of death, even though it has become much rarer in Western countries.

Phagocyte-mediated tissue damage

Phagocytes can damage tissue either by some interruption of phagosome–lysosome fusion or, on a wider scale, through inappropriate triggering of some of their secretory or metabolic functions.

Examples of potentially damaging abnormalities in lysosomal fusion are found, in the case of the neutrophil, in acute gouty arthritis and, in the case of the macrophage, in silicosis. These have already been discussed on p. 15. In silicosis, silica particles are inhaled and deposited in the respiratory bronchioles. They are then phagocytosed by macrophages and come to lie within phagosomes. Silicic acid forms on the surface of the particles and, when phagosome–lysosome fusion occurs, hydrogen bonds form between the silicic acid and the lysosomal membrane. This leads to lysosomal membrane rupture with spillage of enzymes into the cytoplasm. The macrophage then dies and the lysosomal enzymes and the offending silica particle are released into the interstitial tissue. The lysosomal enzymes (including collagenase and elastase) damage tissue, and the released silica is again available for phagocytosis, thus restarting the cycle.

Phagocytic cells may secrete lysosomal enzymes in response to a variety of stimuli. The potential ill effects of such secretion are avoided by protease-inhibiting glycoproteins within plasma and extracellular fluid. As so often happens, the importance of such inhibitors is discovered only when they fail. An example of this is the inherited condition, α_1-antitrypsin deficiency. This protease inhibitor (synthesized in the liver) is encoded by a normal allelic pair of genes. Absence or mutation of both members of this pair renders the affected person homozygous for the deficiency. Such people may develop destruction of the alveolar and bronchiolar walls in the lung leading to **panacinar emphysema**; they may also have an enhanced risk for liver damage leading to **cirrhosis**. Absence or mutation of one member of the pair of genes (the heterozygous state) leads to an increased risk of lung damage by cigarette smoke.

Release of oxygen free radicals by phagocytes is another way in which tissue damage may be brought about. Oxygen metabolites released from activated neutrophils and macrophages may be toxic to a wide variety of eukaryotic cells, including red cells, endothelial cells, fibroblasts, tumour cells, platelets and spermatozoa. Damage to endothelial cells in the pulmonary capillary bed by oxygen-derived free radicals may be the most important pathogenetic mechanism underlying the respiratory distress syndrome that is seen in association with a number of clinical states.

Lodgement of antigen–antibody complexes in various locations may also cause severe tissue damage via free radical release from phagocytes. Experimentally, tissue damage may be avoided by giving superoxide dismutase. Similarly, in experimentally produced antigen–antibody complex-mediated injury in the lung, tissue damage can be reduced by administering catalase, whereas antiproteases have no such protective effect.

FACTORS THAT MODIFY THE INFLAMMATORY REACTION

- Inflammation shows considerable variation depending on factors related to the **injurious agent** and/or the **host**.
- Injury varies according to the amount or dose of the agent, its strength (or, in infection, the virulence of the organism), the duration and the intrinsic nature of the agent.
- The intrinsic nature of the injurious agent may determine pathological changes, e.g. staphylococci promote pus formation while *Corynebacterium diphtheriae* and *Clostridium difficile* cause membranous exudates.
- The most important host factors relate to immune status. This may be affected by mal- and under-nutrition, intrinsic defects in specific adaptive immunity, treatment with immunosuppressive agents and the presence of certain malignant disorders, most notably lymphomas.
- Inflammatory reactions are classified in terms of **duration** (acute or chronic), the **type of exudate** (e.g. serous, fibrinous, purulent, membranous) and **anatomical location**.
- Anatomical location determines the nature of the lesion; for example, the combination of solid tissue and a staphylococcal infection is likely to lead to abscess formation while injury to an epithelium-lined surface causes ulceration.

7 The natural history of acute inflammation I: resolution and regeneration

A spectrum of biological events follows tissue injury and the resulting inflammation. These include:

- a complete return to functional and structural normality (**resolution**)
- the replacement of lost tissue by scar tissue (**healing by repair**)
- persistence of the inflammatory process for weeks, months or years (**chronicity**).

Factors determining which of these will occur include the nature of the injury, the tissue target and the host response. The possible events are shown in *Fig. 7.1*. They involve one or more of the following processes:

- **removal of foreign material** whether living or dead, exogenous or endogenous
- **clearance** of the cellular and other elements of the inflammatory response
- **regeneration** of lost tissue components where this is possible
- **replacement** of lost tissue elements by **connective tissue** with an adequate blood supply.

RESOLUTION

Resolution indicates the return of an inflamed area to the state that existed before the injury that elicited the inflammatory reaction. It implies that no significant tissue loss has occurred: the injury was sufficiently severe to cause inflammation, but not severe enough to cause tissue necrosis. Central to resolution is **complete removal of inflammatory exudate**. This is accomplished largely by proteolysis, but phagocytosis of the exudate by macrophages also plays a part.

The natural history of lobar pneumonia provides a striking example of resolution. This is an acute inflammatory disorder affecting lung

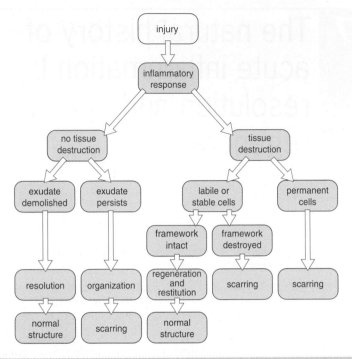

Fig. 7.1   Possible natural history of acute inflammation.

parenchyma and involving large areas of lung tissue in continuity. The sequence of events (*Fig. 7.2*) occurring in this disease is as follows:

- Invasion of the air spaces by *Streptococcus pneumoniae* elicits severe acute inflammation characterized by outpouring of an exudate, initially rich in fibrin and poor in cells, into the affected alveoli.
- This process spreads rapidly through the adjacent air spaces, involving extensive areas of lung tissue. Inflammatory cells migrate into the fibrin-rich exudate; while viable organisms are still present, most of these are neutrophils. The neutrophils engulf and kill most of the organisms, many neutrophils die in the course of this process. The affected lobes of the lungs of patients who die at this stage are **red, fleshy and airless**. Microscopic examination shows the dilatation of alveolar capillaries typical of acute inflammation, and air spaces filled with exudate. There is, however, *no* necrosis of the alveolar septa.
- Once the organisms have been cleared, the nature of the cellular infiltrate changes. Macrophages are recruited to the affected areas and become the dominant cellular element. The fibrin-rich element begins to undergo lysis; this is brought about largely by the action of plasmin, generated

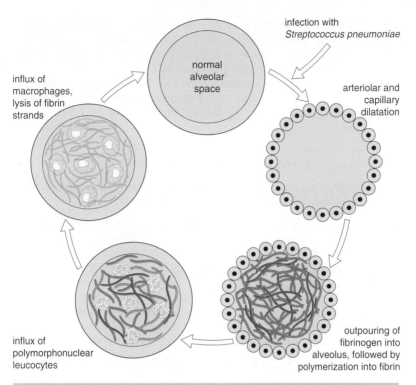

Fig. 7.2 Natural history of lobar pneumonia terminating in resolution.

from plasminogen by plasminogen activator released from infiltrating macrophages.

- The macrophages phagocytose much of the cellular and bacterial debris. Secretion of lysosomal enzymes by reverse endocytosis accounts for the breakdown of the material that has not been phagocytosed. The lysed exudate drains from the lung tissue via the lymphatics; the protein content of this lymph is higher than that draining non-inflamed lung tissue. At the end of the sequence of events, all the exudate should have been removed and the air spaces return to normal both structurally and functionally. Failure to remove the exudate will trigger the process of organization, discussed below.

ORGANIZATION

If demolition fails and the exudate persists, a set of processes known as organization is triggered. The exudate is infiltrated by numerous macrophages, followed by the migration of fibroblasts and new small blood vessels into the exudate. This is more or less identical with what occurs in connective tissue in wound healing. Eventually the exudate is replaced by well-vascularized fibrous tissue and, finally, once the new blood vessels have died back, by dense collagen-rich scar tissue.

We should remember that basic processes like this may occur in a number of different contexts. Thus organization is triggered not only by persisting inflammatory exudate, but also by unlysed blood clot or thrombus and by necrotic areas in tissue that cannot regenerate, such as the myocardium.

Some clinical consequences of organization

Organization of persisting inflammatory exudate can lead to some highly disadvantageous clinical scenarios. Examples include:

- In the peritoneal cavity, persistence of exudate leads to the formation of fibrous tissue strands. These connect either adjacent loops of bowel or the serosal surface of segments of bowel and the abdominal wall. Such adhesions may lead to acute or subacute intestinal obstruction at some future time.
- Organization in other serosal cavities – the pleural cavity or pericardial sac – may cause obliteration of these spaces. In **constrictive pericarditis**, which may follow tuberculosis, the heart becomes ensheathed in a thick unyielding layer of fibrous tissue. This interferes with both diastolic compliance (relaxation of the walls of the heart chambers during diastole) and systolic contraction, and leads to severe congestive failure which can be relieved only by surgical stripping of the fibrous tissue layer.
- In the lung affected by pneumonia, persistence of exudate leads to the affected air spaces becoming filled with connective tissue. This produces a solid meaty consistency instead of the normal spongy one characteristic of the lung; this obviously results in failure to ventilate the affected area and of normal gas exchange.

REGENERATION

Tissue destroyed by injury or inflammation must be replaced, if possible, by new living tissue. Ideally this is accomplished by proliferation of the normal cells of the damaged organ or tissue, to replace those lost.

If this tissue replacement takes place in an orderly fashion, not only are the lost tissue elements replicated but the normal architectural pattern is restored so that the tissue is 'as good as new'. This process, known as regeneration, operates most effectively in non-mammalian species such as the salamander, which can successfully replace amputated limbs.

Successful regeneration depends on two factors:

1) Lost cells must be of a type capable of being replaced by identical cells.

2) The normal architecture of connective tissue and blood vessels in the affected area must be either preserved or restored as it was before injury.

In relation to regeneration, cells can be classified into three basic types:

- **labile cells**
- **stable cells**
- **permanent cells**.

Labile cells

Labile cells are derived by mitosis of stem cells. **Stem cells** are defined as those that:

- are not themselves terminally differentiated
- have no fixed limit on their capacity to divide during the lifetime of an animal
- give rise to daughter cells that can either remain stem cells or embark on a terminal differentiation pathway.

Stem cell populations exist where a replacement mechanism is needed for differentiated cells that cannot themselves divide. The latter often have a rather short life and, hence, a high turnover rate. For example, a fully developed red blood cell cannot divide because it has no nucleus. The epidermis of the **skin** and the epithelium of the **small gut** are other striking examples of cell populations whose size is governed by stem cell activity.

Basically, labile cells fall into two groups:

- **covering epithelia**; these include:
  a) stratified squamous epithelium of the skin, mouth, pharynx, oesophagus, vagina and cervix
  b) transitional epithelium of the urinary tract
  c) gut epithelium
  d) lining epithelium of exocrine gland ducts
  e) endometrial gland epithelium and the lining of the fallopian tubes
- **blood and lymphoid cells**.

In both these categories, cell loss is easily made good.

Stable cells

Stable cells are normally quiescent and have a very low rate of turnover. When they are lost, replacement is carried out by **mitosis of mature cells**; there appears to be no stem cell compartment.

Stable cells include liver cells, renal tubular epithelium, secretory epithelium of endocrine glands, bone cells and fibroblasts. Their loss is followed by a marked upregulation of cell division, and the lost cells are rapidly replaced. For example, if 65% of a rat's liver is removed surgically, a burst of regenerative activity occurs and within two weeks the liver will have attained normal or near-normal size.

Such regeneration involves the upregulation of endocrine, paracrine or autocrine **mitogenic signals**, and possibly also of **receptor function**, **signal transduction** and **expression of DNA-binding proteins**. Many of these alterations in the level of function are regulated by increased expression of certain growth-promoting genes or proto-oncogenes, which will be described in more detail in the section on the origins of cancer (see pp. 483–511).

In liver and renal tubular epithelial regeneration, one of the most potent factors involved is a multifunctional cytokine, **hepatocyte growth factor (HGF) (scatter factor)**. HGF is encoded by a gene on chromosome 7 and resembles plasminogen and other blood proteases. It is produced by various cells including fibroblasts, epithelial and endothelial cells, Küpffer cells in the liver sinusoids and lipocytes (Ito cells) in the space of Disse, also in the liver. Its production is increased by interleukin 1 (α and β) and by a humoral substance known as **injurin**, probably a glycosaminoglycan, which shows increased plasma levels after partial removal of the liver. HGF acts by binding to a high-affinity receptor encoded by a proto-oncogene c-*met*, expressed on a variety of cell types. Interestingly, liver cells show increased expression of c-*met* after liver injury, but this returns to normal soon afterwards. This suggests that normal tissue proliferation may be controlled by changes in the expression of genes coding both for mitogenic signals and their receptors.

Permanent cells

Permanent cells, having been generated in sufficient numbers during fetal life, **never divide in postnatal life and cannot be replaced if they are lost**. Almost all nerve cells are permanent, as are heart muscle cells, the auditory 'hair' cells, and the cells in the lens of the eye. Why these cells should behave in this way is not understood. Permanence seems biologically unhelpful, although in the case of the central nervous system, if neurones regenerated, establishment of the appropriate connections in the central nervous system might be difficult.

Importance of tissue architecture in regeneration

For a tissue to return to normal, the stromal architecture must be maintained or restored. The replacement of lost cells by proliferation is only part of the process leading to regeneration, albeit the most important. If the architectural arrangement of the connective tissue framework of an organ or tissue is destroyed, the arrangement of the regenerating cells will be disturbed; this can have serious consequences for the function of the affected tissue.

The natural history of some cases of liver necrosis is a good example of this. The stable hepatocytes show a striking ability to proliferate by mitosis after an injury that is sufficiently severe to lead to liver cell death. This is demonstrated by the regeneration that follows partial hepatectomy in the rat. In certain cases of either acute massive necrosis or ongoing necrosis of relatively small numbers of cells, the connective tissue framework may either be destroyed or may collapse. In addition, the hepatic stellate cells (Ito cells) in the space of Disse may secrete connective tissue matrix proteins which form septa that grow into the liver acini and produce marked architectural disturbance. In these circumstances, the regenerating hepatocytes grow in the form of disorganized nodules instead of in an orderly fashion. Thus normal hepatic mass may be restored but not normal hepatic architecture.

This sequence of events leads, for example, to marked disturbance in blood flow patterns of the liver. Blood is normally conducted from the terminal branches of the portal vein and hepatic artery to the terminal hepatic venules. Distortion of this flow causes abnormally high pressure in the portal venous system (portal hypertension) and portal blood becomes shunted into the systemic circulation with profound and disadvantageous metabolic effects. This abnormal regeneration pattern and its functional consequences are important parts of the pathological and clinical picture seen in **cirrhosis** of the liver.

Organization of exudate and failure to restore the connective tissue framework to normal result in scarring. **Scarring** is an essential component of wound healing, which provides a useful model to study the events and controlling mechanisms that underlie scarring. This is discussed in Chapter 8.

NATURAL HISTORY OF ACUTE INFLAMMATION I: RESOLUTION AND REGENERATION

- The natural history of acute inflammation includes **resolution** (return to functional and structural normality), **healing** (replacement of lost tissue) and **chronicity**.
- **Healing** involves removal of foreign material and inflammatory debris (**demolition**) and replacement of lost cells by new ones (**regeneration**) or by connective tissue (**scarring**).
- **Failure of demolition** leads to scarring with possible serious functional consequences.
- **Regeneration** depends on the type of cells lost. Cells that cannot divide in postnatal life (**permanent cells**) cannot regenerate.
- Cell populations that are constantly in cycle (**labile**) such as blood and lymphoid cells and covering epithelia are easily replaced, as are cells which normally have a low turnover but can be triggered to divide after cell loss (**stable**). Division of stable cells is triggered by a variety of mitogenic signals.

8 The natural history of acute inflammation II: wound healing

The biological objectives of wound healing are twofold (*Fig. 8.1*):

1) **To restore the integrity of epithelial surfaces**. In this way, the underlying tissues are protected against:
   - an abnormal environment leading to inappropriate drying or wetting of the exposed surface
   - infection
   - entry of non-living foreign material.
2) **To restore the tensile strength of the subepithelial tissue**.

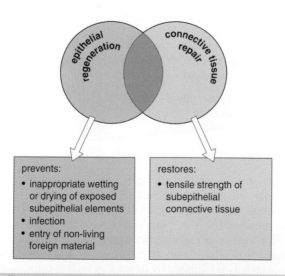

Fig. 8.1   **The basic components of wound healing and their biological purpose.**

HEALING BY PRIMARY OR SECONDARY 'INTENTION'

Whatever the type of wound, the basic healing processes are the same, the differences being largely of **degree** rather than of kind.

Primary intention. By convention, the healing of cleanly incised, easily suturable wounds, where the edges are in close apposition, is termed healing by 'primary intention'.

Secondary intention. Wounds in which there is extensive loss of epithelium, with a large subepithelial tissue defect that has to be filled in by scar tissue, and where the edges cannot be brought together with sutures, are said to be healed by 'secondary intention'.

HEALING OF AN INCISED WOUND

Incision involves the division of:

- epidermis
- dermal connective tissue fibres and matrix
- subcutaneous tissue and, in some cases, deeper tissue layers
- blood vessels.

Severing of blood vessels obviously leads to haemorrhage. This results in accumulation within the tissue defect of platelets and, pre-eminently among the plasma proteins, **fibrinogen** and **fibronectin**. Clotting mechanisms are activated; fibrinogen is converted to polymerized fibrin. This is stabilized by fibronectin binding to it by means of a glutaminase bridge.

The gel formed by fibrin and fibronectin acts in the early stages of healing as a 'glue', which helps to keep the severed edges of the tissue apposed.

Morphological events in healing (*Fig. 8.2*) include:

- those involving the **epidermis**
- those involving the **dermis**.

Epidermal events

Within a few hours of wounding, a single layer of epidermal cells starts to **migrate** from the wound edges, forming a delicate covering over the raw area. This process, called **epiboly**, can be studied *in vitro* using small cubes of excised skin cultured at 37°C. The epidermal cells spread over the five raw dermal faces: eventually, the dermal tissue cube is enclosed by epidermis like a small parcel. The role of cell movement in this process is supported by the fact that epiboly is inhibited by substances such as cytochalasin B that are known to interfere with cell migration.

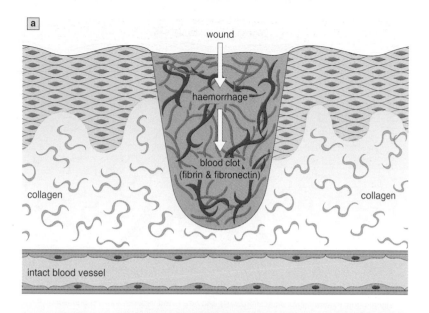

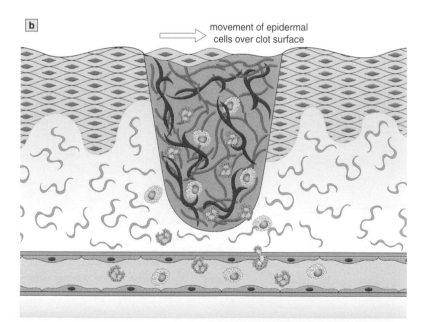

Fig. 8.2a, b

c

regenerated epidermal cells

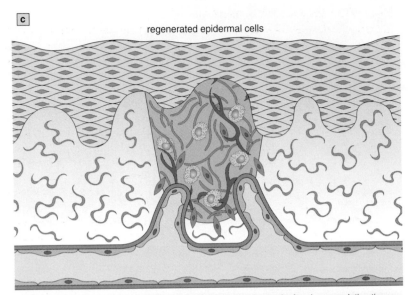

signals from macrophages attract fibroblasts and new blood vessels, forming granulation tissue

d

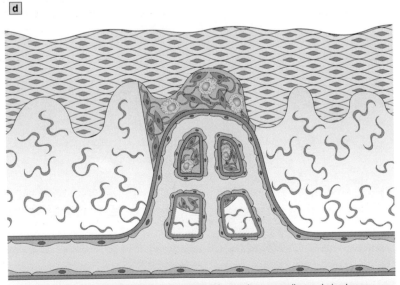

fibroblasts proliferate locally and produce new matrix proteins → a well-vascularized scar

Fig. 8.2 a–d The stages of wound healing.

Mechanisms involved in cell migration

Epidermal cell migration depends on interaction between the keratinocytes at or near the wound edges and the extracellular matrix glycoprotein **fibronectin**. Fibronectins are large two-chained glycoproteins present in plasma and tissues. They act by providing ligands for receptors on many cell types. This ligand–receptor binding mediates cell matrix adhesion. The binding sites often include the tripeptide **arginine–glycine–aspartate** (known as **RGD** sites). The cellular receptors serving as ligands for RGD sequences belong to the **integrin** family and include surface molecules on phagocytes mediating adhesion to endothelial cells (see pp. 58–62).

Differences between plasma and tissue fibronectins are mediated by post-translational modifications, differences in splicing being particularly important. In wounds, the splicing of fibronectin messenger RNA (mRNA) resembles that found in early embryogenesis.

Keratinocytes from normal unwounded skin do not possess fibronectin-binding receptors, being tightly attached to basement membrane laminin and collagen type IV. Those from wounds, however, bind to fibronectin and thus migrate across and, indeed, through the fibronectin-rich matrix.

Epithelial cell proliferation

Epidermal cell movement can provide an initial covering for very small wounds but, mostly, epithelial re-covering cannot occur without epidermal cell **proliferation**.

The new cells come from the epidermal stem cell compartment (the basal cells just above the dermal–epidermal junction). From about 12 hours after wounding, mitotic activity increases markedly in the basal cells, about 3–5 cells from the cut edges. The new cells grow under the surface fibrin–fibronectin clot and for a little distance down the gap between the cut edges to form a small 'spur' of epithelium which afterwards regresses. If the wound has been sutured, similar downgrowth occurs in relation to suture tracks. Occasionally, these may be the basis of keratin-filled dermal cysts – so-called 'implantation dermoid cysts'.

Dermal events

Cellular infiltration

Within the first few hours a mild acute inflammatory reaction occurs with an influx of **neutrophils** into and around the wound (0–1 day after wounding). This is followed by migration of **macrophages** into this area (1–2 days after wounding), a key event as these are the cells that orchestrate the complex interplay of chemical signals that now occurs.

Viewed in an operational sense, the objectives of this dermal phase of healing are:

- **to demolish and remove any inflammatory exudate and tissue debris**

- **to restore the tensile strength of the subepithelial connective tissue**; this involves:
  - a) chemoattraction of fibroblasts, which synthesize and secrete collagen and other connective tissue proteins
  - b) stimulation of these and resident fibroblasts to proliferate and secrete matrix proteins
- **to cause the ingrowth of new small blood vessels into the area undergoing repair**; this involves:
  - a) budding of new endothelial cells from small intact blood vessels at the wound edges
  - b) chemoattraction of these cells into the fibrin–fibronectin gel within the wound.

In a surgical incision, fibroblasts and myofibroblasts appear in the wound 2–4 days after wounding; endothelial cells follow about 1 day later. Initially these endothelial buds consist of solid cores of cells which soon acquire a lumen. Local degradation of the basement membrane of the existing capillary is an essential starting step for the ingrowth of new vessels. Newly formed capillaries have little basement membrane substance and are leaky compared with normal capillaries. The richly vascularized gel containing both inflammatory cells and collagen-producing fibroblasts is called **granulation tissue**. This name, a misnomer, derives from the granular appearance of raw wounds which somewhat resembles the surface of a strawberry.

Collagen production

The ultimate development of tensile strength in a wound depends on:

- **the production of adequate amounts of collagen**
- **the final orientation of the collagen**.

Collagen is the only protein containing large amounts of the amino acids hydroxyproline and hydroxylysine. Within 24 hours of wounding, protein-bound hydroxyproline appears. Within 2–3 days some fibrillar material is present, however this lacks the dimensions and the typical 64 nm banding of polymerized collagen. Within a few weeks of infliction of a surgical wound the **amount** of collagen in the wounded area is normal, although preoperative tensile strength is not regained for some months. This suggests that replacement and remodelling of the collagen formed early in wound healing is an important part of the whole process.

Each type of collagen (there are about 12, of which types I, II and III are the chief fibrillar collagens) consists of three peptide α chains wound round each other in a helical pattern. These chains are synthesized in the rough endoplasmic reticulum of the fibroblast following translation of the mRNA for each one. They then undergo post-translational hydroxylation of the proline and lysine moieties, and the hydroxylysine is then glycosylated.

Chain linkage is accomplished by disulphide bonds. The three chains then become twisted into a helix and the soluble procollagen molecules are secreted into the extracellular environment. Solubility is conferred by the presence of an extra peptide. This is removed extracellularly by a peptidase, and the cleaved molecules assemble into fibres which gain tensile strength by cross-linking. The typical periodicity of the collagen fibres is due to the staggered arrangement of the assembled molecules.

On some occasions, the control mechanisms that determine an appropriate amount of new collagen for healing a given wound are faulty. Excess collagen may be formed and lead to the formation of a bulky scar which stands proud of the surrounding surface. This is known as a **keloid**.

HEALING OF LARGE TISSUE DEFECTS

Large areas of tissue loss can occur in severe trauma or extensive burns or, much less frequently, in relation to certain surgical procedures. **Qualitatively**, there are few differences between the healing of such a wound and that of an incised wound. **Quantitatively**, there are differences, as the formation of granulation tissue and ultimately of scar tissue is on a far larger scale than in incised wounds.

One feature of the healing process in large tissue defects not seen in relation to healing of incised wounds is **wound contraction**.

WOUND CONTRACTION

Within two or three days large open wounds start to decrease in area. This is due to movement of the wound margins and is independent of the rate of epithelial covering.

Wound contraction occurs when relatively little new dermal collagen is being formed. It seems, therefore, unlikely that shortening of collagen fibres at the wound margins is responsible for contraction. It is currently thought that contraction is caused by the action of cells appearing at the margins of the wound in the first few days. On electron microscopy, these cells show features suggesting both fibroblast and smooth muscle differentiation and this has led to the term **myofibroblast** being applied to them. Appropriate antibodies show that the cells contain actin, but no smooth muscle-type myosin has been found within their cytoplasm.

In any circumstances, for a pulling force to be exerted there must be a connection between the object being pulled and whatever is applying the force. In wound contraction, this connection is thought to be fibronectin forming bridges between collagen fibres and receptors on the myofibroblasts.

Strips of granulation tissue from healing wounds can be made to shorten *in vitro* by pharmacological agents that cause actin fibrils to contract. It may be that a similar mechanism causes the contracture of dermal connective tissue seen in conditions such as Dupuytren's contracture.

GROWTH FACTORS AND CYTOKINES IN WOUND HEALING

Cellular events in wound healing depend on 'instructions' which:

- cause cells concerned in repair to **migrate** into the wound.
- cause these cells and also the epithelial cells that must cover the raw surface to **proliferate**.

These instructions consist of chemical signals from a number of sources. Some signals, whose principal function is to upregulate mitosis, are known as **growth factors**. The others, derived chiefly from inflammatory cells, are known as **cytokines**, and have many **regulatory functions** (see *Tables 5.3–5.7*).

GROWTH FACTORS

These are peptides that may reach their specific targets via one or more of three pathways (*Fig. 8.3*):

1) **the endocrine pathway**, where growth factors are synthesized at some considerable distance from their targets and are delivered to them via the bloodstream
2) **the paracrine pathway**, where growth factors are synthesized and released by cells that are in the close neighbourhood of their targets
3) **the autocrine pathway**, in which the same cells both synthesize and use the growth factor.

Growth factors can be divided into two groups depending when they operate in the life of stem cells: a **competence** growth factor can move a cell out of the G0 phase back into cycle, whereas a **progression** growth factor has a mitogenic effect only on cells not in the G0 phase. Competence growth factors typically involved in the healing process are **platelet-derived growth factor (PDGF)** and basic fibroblast growth factor (FGF). Progression growth factors are represented by such molecules as insulin-like growth factors 1 and 2 (the somatomedins) and **epidermal growth factor (EGF)**.

Platelet-derived growth factor

The name 'platelet-derived growth factor' is misleading in two senses. Firstly, although it is stored in the α granules of platelets and released from them when the platelets are activated, PDGF is synthesized and secreted from other cells including:

- endothelial cells
- macrophages
- arterial smooth muscle cells
- cells from certain tumours.

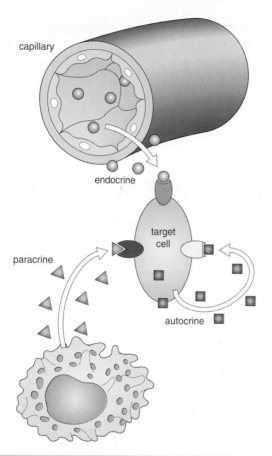

Fig. 8.3   Endocrine, paracrine and autocrine signalling pathways.

Secondly, **PDGF has a number of stimulatory functions** apart from its undoubtedly powerful mitogenic effect. In the context of healing, the most important of these is its ability to cause **chemotaxis** of mesenchymal cells into the wound (*Fig. 8.4*). PDGF also:

- increases intracellular synthesis of cholesterol and also the binding of low density lipoprotein (LDL) by increasing the number of LDL receptors expressed on the target cell
- increases prostaglandin secretion, initially by making more of the starting material (arachidonic acid) available and, later, by stimulating the synthesis of cyclo-oxygenase
- induces changes in cell shape accompanied by reorganization of intra-cellular actin filaments

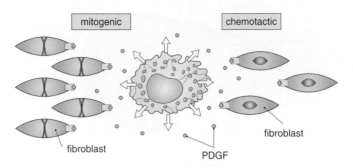

Fig. 8.4   Actions of platelet-derived growth factor (PDGF) in wound healing.

- induces increased synthesis of RNA and protein
- is a potent vasoconstrictor.

Thus PDGF can attract mesenchymal cells into the wound (with the exception of endothelial cells that lack the PDGF receptor) and acts as a mitogen for these cells and a stimulator of protein production. PDGF and other growth factors bind to receptors which, after binding, act as **tyrosine kinases**. Transduction of the signal from the cell membrane is followed, within minutes, by activation of the proto-oncogenes c-*fos* and c-*myc* (see pp. 483–511) and also by the activation of genes encoding production of the contractile protein actin and interferon γ.

Epidermal growth factor (EGF) and transforming growth factor α

EGF is a 53-amino-acid polypeptide, initially found in salivary glands of baby mice, and cleaved from a larger precursor. The purified factor, now known as EGF, also stimulates mitogenesis in connective tissue as well as in epithelial cells. Salivary glands, lacrimal glands and Brunner's glands in the duodenum are all storage sites for EGF, which can be released in saliva, tears and duodenal 'juice'. Thus, literally 'licking one's wounds' may be biologically advantageous, as may tears in corneal abrasion or ulceration. In rodents, EGF may be found in the plasma, but in humans blood-borne EGF is concentrated within platelets, for the most part in α granules. This platelet EGF is derived from synthesis within megakaryocytes.

In experimental wounds EGF application accelerates epidermal regeneration significantly. EGF also has a beneficial effect on the dermal component of healing in experimental wounds, increasing proliferation of dermal connective tissue and the tensile strength of wounds. In humans, also, topical application of EGF accelerates the healing of donor sites for skin grafts.

There is no evidence that EGF is produced by any of the cells taking part in the healing process, although platelets store EGF. However, another factor, known as **transforming growth factor α, (TGF-α)**, shows considerable homology with EGF, and is produced in healing wounds by both

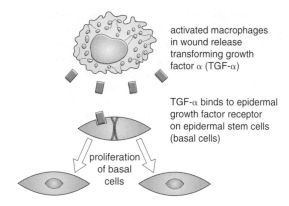

activated macrophages in wound release transforming growth factor α (TGF-α)

TGF-α binds to epidermal growth factor receptor on epidermal stem cells (basal cells)

proliferation of basal cells

Fig. 8.5   Epithelial regeneration in healing skin wounds.

epidermal cells and macrophages. *TGF-α binds to the same receptor on target cells as EGF; it has the same mitogenic effect and thus may be a direct mediator of wound healing (Fig. 8.5).*

Transforming growth factor β (TGF- β)

TGF-β is a polypeptide produced by almost all cell lines in culture. In the presence of EGF it acts as a mitogen, but in some assays also inhibits growth. Macrophages in healing wounds express mRNA for TGF-β as well as for TGF-α. TGF-β is also a powerful chemoattractant for monocytes, and its release from the first wave of inflammatory cells migrating into wounds may recruit additional monocyte–macrophages.

The pattern of expression of growth factors in healing wounds supports the idea that the macrophage plays a leading role in the healing process, as do observations that:

- Wound fluid stimulates cell division and promotes the ingrowth of new vessels.
- Ablation of macrophages in animals slows the process of wound healing.
- Macrophages in wounds also express other growth factors, such as insulin-like growth factor 1.

CYTOKINES

Cytokine (see Tables 5.3–5.7) is the term used for a group of protein cell regulators, including:

- lymphokines
- monokines
- interleukins
- interferons.

Growth factors could also, with justification, be called cytokines: treating them as a separate class of regulator is artificial, if convenient.

The cytokines referred to above are low molecular weight proteins (usually less than 80 kD). They tend to be produced rapidly and locally, and can act in an autocrine or paracrine fashion. They are produced by many cells and have many overlapping actions, mediated by binding to high-affinity receptors on target cells. The response of an individual cell to a given cytokine depends on the cell type, other chemical signals being received at the same time, and the local concentration of the cytokine.

Two cytokines that play a significant role in wound healing are:

- **interleukin 1 (IL-1)**
- **tumour necrosis factor α (TNF-α)** (*syn*. cachectin).

Interleukin 1

IL-1, formerly known as endogenous pyrogen, is a small 17 kD protein which, in healing wounds, is produced by macrophages and activated epithelial cells. IL-1 has many biological actions (see pp. 76, 79–80). In healing these include:

- **a proliferative effect on dermal fibroblasts**
- **upregulation of collagen synthesis by the fibroblasts**
- **an increase in collagenase production**: this may be one of the ways in which the collagen in wounds is remodelled so as to achieve maximal tensile strength.

Tumour necrosis factor α (TNF-α)

This is another monocyte–macrophage product released following tissue injury or infection. *It is the main factor responsible for macrophage-mediated tumour cell killing and is also responsible for the wasting (cachexia) seen in certain chronic bacterial and parasitic infections.* Its biological activity overlaps with that of IL-1, although it lacks the latter's immunoregulatory functions. Its receptor targets, however, differ from those of IL-1; presumably the similarities in actions indicate that they stimulate the same 'second-messenger' systems. The activation of monocytes and macrophages to produce TNF-α may be brought about in a number of ways:

- interaction with fibrin (always present in wounds)
- binding of TGF-β
- the action of interferon γ
- the action of endotoxin.

TNF-α powerfully stimulates ingrowth of new blood vessels in healing wounds; it is not only chemotactic for endothelial cells but is also responsible for the focal degradation of capillary basement membranes that precedes the migration of endothelial cells.

FACTORS INTERFERING WITH WOUND HEALING

Failure to heal satisfactorily may be due to either **systemic** or **local factors**.

SYSTEMIC FACTORS

Nutrition

The patient's **protein intake** is a potent factor in determining success or failure in healing. There may be at least two explanations for this.

1) The undernourished patient shows evidence of **depression of the immune system**; resulting wound infection and its inflammatory response may delay healing.
2) The diet may lack the 'building blocks' needed for collagen synthesis. Sulphur-containing amino acids such as methionine seem to be particularly important; increasing methionine intake alone partially offsets the effects of a low protein intake on wound healing.

Historically, **vitamin C** is most prominent among individual dietary factors affecting healing. It has been known since the seventeenth century that scurvy is associated with poor healing of wounds and fractures. However, it was not until well into the twentieth century that vitamin C and its relation to scurvy was discovered. In experimental wounds lack of vitamin C inhibits the secretion of collagen fibres by fibroblasts, due to a failure of hydroxylation of proline in the endoplasmic reticulum of the fibroblast. In addition, vitamin C concentrations affect the production of galactosamine and hence the deposition of chondroitin sulphate in the extracellular matrix of granulation tissue.

Vitamin A has important functions in relation to morphogenesis, epithelial proliferation and epithelial differentiation. In experimental wounds it counteracts the inhibitory effects of steroids on healing and, applied topically, it accelerates epithelial covering.

Some role for **zinc** in wound healing exists. Zinc accelerates healing of experimental wounds. Zinc deficiency, such as is found in patients who have been on parenteral nutrition for long periods and in those with severe burns, is associated with poor healing: this is reversed by the administration of zinc, which is necessary for the function of many enzymes including nucleic acid polymerases.

Many studies show that **glucocorticoids** inhibit healing and production of fibrous tissue. Indeed, this is used to advantage by administering steroids in situations where inappropriate scarring is taking place, such as in interstitial fibrosis in the lung. It is still not clear whether steroids exert their effect indirectly by damping down inflammation or whether they directly affect one or more of the mechanisms outlined in previous sections.

Age

Age is often stated to be a factor affecting the efficacy of wound healing. It is true that wounds tend to heal more rapidly in the young than in the elderly but it is difficult to be certain that it is age *per se* that is responsible or whether delayed healing in the aged may be due to local vascular factors such as poor arterial perfusion.

Diabetes

Diabetes inhibits healing, especially if control is poor. In uncontrolled diabetes the neutrophil response to injury and infection is impaired. This is reversed by insulin in the ex vivo situation. In addition, diabetics may suffer from poor arterial perfusion and sensory neuropathy. The first of these impairs healing; the second makes repetitive injury more likely to occur. This is particularly noticeable on the soles of the feet where quite trivial injuries may develop into chronic non-healing ulcers.

LOCAL FACTORS

Foreign bodies or infection

Both infection and foreign bodies:

- increase the intensity of inflammation
- prolong its duration
- inhibit healing.

Endogenous materials (e.g. hair, bone fragments) act as foreign bodies if displaced from their normal location.

Excess mobility

Excess movement of a part always prolongs the duration of healing. For example, a cut over a knuckle takes longer to heal than on a site elsewhere on the finger. This is obviously most significant in relation to fracture healing.

Arterial perfusion and venous drainage

The supply and drainage of blood play key roles in healing. Poor arterial perfusion, either from stenosis or occlusion of the supplying vessel, increases the degree of damage caused by a given injury and prolongs or may even lead to failure of healing.

Poor venous drainage of a part also inhibits healing. This is exemplified in chronic ulcers occurring on the anterior surface of the leg, which are very common in the elderly. The use of compression bandages to improve venous return promotes healing.

REPAIR IN SOME SPECIALIZED TISSUES

BONE

The early stages of fracture healing are basically the same as those in wound healing. Thus the tissue defect between the severed ends of bone is made good by well-vascularized connective tissue. Once this stage has passed, new features become apparent because bone, unlike soft tissue, requires mechanical and weight bearing efficiency of a high order. These needs are met by two types of specialized cells:

- **osteoblasts**, which lay down seams of new osteoid (uncalcified bone matrix)
- **osteoclasts**; these multinucleated cells of macrophage lineage resorb bone by releasing proteolytic enzymes and are thus fundamental to bone remodelling.

Stages of fracture healing

Haemorrhage
As the bone fractures, blood vessels tear and the defect in the bone fills with blood clot and blood-derived proteins.

Inflammation
The injury elicits an acute inflammatory response associated with only a mild neutrophil infiltrate. The combination of haemorrhage and inflammatory oedema causes the periosteum to lift from the bone ends, creating a fusiform swelling.

Necrosis
Some degree of necrosis inevitably follows cutting off of the blood supply secondary to blood vessel damage. The morphological changes of tissue damage take 24–48 hours to appear; bone marrow is the first element to be affected. Necrosis of bone itself depends on the anatomy of the local blood supply. Sites such as the **talus, carpal scaphoid** and the **head of femur** are particularly likely to suffer ischaemic necrosis after fracture. A reliable sign of bone necrosis is empty lacunae in bone, marking where osteocytes have disappeared.

Granulation tissue
Macrophages now invade the fracture site and start to demolish the exudate and dead tissue. By about 4 days from the time of fracture, the blood clot and debris are replaced by granulation tissue which extends for some distance both upwards and downwards in the marrow cavity. Within this granulation tissue, small groups of cartilage cells start to differentiate from connective tissue stem cells.

Provisional callus formation

Provisional callus describes a cuff of **woven bone** admixed with **cartilage islands**. This unites the bone ends on their external surfaces but not across the gap between these ends. The callus has a dual origin: the relative contributions of these vary with circumstances.

First and most important is the **periosteum**. Cells on the inner aspect of this membrane proliferate and begin to lay down woven bone. Woven bone lacks the lamellar arrangement of mature bone, the collagen being arranged in short bundles of fibres, each bundle being differently orientated. As a result, it lacks the weight bearing strength of lamellar bone. The periosteal cuffs round each bone end extend until they meet, ensheathing the fracture gap in a single cuff. The efficiency of external callus formation depends on the adequacy of the blood supply in the fractured area. Normally, the amount of cartilage admixed with the woven bone is small in human fractures that are healing well. However, it tends to be greater where the local blood supply is poor or where the fractured bone has been inadequately immobilized.

The second source of provisional callus is the **medullary cavity**, in which fibroblasts and osteoblasts start to proliferate and lay down new bone matrix.

Healing across the fracture gap

Provisional callus extends round the separated ends of the fractured bone but does not bridge the gap between them. After provisional callus formation, the clot filling this gap is invaded, first by granulation tissue and then by osteoblasts. Bone formation within this gap may occur as a result of laying down of bone by osteoblasts within the provisional callus. Alternatively it may be preceded by fibrous tissue formation, this being replaced later by bone. This second process is more likely to occur if the fracture has not been properly immobilized or if there has been infection or a foreign body at the fracture site.

Remodelling

Once union has taken place and weight bearing is occurring, the lumpy new cortical bone is gradually remodelled by resorption and smoothed out. A similar process involves new medullary bone with restoration of a normal marrow cavity. Woven bone, which is quite rapidly formed and much less efficient at weight bearing, is resorbed completely and replaced by lamellar bone. This is a lengthy process: restoration to normal may take up to a year.

NERVOUS TISSUE

Central nervous system

Most neurones cannot be replaced once they have been lost, although there is some evidence to suggest that a limited degree of regeneration can take place in the hypothalamic–neurohypophyseal system. In contrast with the peripheral nerves, where injury is not associated with any marked tendency towards scarring, necrosis within the central nervous system elicits the proliferation of glial cells and the formation of new glial fibres. These, together with the ingrowth of capillaries, may constitute a physical barrier to the regeneration of new neuronal fibres.

Peripheral nerves

When an axon is severed, the nerve cell shows chromatolysis (i.e. it swells and the Nissl granules, which represent zones of the endoplasmic reticulum studded with many ribosomes, disappear). The axon swells and becomes irregular, and its lipid-rich myelin sheath splits and later breaks up. The surrounding Schwann cells proliferate and accumulate some of the lipid released from the damaged myelin.

Soon new neurofibrils start to sprout from the proximal end of the severed axon; these invaginate the Schwann cells, which act as a guide or template for the new fibrils. The neurofibrils push their way down through the Schwann cells at a rate of about 1 mm per day. Eventually they may reach the appropriate end-organ and their myelin sheaths are re-formed as a result of the secretory activity of the Schwann cells; in this way, a degree of functional recovery is attained. In some instances neurofibril sprouting takes place but the fibrils do not grow down existing endoneurial channels, and grow instead in a haphazard fashion. The end- result may thus be a tangle of new nerve fibres embedded in a mass of scar tissue, the whole being called a traumatic or 'stump' neuroma.

NATURAL HISTORY OF INFLAMMATION II: WOUND HEALING

- In wound healing the integrity of epithelial surfaces and the tensile strength of subepithelial connnective tissue is restored.
- The haemorrhage and subsequent clotting of blood associated with wounding trigger part of the healing process.
- In skin wounds the twin processes of migration of epithelial cells from the cut edges and growth factor-stimulated epithelial cell proliferation restore epithelial coverage.
- Dermal and subcutaneous tissue healing involves ingrowth of new capillaries (**granulation tissue**), and proliferation and activation of the collagen-producing fibroblasts. The new collagen produced undergoes remodelling over a period of months before tensile strength is restored.
- In large open wounds the process of wound contraction aids healing.
- Factors inhibiting wound healing may be systemic or local. Systemic factors include poor nutrition, vitamin C deficiency, advanced age, diabetes and high dose steroid hormone treatment. Local factors include infection, foreign bodies, poor arterial perfusion or venous drainage and excess mobility.

Peripheral nerves

9 The natural history of acute inflammation III: chronicity

Inflammatory processes that last for months or years must, *ipso facto*, be termed **chronic**. Many important and common diseases are expressions of chronic inflammation. They are diverse in origin and manifestations, but all share certain structural features that mark a long-lasting process. Whatever the cause and characteristics of chronic inflammation, it represents **failure to complete the natural history of acute inflammation** outlined in Chapters 7 and 8.

Chronicity may be defined in terms of:

- **Duration.** Any inflammatory process lasting for more than a few weeks is regarded as chronic.
- **Morphological appearance.** The main types of chronic inflammation have a characteristic microscopic appearance, which serves to indicate that they are chronic.
- **Biological processes involved.** These can be correlated with the microscopic appearances that are the expression of these processes.

CLASSIFICATION

Chronic inflammatory disorders are difficult to classify because they are so heterogeneous. This difficulty may be eased slightly by considering them as members of several major groups, as described below.

Following significant acute inflammation
In conditions in which there has been a significant phase of acute inflammation (e.g. chronic peptic ulcer, chronic osteomyelitis) formation of an inflammatory exudate and infiltrate continues, accompanied by attempts at healing.

Tissue damage caused by non-living agents

Where tissue damage has been caused by non-living foreign material the irritants can persist within the tissue for a long time. If the material is cyto-toxic, the inflammatory response is dominated by the macrophage and by evidence of repair (e.g. pulmonary silicosis).

Granulomatous inflammation

The acute inflammatory phase is short lived and mild, and the process is predestined by the nature of the injury to be chronic. The lesions in this group are characterized by focal accumulation of macrophages and lympho-cytes. Necrosis of a greater or lesser degree may occur and there may be extensive scarring. Cell-mediated immune reactions play a dominant role in the pathogenesis of this group, which includes such important conditions as **tuberculosis** and **leprosy**. This form of inflammation is known as granulo-matous inflammation and is discussed in a later section.

Antibody-mediated inflammation

Chronic inflammation is dominated by the humoral effector arm of the immune system, such as occurs in immune complex-mediated disorders (see pp. 202–204).

Autoimmune reactions

Chronic inflammatory disorders occurring as a result of autoimmune reactions are associated with autoantibodies in the plasma (e.g. rheumatoid disease, Hashimoto's thyroiditis).

Chronic duct obstruction

Duct blockage may result in chronic inflammatory disorders because of failure of drainage of the normal secretions of exocrine glands. This is seen in chronic pancreatitis or chronic inflammation in salivary glands (sialoadenitis).

NON-SPECIFIC CHRONIC INFLAMMATION

Non-specific chronic inflammation occurs as a complication of an acute inflammatory process. It is the expression of **failure of the normal sequence of events** where the acute inflammatory reaction elicited by injury terminates in either resolution or repair.

Several objectives, listed below, must be attained if complete healing of acute inflammation is to occur. Chronicity results from failure to reach one or more of these.

- **Elimination of the injurious agent.** Persistence of injury is one of the most important factors in causing chronicity.
- **Removal of the exudate** and any foreign material that is present. If suppuration has occurred, the pus *must* be drained adequately.

- **Adequate arterial perfusion and venous drainage**. A classical clinical situation in which these factors are involved is chronic stasis ulceration of the lower limbs. In about 80% of patients with chronic leg ulcers there is evidence of vein disease and in about 33% there is also evidence of arterial disease. In about 40–50% of cases, venous ulceration is associated with evidence of previous deep vein thrombosis and in almost all cases there is incompetence of the communicating veins. *Thus there is a strong association between venous ulceration and failure of the calf pump due to vein abnormalities.* This is not uncommon, about 0.2% of the adult population being affected. In many cases the ulcers are chronic so this condition is important in terms of morbidity and the health-care resources needed.
- In appropriate anatomical locations, **drainage of exocrine gland secretions must be maintained** or re-established.

If all these conditions are not met, a type of pathological process is likely to develop in which there is a mixed morphological picture, well exemplified by chronic peptic ulcer.

Chronic peptic ulcer

This arises from a condition in which there is an imbalance between factors that promote acid and peptic digestion of the mucosa in the stomach and duodenum (**injury**) and those that protect the mucosa from such digestion (**defence**).

Table 9.1 describes the morphological features of a chronic peptic ulcer from the mucosal surface outwards, and relates these to the biological processes operating in the lesion (*Fig. 9.1*). Chronic peptic ulceration shows evidence of all the biological processes involved in an acute inflammatory response to injury, terminating in repair by scarring; however, in contrast with what occurs in acute inflammation brought to a successful conclusion, **these processes are not sequential but concurrent**. In the peptic ulcer model, chronicity is due to **persistence of injury**, associated in most cases with infection by *Helicobacter pylori*. The zonal pattern described in relation to ulceration occurs in other chronic inflammatory lesions, such as chronic abscesses. In abscesses, the mechanism that can trigger chronicity is failure to drain pus.

THE MACROPHAGE IN CHRONIC INFLAMMATION

As in healing, the macrophage plays a dominant role in the natural history of chronic inflammation. Its importance in both these areas rests on the fact that it is a cell with power to:

- phagocytose and scavenge living (microorganisms) and non-living foreign or effete material (tissue debris, 'old' or abnormal red blood cells, immune complexes, modified lipoprotein)

Table 9.1 Morphological features of chronic peptic ulcer (from mucosa outwards) and their correlates in terms of process

Morphological features	Related biological processes
Loss of surface epithelium, underlying mucosal glands; stroma, muscularis mucosae and some of the muscularis propria. Epithelial and other debris is admixed with fibrin to form a greyish-white slough which can be seen on endoscopic examination.	Injury of sufficient severity to cause death of gastric or duodenal mucosa
Immediately beneath this is a zone of acute inflammation infiltrated by neutrophils and some macrophages	Typical acute inflammatory response to injury, which in this case is persistent
Beneath this is a zone of vascular granulation tissue in which numerous large activated macrophages, lymphocytes and plasma cells are present. Many of the macrophages contain phagocytosed debris	The macrophage infiltrate is a reflection of: • attempts at demolition of the exudate • the role of the macrophage as a secretory cell which orchestrates vascularization and repair The lymphocytes and plasma cells are evidence of tissue immune reactions elicited by local antigens.
A zone of scar tissue well vascularized in its more superficial part and consisting, more deeply, of dense fibrous tissue. Arteries in this 'ulcer bed' show intimal thickening due to hyperplasia of smooth muscle cells producing connective tissue matrix proteins. This is known as **endarteritis obliterans** and is seen in many chronic inflammatory lesions. Nerve bundles in this area are also unduly prominent	This zone represents healing by repair. The process is clearly unsuccessful as necrosis and inflammation still continue. The changes in arteries and nerve bundles suggest the local release of growth factors

- kill many microorganisms
- synthesize and release tissue-damaging products
- synthesize and release mediators of acute inflammation and fever
- present antigens to both B and T lymphocytes and thus initiate immune responses
- become activated by signals released from lymphocytes following such antigen presentation
- release mediators that are chemoattractant for cells involved in repair and angiogenesis
- release growth factors

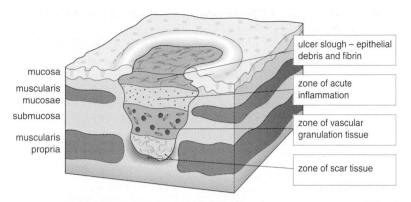

Fig 9.1   The architecture of chronic inflammation as exemplified by a chronic peptic ulcer.

- regulate its own activities to a certain extent through the operation of autocrine loops.

Secretion of a wide range of products is an important part of the macrophage's functional repertoire. Some of the secretion products of macrophages relevant to chronic inflammation and their main actions are shown in *Tables 5.3–5.7.*

LOCAL IMMUNE RESPONSE

A common feature of chronic inflammation is the presence of both B and T lymphocytes in the lesion. These cells represent a local immune response to antigens released at the site of injury and inflammation; they reach such areas by emigrating from local microvascular channels. In some situations it has been demonstrated clearly that infiltrating lymphocytes react with anti-gen present in the lesions. This implies that there is a selective mechanism that determines which lymphocytes remain within the chronic inflammatory lesion and which migrate back to the blood or lymph. In the case of the T cells, this involves the 'specific fit' of the T-cell receptors, and in B cells the configuration of surface immunoglobulin in relation to the local antigens (see pp. 162–164, 167–168).

The plasma cell

The plasma cell is a reliable marker of chronicity in inflammation; it represents terminal functional differentiation of a B lymphocyte (see pp. 147–149) that is now producing large amounts of immunoglobulin.

The plasma cell measures 10–12 μm in diameter. It has a single, slightly eccentrically placed, nucleus in which the chromatin appears to be fragmented and concentrated at the nuclear membrane, giving a clock-face or cartwheel appearance. There is a prominent perinuclear halo, known as the **hoff**, which is the site of the Golgi apparatus. In sections stained with haematoxylin and eosin, the cytoplasm is markedly basophilic, indicating abundant secretion of RNA. This can be confirmed by treating sections with pyronin, which stains the RNA red. On electron microscopic examination, the structure mirrors the predominantly secretory function of the plasma cell, with much rough endoplasmic reticulum and a prominent Golgi apparatus.

The role of the plasma cell is to produce specific immunoglobulin (see pp. 140, 151–157); this can be confirmed by using appropriate fluorescein and peroxidase-linked antibodies which bind to the immunoglobulin in the plasma cell cytoplasm.

NATURAL HISTORY OF ACUTE INFLAMMATION III: CHRONICITY

- Chronic inflammation (CI) can be defined in terms of **duration**, **typical pathological changes** and the **biological processes** involved.
- Chronic inflammation may follow:
  — acute inflammation
  — tissue damage caused by non-living agents
  — duct obstruction
  — autoimmune processes
  — immune complex deposition.
  In addition there is **granulomatous** chronic inflammation, characterized by focal aggregates of macrophages and lymphocytes, which is always chronic.
- Where there has been significant acute inflammation, chronicity represents failure for this process to terminate in either resolution or repair because of failure to eliminate the injurious agent or remove exudate or foreign material.
- Macrophage biology is important in chronic inflammation since macrophage products are microbicidal, can cause tissue damage, mediate inflammation and fever, and play roles in repair, new blood vessel formation and remodelling of connective tissue.
- A local immune response in the form of lymphocytes and plasma cells is a common microscopic feature of 'non-specific' chronic inflammation.

10 The immune system

It has been known for many centuries that a non-fatal attack of certain infectious diseases results in a diminution of the individual's susceptibility to that disease in the future. This increased resistance against specific infectious agents is known as **acquired specific immunity**. It is the basis of many successful immunization programmes, some of which have led to the virtual eradication of some highly lethal infectious diseases such as poliomyelitis and smallpox.

While this has clearly been beneficial, the biological implications of acquired specific immunity are much more far reaching, as will be seen in later sections dealing with hypersensitivity and autoimmune disease.

The specific immune system present in most vertebrates is capable of:

- **recognition** of what is foreign to the host, i.e. the ability to distinguish between **self** and **non-self**
- mounting a highly **specific response** to what is recognized as foreign
- **memory**: the existence of memory in the immune system can be inferred because a **subsequent encounter** with what has previously been recognized as foreign evokes a response that is both greater in degree and much quicker than that occurring on a **first encounter**.

What does immunity mean?

Difficulties arise when the word immunity is used to describe the whole range of activities of the immune system, since the commonly accepted meaning of the term is **a state in which there is absolute or relative freedom from some harmful condition**.

On the whole, the altered reactivity of a host following an encounter with some foreign species is extremely beneficial to the host in that it constitutes a powerful defence against the effects of pathogenic microorganisms (*Fig. 10.1*). However, the same mechanisms that operate to protect the host

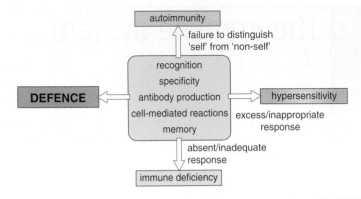

Fig. 10.1 **Properties of the immune system: normal and abnormal.**

can be turned against it and cause serious damage to tissues. In this case, despite the dictum of Humpty Dumpty who declared that 'a word means precisely what I choose it to mean, neither more nor less', the use of the word **immunity** seems less appropriate. Harmful events mediated through the immune system need to be identified in some other way; this problem is explored in subsequent chapters.

COMPONENTS OF THE IMMUNE REACTION

ANTIGENS

To generate an immune response, the cells making up the immune system must encounter a molecule that can be recognized as being of the '**non-self**' variety. Such molecules are known as **antigens**. They are usually protein, polypeptide or polysaccharide in nature. The chemical sites on the cells of the immune system or on the specific globulins (antibodies) that are responsible for **recognition** of foreign chemical species are very small, binding to only a few amino acids or sugar residues. This means that the part of an antigen eliciting specific recognition is correspondingly small. Most antigens in fact consist of many such areas, which are called determinants or **epitopes**. Each is capable of evoking a specific response.

The ability of a chemical species to function as an antigen is related, in part, to its size. Most antigens have a molecular weight in excess of 10 000. About 2500 seems to be the limit below which foreign substances cannot elicit a response from the immune system. However, it is possible for certain small molecules, which cannot act as antigens by themselves, to bind to a carrier, usually a protein. The resulting complex can produce an immune response in which the antigenic determinant is the small 'passenger' molecule, known as a **hapten**. The antibodies formed in response to the hapten–

carrier complex can react specifically in solution with the free hapten (e.g. in sensitivity reactions to certain drugs) (*Fig. 10.2*).

Because of the 'foreignness' inherent in the concept of antigens, it is tempting to view them as chemical species derived entirely from the environment (**exogenous**). It is true that such exogenous antigens are involved in a wide spectrum of human diseases, including all infections and many hypersensitivity reactions such as asthma and hay fever. However, many antigens exist that are 'native' to the host; these **endogenous** antigens play an important part in many of the functions of the immune system in both health and disease. They may be classified as: **heterologous, autologous, homologous (iso-antigens)**.

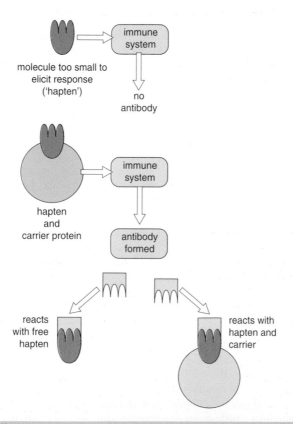

Fig. 10.2   Haptens.

Some molecules are too small to elicit a response from the immune system. Such molecules, known as haptens, can bind to a carrier protein and together produce an immune response in which the antigenic determinant is the hapten.

Heterologous antigens

These are antigens common to species that are unrelated phylogenetically. The existence of such antigens can lead to curious cross-reactions which may be important in the genesis of certain diseases. One such example is the cross-reactivity that exists between the M proteins of certain strains of β-haemolytic *Streptococcus pyogenes* and determinants present in heart muscle and many other human tissues. As there is a known association between infections with these streptococcal strains and acute rheumatic fever, cross-reactivity between the bacterial and human antigens has been implicated in the pathogenesis of the disease. Absolute proof that this is the mechanism responsible is still lacking.

Autologous antigens

These are the host's own normal constituents which, normally, are recognized as 'self'. Thus they do not elicit an immune response, a state known as **tolerance**. Tolerance can be broken down in several ways (see pp. 210–215) and immune reactions can be mounted against native tissue constituents. Disorders associated with this partial breakdown in the ability to distinguish between 'self' and 'non-self' are known as **autoimmune diseases**.

Homologous antigens

These molecules, also known as **iso-antigens**, are the determinants that distinguish the tissue components of one individual from another. Their expression is genetically controlled, as can be seen from the mode of inheritance of one important antigen set: the ABO blood group system.

The consequences of an encounter between host and antigen include one or more of three basic reactions (*Fig. 10.3*): **antibody formation, clonal proliferation** and **specific tolerance**.

Antibody formation

This is the production of globulins possessing the ability to bind **specifically** to the antigenic determinant that has been introduced. Antibodies are produced by **plasma cells**, the fully differentiated form of **B cells**, one of the two major classes of lymphocytes.

The essential role of antibodies is in **defence** of the host against infections by extracellular, pathogenic microorganisms such as staphylococci and streptococci. In this type of response, known as the **humoral** type, bacterial toxins may be neutralized, complement-mediated cell lysis brought about, phagocytosis assisted through specific opsonization, and the entry of viruses to certain cells prevented.

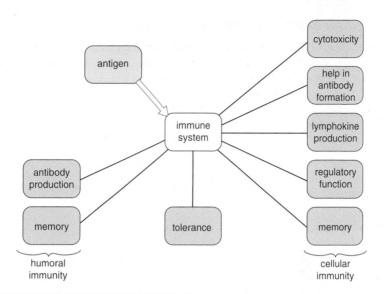

Fig. 10.3   Consequences of an encounter between antigen and host.

CLONAL PROLIFERATION

This is the expansion of a clone of another class of lymphocytes, the **T cells**. These have a wide range of biological activities including the ability to:

- directly lyse foreign cells whose antigenic make-up has been modified by viral infection, and certain tumour cells
- release a range of **non-antigen-specific** soluble products (**lymphokines**); some activate macrophages and others either 'help' or 'suppress' the function of one or both of the lymphocyte classes.

Antigen-induced proliferation of this class of lymphocyte and the resulting range of activities is known as **cell-mediated immunity**. In defence against infection, this is most effective against **organisms that grow intra-cellularly** such as viruses, certain bacteria (e.g. the organisms responsible for tuberculosis and leprosy) and fungi.

SPECIFIC TOLERANCE

Specific tolerance to a given antigen can be induced when the antigen is introduced during fetal or very early neonatal life. A second exposure to such an antigen is not followed by antibody production or proliferation of sensitized lymphocytes.

CELLULAR BASIS OF IMMUNE REACTIONS

The response of the immune system following exposure to foreign molecules, to which the host is not tolerant, has a dual nature. This is expressed by one or both of the following:

- the production of immunoglobulins reacting specifically with the antigen (**antibodies**)
- the proliferation of lymphocytes with a variety of other functions, some of which were listed above.

The effector cell line in both reactions is the small lymphocyte. When animals are depleted of small lymphocytes by repeated drainage of the thoracic duct, both sets of functions are lost.

Small lymphocyte classes: T and B cells

Recognition of functions as different as the **production of specific antibody globulins** on the one hand and the wide range of activities characteristic of **cell-mediated immunity** on the other suggested that these might be carried by at least two distinct lines of small lymphocytes. The truth of this proposition began to emerge with the studies carried out by Miller in the mid-1960s on the role of the thymus. Miller found that neonatal thymectomy resulted in:

- a fall in the number of circulating lymphocytes
- loss of the ability to reject a tissue graft from a different strain of the same species (an allogeneic graft)
- a reduction in the antibody response to some antigens
- death of affected animals from a wasting disease after 3–4 months (this was probably related to an inability to resist infection, as neonatally thymectomized animals kept under germ-free conditions did not succumb to this disorder)
- an increased susceptibility to viral infection
- retention of the ability to mount an unimpaired antibody response to certain antigens and no alteration in plasma concentrations of immunoglobulins.

These data can be interpreted in the light of a series of elegant experiments in which immunological competence (e.g. the ability to reject allogeneic grafts) is first destroyed and then restored. For instance, if immunological competence is destroyed in an adult mouse by irradiation of the bone marrow, it can be restored by transfer of bone marrow cells from an animal of the same species. If, in addition to irradiation of the bone marrow, the thymus is also removed, immunological competence cannot be restored by transfusion of bone marrow cells, although it can be by transfusion of adult spleen or lymph node cells.

Thus the role of the thymus appears to be in **processing** a population of small lymphocytes derived from the bone marrow. In the absence of the

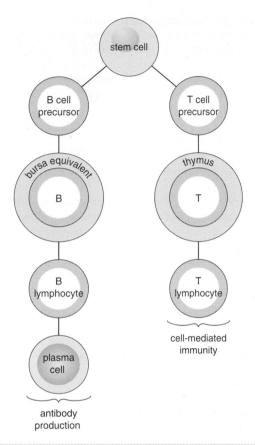

Fig. 10.4 B- and T-cell compartments of the immune system.

thymus these cells cannot develop their normal range of functions. Small lymphocytes processed in this way are known as **T lymphocytes** or thymus-derived cells (*Fig. 10.4*).

T lymphocytes

Despite having a wide range of activities, T cells cannot produce antibody. Another lymphocyte population is the precursor for the mature antibody-producing cell or plasma cell. Animals retain the ability to produce antibody following neonatal thymectomy. This suggests that the bone marrow precursors of plasma cells are processed in some place other than the thymus. The only species in which such an organ has been identified with certainty is the chicken, in which there is a localized mass of lymphoid tissue in relation to an outpouching of the cloaca. This is known as the bursa of Fabricius, and the small lymphocytes that are coded to transform into antibody-producing plasma cells on encountering the appropriate antigen are called **bursa-derived** or **B lymphocytes** (*Fig. 10.4*). There is no precise single homologue of the bursa in mammals; processing of B-cell precursors is believed to take place in the haemopoietic system, and some also occurs in **mucosa-associated lymphoid tissue** (**MALT**) (e.g. Peyer's patches in the intestine, pharyngeal tonsil, etc.).

T-cell functions

In defence against infection, T cells function in two ways:

1) On their own they act against pathogens that can survive and grow intracellularly.
2) In cooperation with B cells and antigen-presenting cells, they play a vital part in the upregulation or downregulation of the immune response. In upregulation the subset of T lymphocytes responsible is the **T helper cell** and in downregulation it is the **T suppressor cell**. These subsets can be distinguished from each other by the possession of different antigens, and are thus identified by using specific antibodies.

T lymphocytes also play an important part in the rejection of allogeneic grafts. There is considerable evidence that T cells may also recognize certain tumour cells as non-self and destroy them in the same way as the cells of an incompatible graft. This variety of **surveillance** may also serve to suppress cells that have not undergone malignant transformation but may have been altered by viruses or spontaneous mutation.

T cells are responsible for a variety of inflammatory responses occurring after second and subsequent exposures to certain antigens or haptens. The archetype of this variety of T-cell activity is the set of skin reactions characterized by local redness and swelling 24–48 hours after intradermal injection of antigens derived, for example, from the organisms responsible for tuberculosis or leprosy. This is known as **delayed hypersensitivity**, in contrast with the virtually immediate reactions due to antibody which, in sensitized subjects, may follow second and subsequent exposure to certain antigens.

Delayed hypersensitivity can be transferred from sensitized to normal individuals only if lymphocytes are transferred, whereas the immediate type of hypersensitivity can be transferred via the medium of cell-free serum. Delayed hypersensitivity, originally defined in terms of the skin reactions described above, plays an important part in the production of many serious pathological lesions, such as those of tuberculosis.

Mode of action of the T cell

The functions outlined above are carried out either through:

- **cell-to-cell contact**, in the course of which virally infected cells, allogeneic graft cells or transformed cells are destroyed by the T cells

- **synthesis and secretion** of a number of active compounds known as **lymphokines**, which are concerned primarily with mediating interactions between cells – T cells with B cells, and T cells with macrophages.

B cells

B-cell function

The B cell operates by producing antibody. Before the synthesis and secretion of such antibody takes place the small lymphocyte must undergo a series of morphological and functional transformations and mature into the **plasma cell** (see pp. 135–136).

Lifespan and circulation of small lymphocytes

The differing immunological roles of the T and B cells are also reflected in other characteristics. Most circulating lymphocytes are T cells (70–80%) and this is likely to be an expression of their **long life** (a lifespan in humans of 5–10 years). It is presumably for this reason that thymectomy in adult life does not, as a rule, deprive the subject of immunological competence, as a long-lived population of memory T cells has already been established. B cells have a much shorter lifespan, although again it seems likely that there is a fairly long-lived subset of memory B cells.

The differing immunological functions of the two sets of lymphocytes are also mirrored in terms of their **relative mobility**. The primary role of the B cell is to produce large amounts of specific immunoglobulin. This is discharged into lymph and thence into the bloodstream from the secondary lymphoid tissue (lymph nodes, MALT and spleen), where there are large concentrations of B cells.

Some aspects of T-cell function require cell-to-cell contact, and lymphokine-mediated T cell–B cell interaction requires relatively close proximity of the interacting cells. Thus the T cell must be mobile and able to travel constantly between the blood and the secondary lymphoid tissue where antigens are trapped by macrophages. The bulk of this traffic occurs via postcapillary venules in the lymph nodes. These venules can be recognized by their high, rather cuboidal, endothelium. T cells emigrate via interendothelial cell gaps from the blood into the lymph node tissue where they can come into contact with antigens processed by macrophages and other antigen-presenting cells (APCs), and thus become stimulated to divide and differentiate.

NORMAL ANATOMY OF THE IMMUNE RESPONSE

Immune responses result from a series of cellular interactions occurring, for the most part, within the **peripheral lymphoid tissue**. The latter consists of a number of different elements:

- **Lymph nodes** that respond to antigens within the tissues reaching the nodes via lymphatics.

- The **spleen** responds to antigens within the blood.
- **Mucosa-associated lymphoid tissue** (**MALT**) responds to antigens at mucosal surfaces. This functional characteristic dictates the siting of 'native' MALT, normally found principally in the alimentary tract. In disease, MALT also occurs in salivary glands, lacrimal glands, the lactating breast and the genitourinary system. MALT is distributed in **two forms**: component cells may be distributed diffusely within the tissue compartment immediately beneath epithelia or they may be arranged in well-formed follicles (Peyer's patches).

LYMPHOCYTE 'TRAFFIC'

Expansion and activation of clones of lymphocytes sensitive to a particular antigen, and recruitment of these cells to required tissue locations, demands a series of pathways through which lymphocyte trafficking occurs. These pathways consist of:

1) An **extensive network of lymphatics**, some of which drain tissues and enter lymph nodes (**afferent** lymphatics) and others which drain nodes (**efferent** lymphatics). Lymph eventually enters the thoracic duct, from which it enters the bloodstream via the left subclavian vein.
2) The **blood**. Lymphocytes within the blood leave it again by migrating across vascular endothelium.

In **lymph nodes**, migration takes place across the so-called 'high endothelial venules' (HEVs), postcapillary venules lined by endothelial cells that are taller than normal. Migration of lymphocytes is mediated by adhesion to this endothelium. This is due to a binding reaction between adhesion molecules on the surface of the lymphocytes and complementary molecules (so-called **addressins**) on the surface of the endothelium of the HEV. The lymphocyte surface ligand is one of the selectin family, **L-selectin**. Its amino-terminal domains recognize oligosaccharides of the HEV addressin. The rest of the molecule consists of an epidermal growth factor-like sequence, several repeats of structures homologous with complement-binding proteins, a transmembrane domain and a short intracytoplasmic 'tail'.

In **MALT**, lymphocytes leave the blood by binding to an endothelial selectin which reacts with a lymphocyte surface ligand, **CD44**. This ensures that lymphocytes whose function is protection of mucosal surfaces by synthesizing dimeric IgA will leave the bloodstream at functionally appropriate sites.

At sites where there is inflammation within tissues, lymphocytes leave the **microvasculature** via similar adhesion mechanisms involving interactions between surface sugars, integrins, selectins and adhesion molecules of the immunoglobulin gene superfamily such as ICAM-1 and VCAM.

FUNCTIONAL ANATOMY OF THE LYMPH NODE

A normal lymph node consists of two sets of channels (lymphatics and blood vessels) and a number of functional cell compartments. It has a fibrous capsule from which septa penetrate into the substance of the node.

Anatomy of lymph flow

Just within the capsule is the marginal sinus surrounding the node parenchyma. Afferent lymphatics penetrate the capsule, entering the marginal sinus. From the latter, cortical sinuses are derived; these penetrate into the node and break up into a series of fine branching channels. These fine channels join to form larger sinuses (medullary sinuses), and in turn the medullary sinuses join to form a single efferent lymphatic channel.

The sinuses, lined by phagocytic endothelial cells, also contain a resident population of macrophages. These two cell populations act as a filter for antigens in the afferent lymph.

Anatomy of nodal blood flow

Blood enters the lymph node at the hilum via a single artery. This branches, forming successive generations of vessels of decreasing size until a fine network of capillaries has been formed. These drain into the high endothelial venules in which migration of lymphocytes from the blood occurs. The high endothelial venules fuse to form larger veins, which ultimately unite in the region of the hilum to form a single draining vein.

The cell compartments of the lymph node (*Fig. 10.5*)

Three types of lymphoid cells are concerned with the regulation and mediation of immune responses:

- B lymphocytes
- T lymphocytes
- APCs (antigen-presenting cells).

The two lymphocyte populations are functionally and anatomically distinct. Each shows a spectrum of cells in different stages of differentiation and activation.

The B-cell compartment

Most B cells are situated in the peripheral part of the node (**cortex**). The cells form rounded aggregates (**follicles**). In unstimulated nodes, these follicles are small and show no division into functional zones. When stimulated by antigens, they enlarge and separate into two zones:

1) the **follicle centre**, which on low-power examination appears somewhat paler and more open than the second zone
2) the **mantle zone**, which partially surrounds the follicle centre, usually

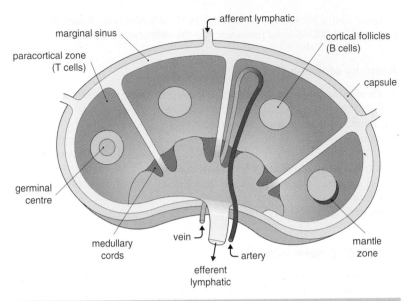

marginal sinus

afferent lymphatic

paracortical zone
(T cells)

cortical follicles
(B cells)

capsule

germinal
centre

medullary
cords

vein

artery

efferent
lymphatic

mantle
zone

Fig. 10.5   Basic anatomy of a normal lymph node.

on its capsular aspect; mantle zone lymphocytes show both IgM and IgD on their surfaces.

The principal cell components of the follicle centre are centroblasts and centrocytes.

Centroblasts are large, actively dividing, cells with rounded nuclei in which there are usually at least two nucleoli, touching the inner aspect of the nuclear membrane. The cytoplasm is small in amount and the cells tend to be clustered in the part of the follicle that is furthest from the node capsule.

Centrocytes are smaller than centroblasts and tend to have rather irregularly shaped nuclei with a chromatin pattern rather coarser than that of the centroblast. Nucleoli are inconspicuous. In the course of B-cell proliferation elicited by antigenic stimulation, many B cells are eliminated by the process of programmed cell death (**apoptosis**). The cell fragments are engulfed by macrophages, present in large numbers within the follicle centres. These cells showing lymphocyte debris within their cytoplasm are known as **tingible body macrophages**.

Differentiation of B cells within follicle centres is driven by encounters with antigen and is expressed in a series of morphological changes in the small 'virgin' (in the sense of not having encountered antigen) B lymphocytes at the margins of the follicle centres. Antigen-dependent B-cell differentiation and proliferation may take one of two forms:

1) If the immune response is a **primary** one, small B cells may be transformed directly into **immunoblasts**, differentiate into IgM-

secreting plasmacytoid lymphocytes or plasma cells, and produce the IgM characteristic of the primary response. The immunoblast is a large cell with a somewhat vesicular nucleus, a large centrally placed nucleolus, and abundant cytoplasm which is basophilic in sections stained with the Giemsa stain.

2) In the **late primary** or in a **secondary** response, differentiation and proliferation occur within the follicle centre. The small B cells become converted to **centroblasts**. The appearance of the centroblast in the follicle centre is followed by that of the **centrocyte**. Two populations of centrocytes exist, one composed of small cells and the other of larger cells. Ultimately these cells differentiate into immunoblasts from which plasma cells and B 'memory' cells are derived. *Lymphomas of follicle centre cell origin can express any of these differentiation patterns.*

The T-cell compartment

The T-cell compartment is co-terminous with the cortical tissue lying *between* the follicles and is termed the **paracortex**. The high endothelial venules are situated in this area. In haematoxylin and eosin-stained sections, mature T cells appear as small lymphocytes morphologically indistinguishable from B cells. Cells that have encountered antigen and undergone transformation are, of course, much larger, both B and T variants being present in the paracortex.

Antigen-presenting cells (APC; accessory cells)

There are two types of APC within lymph nodes: **dendritic cells** and **interdigitating reticulum cells**.

Dendritic cells

These are small cells with elongated cytoplasmic processes forming a meshwork within the follicle centre. They trap immune complexes, which are formed as the result of the reaction between quite small amounts of immunogen, homospecific circulating antibody and C3. The dendritic cells express large numbers of receptors for IgG Fc and iC3b, and these enable the cells to trap the newly formed complexes effectively. The importance of complement in antigen localization in follicle centres is shown by the failure of such localization in animals that have been C3 depleted. These complexes act as powerful immunogens and cause a marked degree of B-cell proliferation and activation within the follicle centre.

Dendritic cells within the skin (Langerhans' cells) can process antigen and then travel in the lymph as so-called 'veiled' cells, delivering antigen to the T cells in the paracortical areas of lymph nodes.

Interdigitating reticulum cells

The second type of APC, found within the paracortex, is known as the interdigitating reticulum cell. These cells have pale nuclei and abundant cytoplasm; their sole function is the stimulation of T cells within the paracortical areas of the node. They express large amounts of surface glyco-protein coded by the MHC, and also leucocyte common antigen and the β-integrin p150,95.

THE SPLEEN

Lymphoid tissue in the spleen is concentrated in the white pulp (Malpighian corpuscles) and is arranged for the most part around arterioles. This peri-arteriolar lymphoid sheath is divided into T- and B-cell zones. The T cells are adjacent to the central arteriole, helper cells making up 70% and sup-pressor cells 30% of the T-cell population. B cells are segregated from T cells and consist of a germinal centre surrounded by a mantle zone.

FUNCTIONAL ANATOMY OF MALT

MALT is characterized by two functions:

- **transport of immunoglobulins to luminal surfaces**, as for example in the gut or respiratory tract
- a **specific pool of lymphocytes which appear to 'home' on to MALT**.

In the gut, where the functional anatomy of normal MALT has been most studied, it is clear that there are three cell compartments:

1) Peyer's patches in the small intestinal mucosa and their homologues in the large gut
2) lymphoreticular cells diffusely distributed in the lamina propria of the gut mucosa
3) intraepithelial lymphocytes, which are chiefly suppressor T cells (expressing CD8).

Peyer's patches

Each patch shows a B-cell follicle centre partially surrounded by a mantle zone, thickest on the mucosal side of the follicle centre. Surrounding this mantle is another zone of small B lymphocytes, known as the **marginal zone**, which is also thickest on the mucosal aspect of the patch. Marginal zone lymphocytes stretch up to involve specialized epithelium (**dome epithelium**) over the patch, which can sample gut luminal constituents.

MALT cell population of the lamina propria

The mucosal lamina propria contains a mixed cell population consisting of macrophages, plasma cells and small lymphocytes. Mucosal plasma cells secrete equal amounts of both classes of IgA, two-thirds of which is in dimeric form which can bind to the secretory component, the complex being transported across into the gut lumen. Other immunoglobulin subclasses are also synthesized within plasma cells in the lamina propria but in considerably smaller amounts than IgA.

Intraepithelial T lymphocytes

Normally, lymphocytes are found between the epithelial cells lining the gut lumen. These lymphocytes consist essentially of suppressor-type T cells, differing in some respects from T cells outside the gut. The function of this intraepithelial T-cell population remains to be clarified.

IDENTIFICATION OF T AND B LYMPHOCYTES

There are no **morphological** differences between T and B lymphocytes. However, these cells possess a number of different surface markers and also respond to different sets of chemical species by polyclonal proliferation. This makes it possible not only to distinguish between the two groups, but also to identify T-cell subsets such as helper and suppressor cells.

The outstanding feature of the B-cell surface is the presence of immunoglobulin, identified by either immunofluorescence or immuno-peroxidase techniques using antibodies prepared against these immuno-globulins. T cells are identified by the immunohistological demonstration of a surface molecule known as CD3, which transduces the signal that specific antigen has been recognized to the inside of the T cell (see pp. 162–163). Other differences in cell markers, as determined by using monoclonal anti-bodies, define specialized T-cell subsets such as **cytotoxic cells** (**CD8+**) and **helper cells** (**CD4+**). Normally each B lymphocyte is programmed to make immunoglobulin of only one specificity and it is this immunoglobulin on the B-lymphocyte surface that acts as specific receptor for antigen.

In addition to the possession of recognizable surface components, T and B lymphocytes respond to different sets of stimulating agents which cause them to proliferate and become larger and more primitive in appearance (this response is known as **blast transformation**).

ANTIBODIES (IMMUNOGLOBULINS)

Antibodies can be defined both in operational and chemical terms. In the **operational** sense they are molecules binding specifically to appropriate antigen. In doing this, they perform a range of tasks of great biological significance, even though these may not all be beneficial. Depending on the class of antibody involved, these operations include:

- **agglutination and lysis** of bacteria (IgM)
- **opsonization** of such organisms

- **initiation of the 'classical' complement pathway** through the ability to bind the C1q component of complement avidly (IgM_1)
- **blocking entry of microorganisms** from the respiratory tract, gut, eyes and urinary tract into tissues that lie deep to the epithelia (IgA)
- **killing of the infected cell** via antibody-dependent cell-mediated cytotoxicity, in which antibody bound to antigen (e.g. viral antigen expressed on the surface of an infected cell) binds to Fc receptors of killer cells
- **neutralizing bacterial toxins** and some of the bacterial products that otherwise enable the bacteria to avoid the effects of specific immunity.

From the **chemical** point of view it has long been known that the antibody activity of the plasma resides in its **globulin** fraction, i.e. the group of plasma proteins migrating most slowly on electrophoresis; antibodies are, in fact, also termed **immunoglobulins**.

STRUCTURE OF ANTIBODY

Immunoglobulin has a Y-shaped, four-chain structure. In the monomeric form, characteristic of three of the five major classes of immunoglobulin, the molecule consists of four polypeptide chains held together by disulphide bonds (*Fig. 10.6*). Two of these chains have a molecular weight of 22 000 and are known as **light chains**. The other two have molecular weights ranging from 55 000 to 72 500, depending on the immunoglobulin class, and are called **heavy chains**. *Each monomer has a pair of identical heavy chains and a pair of identical light chains.*

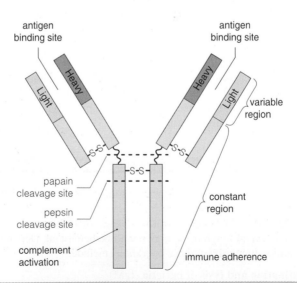

Fig. 10.6   A monomeric immunoglobin molecule.

Table 10.1   Immunoglobulin classes

Immunoglobulin class	Heavy chain
IgA	alpha (α)
IgG	gamma (γ)
IgD	delta (δ)
IgE	epsilon (ε)
IgM	mu (μ)

The chemical and biological differences between the five classes of immunoglobulin are due to differences in their heavy chain structure and whether or not they exist as monomers (IgG, IgD, IgE), dimers (IgA) or pentamers (IgM). The heavy chain classes are shown in *Table 10.1*.

Two different classes of light chain exist and are known as kappa (κ) and lambda (λ). Pairs of one or other of these are found in all five classes of immunoglobulin.

Relationship between structure and function in the immunoglobulin molecule

Treatment of a monomeric immunoglobulin molecule (such as is illustrated in *Fig. 10.6*) with the proteolytic enzyme papain, cleaves it just above the disulphide bridges between the heavy chains and thus splits it into three fragments. The two fragments containing the light chains are identical. Each can bind specifically to antigen and is known as the **Fab** (**fragment antigen binding**). With soluble antigen, the union between these fragments and the antigen leads to the formation of a soluble complex, due to the fact that binding is **univalent**.

The third fragment cannot bind to antigen, is easily crystallizable and is known as **Fc** (**fragment crystallizable**). It is, however, the site of important functions such as **complement activation** and **immune adherence** to receptors on the surface of neutrophils and macrophages. Treatment of an immunoglobulin molecule with another proteolytic enzyme, pepsin, cleaves the molecule below the disulphide bond, as shown in *Fig. 10.6*, with the production of a divalent F(ab)$_2$ fragment and a dimer consisting of only part of the Fc portion (pFc).

Diversity of antibody in relation to its structure

One of the most remarkable features of the antibody system is that each antibody has a combining site that matches with the epitope with which it binds **specifically**. Thus huge numbers of combining sites must exist. This diversity is the expression of the great variability in the amino acid sequence which exists at the *N*-terminal or antigen-combining portion of both light and heavy chains; these portions of the chains are known as the **variable** regions.

Both light and heavy chains possess units of about 110 amino acids which are known as domains. These portions of the chain are usually folded, the folded loops being bridged by disulphide bonds. When amino acid sequencing is carried out on a monoclonal immunoglobulin such as the proteins secreted by myeloma cells, the light chain is shown to have two domains: a variable one at the amino terminal end (V_L) and a constant one (C_L), each occupying about half the length of the chain. The heavy chain also has a variable domain at its amino terminal end (V_H). As this is about the same length as the variable domain found on light chains, only a quarter of the heavy chain is variable. The remaining three-quarters are divided into three constant domains (C_H1, 2, 3) (four in ε chains).

To form the combining site, the polypeptide domains in the light and heavy chains are folded into their unique shape by weak non-covalent chemical forces determined by the amino acid sequences of each variable domain. As the amino acid sequence determines the shape of the combining site, it is necessary only to vary this sequence to create a specific antibody, and thus it is easy to conceive how a vast number of antibody molecules can come into being.

The genetic basis of combining site diversity

If a very large number of different combining sites can exist, does this mean that there is an equally vast array of genes coding for each of the possible amino acid sequences? Strict adherence to the one gene–one polypeptide view would mean just this, but in fact a quite different set of circumstances exists in relation to immunoglobulin chains. For each chain the variable and constant regions are coded for by a different gene. The complete gene coding for a heavy or light chain is not present in the germ cell line. Instead portions of each chain's gene are brought together during early development of the B cell, being physically translocated at this phase.

To encode the variable portion of a human κ light chain, two gene portions are required: a large V region and a small J region. The constant region is encoded by a single gene. There are about 70 V genes and five J genes. During B-cell development, translocation leads to one V gene joining with one J segment. After transcription, the VJ region transcript is spliced with the transcript of the constant region and this VJC messenger RNA is translated in the endoplasmic reticulum to form the κ light chain. Much the same occurs in relation to the arrangement of the genes coding for the variable regions of the λ light chains and the heavy chains. In addition to the V and J genes mentioned above, the heavy chains have a D segment.

IMMUNOGLOBULIN CLASSES

Immunoglobulin G (IgG)

IgG is, quantitatively, the most important of the five main immunoglobulin classes, constituting about 70–80% of plasma immunoglobulin. It is monomeric and has the four-chain structure described above. It diffuses readily into the extravascular compartment and thus plays an important part in the neutralization of toxins and in bacterial opsonization. However, to accomplish this, more than one IgG molecule needs to bind to a small area on the bacterial cell wall so that multiple Fc fragments may be presented to the receptors on phagocytic cells. The coating of certain target cells with IgG can also attract cells of the lymphoid system that have Fc receptors but which are not specifically sensitized to any epitope on the target. These cells can kill the antibody-coated targets and are known as **K** or **killer cells**.

Two molecules of IgG bound closely together on a surface can activate complement by the rearrangement of part of the Fc fragment. This expression of biological activity varies within the IgG class; variations in the C_H2 region and four subclasses of IgG have so far been identified. IgG_1 and IgG_3 molecules readily activate complement when bound to antigen; IgG_2 antibodies are less efficient than this, and IgG_4 does not activate complement at all.

Of all the immunoglobulins, only IgG crosses the placental barrier and thus is the most important of the antibody classes in protecting newborn infants against infection.

Immunoglobulin A (IgA)

IgA appears selectively in the seromucous secretions of the gastrointestinal and respiratory tracts, and in tears, sweat, bile and breast milk. Basically, it has the same four-chain structure as IgG, with higher molecular weight heavy chains. IgA is dimerized by linkage in plasma cells to a small cysteine-rich protein known as the **J chain**. This dimer is then released into the lamina propria of the gut mucosa or the subepithelial tissues of the respiratory tract. It is then transported across the surface epithelium into the lumen. While crossing the epithelium, the IgA becomes stabilized against proteolysis by attaching to a peptide known as the **secretory component**, secreted by epithelial cells.

The fact that dimerization takes place *within* the plasma cells ensures against the formation of dimers of **mixed specificity**, such as might occur if the process took place in the lamina propria. This avoids dilution of the antigen-combining efficiency of the molecule.

IgA acts by inhibiting adherence of coated microorganisms to mucosal surfaces and thus prevents them from entering the tissues. Both bacteria and viruses may be affected in this way; oral polio vaccines probably induce immunity by sensitizing the IgA-producing plasma cells in the mucosa of the gut. The role of the relatively large amounts of **monomeric IgA** in the plasma is still not clear.

Immunoglobulin M (IgM)

IgM is the largest immunoglobulin, with a molecular weight of 900 000. It consists of five basic four-chain units joined together to form a 20-chain molecule. This is held together by disulphide bonds between the five Fc fragments and by a J chain, identical with that involved in the dimerization of IgA. The μ chain of IgM is the heaviest immunoglobulin chain; about 10% of its weight is accounted for by carbohydrate. Because of its pentameric structure, **IgM has ten potential antigen-combining sites**, but in practice, perhaps because of some inherent rigidity in the pentamer, only five of these are usually involved in antigen binding at any one time. The multiple binding sites give IgM the ability to bind with great strength to antigenic surfaces on which there is a repetitive epitope pattern.

IgM antibodies are the first to be formed after immunization. Once IgG synthesis starts, the level of IgM falls. When antibodies are made that react with the antigen-combining sites on IgM (anti-idiotype antibodies), they are also found to react with the IgG antibodies appearing later against the same antigens. These results have been interpreted as suggesting that the differentiating clone of lymphocytes responding to an antigen first uses a pair of V_L and V_H gene segments in combination with a pair of C_L and C_H gene segments to produce the IgM antibody. Later, the same variable gene segments are used with C_L and C_H segments to produce IgG antibodies that have the same specificity as the IgM.

In **complement activation** and consequent bacterial killing, IgM is the most effective immunoglobulin. Its very large size means that the molecule can cross capillary walls only with great difficulty and IgM **does not cross the placental barrier in significant amounts**. Thus, if IgM is detected in cord blood or in blood taken from a neonate, it is reasonable to assume that this represents an immune response by the child itself and that intrauterine or neonatal infection has occurred. The inability of IgM to cross the placenta has direct relevance to the rarity of haemolytic disease of the newborn due to ABO group incompatibility.

Carbohydrate antigens such as A and B blood group substances elicit a prolonged response by IgM antibodies, and the usual switch-over to IgG production does not occur. Most people produce antibodies to blood groups that are not their own as a result of stimulation by plant carbohydrates resembling blood group substances. If IgM antibodies crossed the placenta, incompatibility between the ABO blood groups of mother and baby would inevitably lead to immune haemolysis of the infant's red cells.

Immunoglobulin D (IgD)

IgD is present in the plasma in only very small amounts. For a long time its function was uncertain, but it has been found that about half of all B lymphocytes have IgD on their surface, often in association with monomeric IgM. Both the coating immunoglobulin molecules appear to have the same idiotypic determinants (i.e. they have the same V_H and V_L regions on their respective light and heavy chains). It seems likely that they function as mutually assisting antigen receptors for the control of B-lymphocyte activation and suppression.

Immunoglobulin E (IgE)

IgE is present in only minute amounts in the plasma of most people. It can bind (via its Fc portion) to receptors on tissue mast cells, these cells having between 100 000 and 500 000 Fc receptors on their plasma membranes. When the appropriate antigen binds to the Fab portions of adjacent IgE molecules, a series of events is started similar to that occurring when chemotactic signals bind to receptors on the neutrophil surface. In the tissue mast cell, however, activation leads to a discharge of the cell granules, which include **histamine**, **leukotrienes** (products of arachidonic acid metabolism via the lipo-oxygenase pathway) and a factor chemotactic for eosinophils (*Fig. 10.7*). The release of these active compounds causes a local inflammatory reaction and, if the IgE antibody is bound to mast cells in the neighbourhood of bronchial smooth muscle, contraction of this smooth muscle. This reaction may be helpful in combating certain parasitic infestations.

Some people have a genetically determined predisposition to produce large amounts of IgE-type antibody. This renders them more liable than others to a variety of unpleasant and even dangerous clinical expressions of large-scale release of mast cell granule contents, such as **asthma**, **hay fever** and **urticaria**. The antigens that trigger these reactions are called **allergens**, and those with a constitutional predisposition to respond in this way are often spoken of as being **atopic**. This problem is explored in Chapter 11.

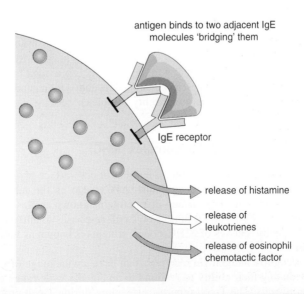

Fig. 10.7 IgE-mediated degranulation of mast cells.

THE IMMUNE RESPONSE

The induction of a response to any antigen depends primarily on the **recognition** of a specific epitope by genetically programmed lymphocytes. This is followed by a monoclonal form of **cell proliferation**. Next **differentiation** occurs, which may lead to one or both of the following:

* antibody production
* initiation of one or more of the activities of the T-cell system.

In addition there will be an increase in the number of cells programmed for recognition (or **memory cells**); this feature is responsible for the increased speed and magnitude of the reaction that takes place as a result of a subsequent exposure to the antigen concerned. The functioning of such a system depends both on the nature of the antigenic **signal** and on the mechanisms that exist for the **reception** of such a signal.

THE SIGNAL

While both B and T cells may respond to the same antigen, the way in which this signal is presented is fundamental. B cells recognize an antigen irrespective of the form in which it is presented. Thus they can bind free antigen in solution, antigens present on the membranes of cells, and antigens insolubilized in various ways.

In contrast, the vast majority of T cells only bind antigen that is associated with the surface of a cell. Helper T cells and those that secrete lymphokines recognize foreign antigens that have been processed (with the exception of **superantigens**, see below) and then presented to them on the surface of macrophages and, perhaps, other accessory cells such as dendritic cells. In addition, however, a second signal is required. This is provided by a glycoprotein on the surface of the presenting cell that is coded for a gene sequence within the **MHC** (major histocompatibility complex).

The major histocompatibility complex (MHC)

The MHC is a set of genes encoding a number of cell surface glycoproteins of great importance in **cell recognition**. APCs such as the macrophage chiefly express MHC-coded surface glycoproteins known as class II histocompatibility antigens. The limitation of T-cell responses to antigens associated with specific classes of MHC-coded proteins is known as **haplotype restriction**.

T cells recognize antigen via receptors that have a wide range of variable regions mediating their ability to respond to an equally wide range of antigenic determinants. The T-cell repertoire develops during T-cell processing within the thymus:

- cells that are selected for restriction to MHC class I molecule recognition almost all become cytotoxic T cells (CD8+)
- those showing MHC class II restriction become T helper cells (CD4+).

Antigens expressed in association with MHC-coded proteins are processed within APCs and are then expressed on the surface membranes of the APC.

MHC class I proteins consist of a heavy α chain and a β_2-microglobulin light chain. MHC class II-coded proteins consist of α and β chains of more or less equal size. Both types of molecule show some common features. Each has:

- two immunoglobulin-like domains
- a peptide-binding site formed by an eight-stranded β-pleated sheet and two α-helical regions.

Processed antigens are presented to the T cells within 'binding grooves' within MHC-coded proteins. This groove is formed by the α-helices and the β-pleated sheet portion in the outer domains.

A large number of possible alleles per locus exists in respect of the MHC genes; this has important implications in finding compatible donor grafts for patients requiring transplants (see pp. 223–225).

Superantigens and the MHC

A few antigens can bind to MHC class II proteins without first being processed within APCs. These are known as **superantigens**. They are implicated in several disorders including **rabies**, acute T-cell responses to bacterial toxins, such as those of *Staphylococcus aureus* which may cause the **toxic shock syndrome** or **severe food poisoning**, and **acquired immune deficiency syndrome**. It is also suggested that superantigens may be implicated in certain autoimmune diseases such as rheumatoid arthritis.

Superantigens bind to MHC class II proteins outside the usual binding groove. The staphylococcal antigen that causes food poisoning (enterotoxin B) binds to the α_1 domain of the human MHC class II molecule and in so doing creates a novel binding site for the T-cell receptor. Whole T-cell subpopulations can be activated by superantigens, independent of antigen specificity. These T cells share a common Vβ chain configuration.

Antigen processing

With the exception of superantigens, T cells recognize antigens that have been processed in some way within the APCs.

Processing within cells expressing MHC class II proteins *(Fig. 10.8)*

Exogenous soluble protein antigens are endocytosed by APCs. Within the endosome these proteins undergo unfolding and a limited degree of proteolysis as the early endosome undergoes progressive acidification.

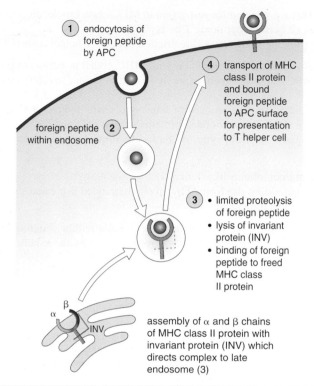

Fig. 10.8   Processing and presentation by antigen-presenting cells (APCs) of antigens in association with MHC class II proteins.

Antigen processing in these cells is blocked by treating them with chloroquine, which prevents acidification. This altered protein is later presented to the T cells in combination with the MHC class II proteins. A similar series of operations is involved in the case of microorganisms, whose antigens undergo proteolysis within phagolysosomes.

Meanwhile, the class II molecules are being assembled within the endoplasmic reticulum. α and β chains are complexed with a membrane-bound invariate chain with two functions:

1) it dictates the folding of the class II molecule.
2) it prevents premature binding of proteins to the class II molecule before the latter reaches the location of the intracellular processed antigen.

The vacuole containing the complex of class II and invariant chains now fuses with the endosome containing the partially proteolysed antigen. Cathepsins B and D, derived from the endosome, degrade the invariant chain. This frees the class II binding groove and allows the processed antigen to bind to the class II protein. The antigen–class II protein complex is now transported to the cell surface.

Processing within cells expressing MHC class I proteins (*Fig. 10.9*)

Virally coded proteins, presented on the surface of cells expressing class I MHC-coded proteins, can also pass through this process of proteolysis with the formation of peptides, some of which are recognized by T-cell receptors. The proteins are degraded to peptides following conjugation with ubiquitin by a complex of peptidases known as a proteosome. With certain viral coat proteins, proteolytic degradation takes place within the lumen of the endoplasmic reticulum where there is a set of resident proteases. The peptides are then translocated into the endoplasmic reticulum of the infected cell by a transporter mechanism known as TAP1 and TAP2. In the endoplasmic reticulum the peptides cooperate with β_2-microglobulin and complex with newly formed class I heavy chains bound to membranes. The peptide MHC class I-coded protein complex is transported across the Golgi apparatus, where it acquires some carbohydrate side-chains. The complex is then presented on the cell surface.

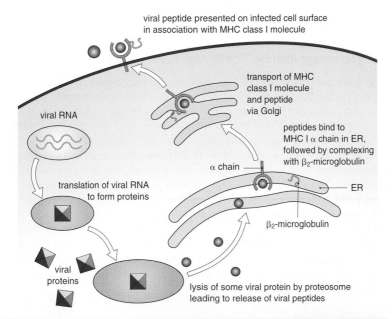

Fig. 10.9 Processing and presentation of viral antigens in association with MHC class I proteins.

ER, endoplasmic reticulum.

Other molecules concerned with antigen presentation

A third group of antigen-presenting molecules may exist in the form of certain class I-like β_2-microglobulin-associated proteins. Some of these are encoded by a gene on chromosome 1 (unlike MHC genes which are situated on chromosome 6). One of these molecules, CD1b, presents lipids from the mycolic acid in the cell wall of *M. tuberculosis*. It has been suggested therefore that T cells may also recognize non-protein microbial antigens.

KEY POINTS: ANTIGEN PRESENTATION AND THE MHC

- Class I MHC molecules are present on virtually all nucleated cells in the body and signal to cytotoxic T cells.
- Class II molecules are particularly associated with professional APCs, B cells and macrophages, and signal to T helper cells. Their expression may be induced in endothelial and some epithelial cells by IFN-γ.
- The 'professional APCs' (B cells, macrophages, dendritic cells, Langerhans' cells in the basal layer of the skin and, under certain circumstances, endothelial cells) present antigen more efficiently – partly because of their ability to process endocytosed antigens and partly because they possess cell surface proteins binding to counterstructures on the T-cell surfaces.

THE RESPONSE

Antigen recognition by T cells and T-cell activation

The 'eyes' used by T cells to 'see' the antigens presented to them are **receptors**. The antigen-specific T-cell receptor is a membrane-bound two-chain molecule (most commonly an α and a β chain) linked by disulphide bonds. Each chain is folded into two immunoglobulin-like domains, one with a relatively constant structure, the other with a high degree of variability.

A less common type of receptor (TCR1) has γ and δ chains. In peripheral blood this receptor is found on only 0.5–15% of T cells. In the intestinal epithelium and skin it is more common. $\gamma\delta$ T-cell receptors are particularly concerned with the recognition of mycobacterial antigens, especially the mycobacterial heat shock protein hsp65 which cross-reacts with a self-antigen.

The gene segments encoding the T-cell receptor β chains have V, D, J and constant segments, just as in the heavy chain of immunoglobulin. These segments undergo rearrangement to form a continuous VDJ sequence, as happens in the development of B cells.

The CD3 complex

Binding of antigen to an antigen-specific T-cell receptor is in itself insufficient for T-cell activation. In normally functioning T cells, the T-cell receptor is closely linked with a molecule known as CD3, which is made up of five peptide chains (γ, δ, ε, ζ and η). CD3 transduces the signal received by the T-cell receptor to the interior of the T lymphocyte (*Fig. 10.10*). Two of the chains (γ and ζ) are associated with the Fc receptors I and III on natural killer (NK) cells and function as signal transducers in these cells as well.

Adhesion of T cells to APCs precedes antigen recognition

Antigen recognition by the T-cell receptor is preceded by a non-specific phase during which T cells adhere to APCs. Because APCs can present many different determinants on their surfaces and any T-cell receptor can 'see' only a few of these, the adhesion phase permits the T-cell receptor to '**sample**' what is being presented. If appropriate antigens are not present, adhesion between T cell and APC is broken.

Adhesion between T cells and APCs is mediated via a ligand–receptor bond. The adhesion molecules on the T cells are LFA-1 (an integrin; see

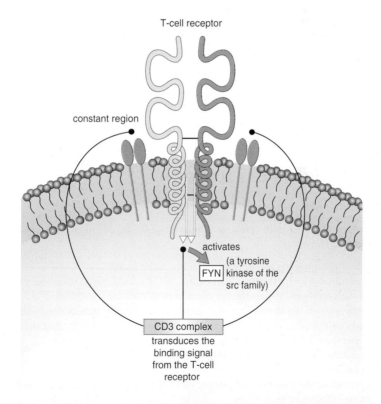

Fig. 10.10   The T-cell receptor is associated with the CD3 complex, which mediates transduction of the binding signal received from the receptor.

pp. 61–62) and CD2. CD2 binds to LFA-3 (another integrin) on the surface of the APC, and LFA-1 binds to ICAM-1 (see p. 61).

T-cell activation requires co-stimulatory signals

Another important bond between T cells and APCs is that between CD28, expressed on the surface of all T helper cells and most cytotoxic T cells, and B7, a molecule that can be induced on APCs and is normally expressed at low densities on B lymphocytes. B7 is an important co-stimulatory signal for T-cell activation, the other being IL-1.

Two signals are required before a resting T cell can be activated.

- The first is the complex formed by the T-cell receptor, the antigen and the MHC-coded protein.
- The second is either B7 or IL-1. A T cell that is already activated will respond to a single signal.

Signal transduction is accomplished by tyrosine phosphorylation and subsequent activation of the phosphatidylinositol pathway

Activation of the T cell involves phosphorylation of CD3, carried out by two protein tyrosine kinases, both of which are related to the src proto-oncogene family (see pp. 487, 490). This is followed, within 15 seconds, by phosphorylation and activation of phospholipase Cγ which activates the phosphatidylinositol pathway, releasing inositol triphosphate and diacyl glycerol from PIP-2. Thus there is much in common between T lymphocyte activation after antigen recognition and neutrophil activation after binding of a chemotactic signal.

THE EFFECTS OF T-CELL ACTIVATION

T helper cells

T helper (CD4+) cells play a dominant role in cell-mediated immune response. They:

- select the antigens and epitopes that are recognized
- determine which effector mechanisms will be used in the response to the chosen epitopes; these effector mechanisms include: cytotoxic T lymphocytes (CD8+ or T_C cells), antibody and cells such as mast cells and eosinophils, and activation of macrophages and induction of delayed hypersensitivity such as occurs in granulomatous inflammation
- assist the proliferation of appropriate cell types via the release of cytokines
- upregulate the functions of phagocytic cells such as macrophages and other effector cells.

When 'virgin' T cells are stimulated they differentiate into T_H subsets. In the short term T_H0 cells arise which synthesize and release cytokines such as

Table 10.2   Cytokines released by T$_H$1 and T$_H$2 subsets

Cytokine	T$_H$1-produced	T$_H$2-produced
IL-2	+	0
IFN-γ	+	0
IL-4	0	+
IL-5	0	+
IL-6	0	+
IL-10	0	+

IL-2, IL-4, IL-5 and IL-10 and IFN-γ. In the longer term, as in chronic inflammation, two specialized subsets T$_H$1 and T$_H$2 differentiate:

- T$_H$1 cells promote macrophage activation and tend to respond well to the antigens presented by macrophages.
- T$_H$2 cells tend to promote the production of antibody and stimulate the activities of mast cells and eosinophils.

Both these subsets express some cytokines (IL-3, TNF-α and GM-CSF) in common. Expression of other cytokines is restricted to one or other T helper cell subset (*Table 10.2*).

The cytokines expressed by these subsets can oppose each other; the relative dominance of one or another in certain pathological situations, for example in tuberculosis, may have profound implications for the natural history of the disease.

Amplification of T-cell responses

The expansion of appropriate clones of T cells that follows antigen recognition depends on the synthesis and release of the cytokine IL-2, which acts as a growth factor. IL-2 acts by binding to high-affinity receptors which are not present on the surfaces of resting T cells but are expressed within a few hours of T-cell activation following the T-cell receptor recognition of antigen. The importance of IL-2 production following antigen recognition is underlined by the effectiveness of the drug cyclosporin A, widely used in preventing rejection of allogeneic transplants. Cyclosporin blocks the transcription of the IL-2 gene, normally following T-cell activation (see *Fig. 13.4*).

T-cell-mediated cytotoxicity

Cytotoxic (CD8+) T cells also synthesize and release cytokines. The output of cytokines in many instances resembles that of T$_H$1 cells; cells whose cytokine range is similar to that of T$_H$2 cells are thought to have regulatory rather than killing functions.

Killing of cells by lymphocytes takes place under three sets of circumstances; in each case a different population of lymphoid cells is involved:

1) MHC-restricted T lymphocytes (mainly CD8+) recognize specific antigens (for example, virally coded proteins) on the surface of cells. Binding takes place via the T-cell receptor as described previously.
2) Certain epitopes are recognized by receptors on NK cells. These cells are derived from large granular lymphocytes constituting about 5% of blood lymphocytes in humans. They do not express CD3 but do express CD16 (an FcγIIIb receptor) and CD56, an adhesion molecule. Expression of class I MHC-coded proteins on the surface of a cell appears to protect it from NK cell-mediated lysis.
3) When a cell is coated with antibody recognized by lymphoid cells with the appropriate Fc receptors, binding occurs between the 'target' cell and the lymphocyte, and the former is lysed. This is known as **antibody-dependent cell-mediated cytotoxicity** (ADCC) and is carried out by killer (K) cells. The term 'K cell' is an operational one, i.e. a lymphoid cell that kills by ADCC, and covers several different cell types including both CD8+ and NK cells. *ADCC is not confined to lymphoid cells – monocytes may also be cytotoxic to cells coated with antibody, and eosinophil-mediated damage to antibody-covered schistosomes is also well recognized.*

Mechanism of lymphocyte-mediated cytotoxicity

The basic mechanisms involved in lymphocyte cytotoxicity are believed to be similar in the three circumstances listed above. Most of our knowledge is derived from studies of NK cell activity.

- The cytotoxic cells adhere to appropriate ligands on target cells.
- The contents of vesicles in the cytotoxic cells are released into the space between the cytotoxic cell and its target. This process is calcium dependent.
- The vesicle contents so released contain **perforin**, a protein structurally resembling complement component 9. The perforin becomes inserted into the membrane of target cells where it polymerizes to form a transmembrane channel rather similar to that of the complement membrane attack complex.

Complement membrane attack complex damages cells by causing lysis of their membranes. This is not the case with perforin, which instead induces **apoptosis** (programmed cell death) (see pp. 39–42).

Other factors that may cause cell damage are present in cytotoxic lymphoid cells. These include:

- a set of serine proteases known as **granzymes**; this contains a subset, the **fragmentins**, which are also thought to induce apoptosis
- tumour necrosis factor α
- adenosine 5′-triphosphate (ATP).

B-CELL ACTIVATION

Specific activation of B cells, resulting in a clone of antibody-producing cells, involves recognition of homospecific antigen and, with most antigens, assistance from T cells.

Some antigens can trigger B-cell responses independently of T cells (**thymus-independent antigens**). They are all polymers and include such molecules as pneumococcal polysaccharide, dextran, bacterial lipopolysaccharide, levan and others. The antibody response to these is unusual, consisting almost exclusively of IgM; very few memory cells are produced, and tolerance is readily induced. The recognition process is mediated by surface immunoglobulins on the appropriate B cells. The variable domains of

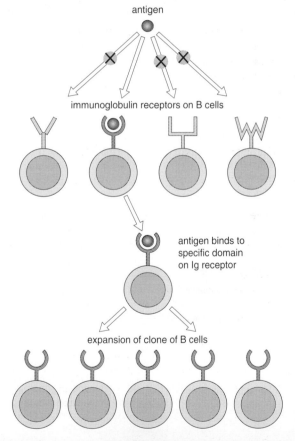

Fig. 10.11 Clonal selection in the immune response: result of the first exposure of B cells to antigen.

Some of the clone will become memory cells and some effector cells.

these surface immunoglobulins fit precisely with the antigenic determinant. Thus each lymphocyte is genetically programmed to bind one antigenic determinant. It is this specificity of the variable regions of the surface immunoglobulins that determines which clone of B cells will proliferate and differentiate (*Fig. 10.11*).

All B cells express IgM on their surface and about 70% express IgD. Only a relatively small proportion of B cells expresses immunoglobulins of other classes, and IgM is also expressed on these cells. The nature of the immunoglobulin receptors on the B-cell surface has important implications for future production of the antibody classes. When stimulated by the appropriate antigen, B cells bearing IgM or IgM and IgD on their surface give rise to clones of cells that, when differentiated into plasma cells, produce IgM only. If immunoglobulin of one of the other classes is present in addition to surface IgM, then class switching occurs and IgG, IgA or IgE antibodies are produced, depending on which is present on the unstimulated B-cell surface.

B- and T-cell cooperation (*Fig. 10.12*)

As already stated, most antigens fail to trigger proliferation and maturation of B-cell clones without the participation of T helper cells. Cooperation between T helper cells and B cells is a two-way process in which:

- Specific antigen is presented to the T_H cells by B cells, the processed antigen being presented in association with MHC class II coded proteins.

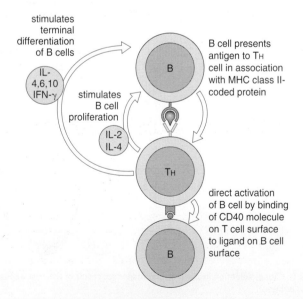

Fig. 10.12   Cooperation between B and T_H cells.

- The same B cells receive signals from the stimulated T_H cells which cause proliferation and differentiation into cells that produce and export antibody.

Within B cells, antigen bound to surface immunoglobulin is internalized and processed and is then presented on the B-cell surface in association with MHC class II proteins.

Part of the T cell-mediated activation of B cells which then ensues is direct. Activating signals on the B-cell surface are 'triggered' by binding to appropriate ligands which are expressed on the T-cell surface after antigen has been presented. The most powerful of these activating signals is known as CD40.

In addition the T cell exerts powerful effects on B cells through its expression of cytokines, including IL-2 and IL-4 which stimulate B-cell **proliferation**, and IL-4, IL-6, IL-10 and IFN-γ which promote terminal **differentiation** into antibody-producing cells.

KEY POINTS: HOW AN IMMUNE RESPONSE IS ELICITED

In most instances, mounting an immune response requires uptake and processing of antigen by an APC such as the macrophage and the expression of the antigen or part of it on the surface membrane of this cell in association with a MHC-coded protein.

Following reception of the appropriate signals, selected B- and T-cell clones proliferate and mature. The signals are usually multiple. In the case of B cells, they consist of the antigen itself, which binds to surface immunoglobulins, together with membrane-bound and soluble factors of T helper cells. In the case of T cells, the signals are antigen (expressed on the surface of the APC) surface proteins (coded by the MHC), and IL-1 (a soluble product released by the APC).

COMPLEMENT ACTIVATION

No account of the functional component of the immune response would be complete without some further consideration of the role of complement, which has been alluded to in the section dealing with acute inflammation (see pp. 66–69).

The complement system consists of sets of proteins and is involved in acute inflammation, phagocytosis and clotting, as well as in immune and hypersensitivity reactions. Some of the proteins become activated sequentially to carry out complement's biological functions including:

- killing of bacteria by membrane lysis
- promotion of phagocytosis by opsonization
- mediation of vascular and cellular pathways of acute inflammation

- processing of immune complexes, thus preventing precipitation and promoting the removal of immune complexes from tissues and blood
- assistance in binding of antigen to APCs and B cells.

Other complement proteins group into superfamilies sharing genetic and functional characteristics. Such a grouping encompasses the **complement control proteins**, six proteins inhibiting stable formation of the pivotal convertase complexes in both classical and alternate pathways of complement activation (*Fig. 10.13*). This superfamily consists of:

- factor H
- decay accelerating factor (CD55), which promotes breakdown of the C3 convertase formed in the course of classical pathway activation
- C4-binding protein
- membrane co-factor protein (CD46), which promotes the cleavage of C3b
- complement receptors 1 and 2.

These proteins are encoded by a closely linked gene cluster on chromosome 1; all share a common 60-amino-acid domain known as a short consensus repeat, which may be repeated many times in an individual member of the group.

In the course of complement activation, each activated component becomes able to activate several molecules of the next protein in line. Thus a marked amplification of the original step occurs, one activated molecule of C1 leading to a cascade in which thousands of molecules of the proteins

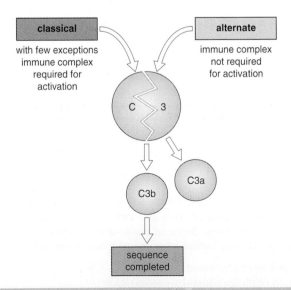

Fig. 10.13   **C3 cleavage is the pivotal event in complement activation.**

'further down the line' are activated. *Complement activation occurs through the operation of one or both of two pathways, which ultimately converge after activation of C3.* The first of these is known as the **classical** and the second as the **alternate** pathway of activation.

THE CLASSICAL PATHWAY

Each of the nine protein components in the classical pathway is designated by a number prefixed by C. C1 consists of a trimolecular complex made up of subunits C1q, r and s. For classical activation to occur (*Fig. 10.14*), bound IgG or IgM antibodies are essential, because **C1q** binds to the CH_2 of the Fc portion of these immunoglobulins. C1q has a collagen-like stem from which grow six peptide chains, each with a terminal subunit binding to Fc. For activation, at least two of the subunits must bind to CH_2; this is much more easily accomplished with the pentameric IgM than with monomeric IgG.

Thus IgM antibodies to red cells have much greater haemolytic potential than IgG: 'one hit' provides sufficient Fc binding sites to activate C1q. In the

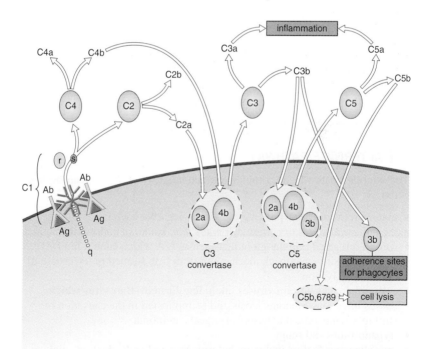

Fig. 10.14 Complement activation: the classical pathway.

case of IgG a greater number of hits is required for antibody molecules to be bound close enough to each other to provide the dual binding sites required for C1q activation. C1q forms a calcium-dependent complex with the r and s components; activated C1 acquires esterase activity, binding first C4, which is cleaved into C4a and C4b, and then C2, which is cleaved into C2a and C2b. C1 activation is regulated by C1 inhibitor. The C4b2a complex is the convertase for the cleavage of C3, which leads to release of **C3a** (chemotactic for phagocytes and causing histamine release from mast cells) and **C3b**, bound to the surface membrane of the cell to which the antibody is attached. Formation of the C4b2a complex is inhibited by C4-binding protein.

C3b exhibits **immune adherence** binding to a receptor on the plasma membrane of both neutrophils and macrophages. In this way it acts as an **opsonin**.

The final phase of complement activation is the formation of a membrane attack complex. This phase starts with non-enzymatic binding of C5 to C3b. C5 is then cleaved by the convertase C4b2a3b. One of the cleavage products, C5a, is strongly chemotactic for phagocytic cells. The other, C5b, then forms a trimolecular complex with C6 and C7, also chemotactic for phagocytic cells. The final binding of one molecule of C8 with six of C9 leads to lysis of the cell membrane to which the antibody had originally bound.

The fundamental difference between classical and alternate pathways of complement activation is that the latter does not require the presence of immune complexes, but there are some circumstances in which classical pathway activation occurs in the absence of such complexes. Such activating factors include certain polyanions, microorganisms (including *Mycoplasma*) and retroviruses (not including human immunodeficiency virus).

THE ALTERNATE PATHWAY

The alternate pathway of complement activation (*Fig. 10.15*) can be triggered by:

- many strains of Gram-positive and Gram-negative bacteria
- the polysaccharides of certain cell walls (e.g. bacterial endotoxins)
- some aggregated immunoglobulins such as IgA which cannot bind C1q, and by a positive feedback mechanism from C3b formed in the course of classical activation
- cells infected by certain viruses, including Epstein–Barr virus which causes infectious mononucleosis and is implicated in the causation of Burkitt's lymphoma and nasopharyngeal carcinoma
- trypanosomes and fungi
- miscellaneous factors including heterologous red cells, dextran sulphate and certain carbohydrates.

In the **classical pathway**, C3 is activated by the formation of the convertase C4b2a. In the **alternate pathway**, the convertase is formed by the

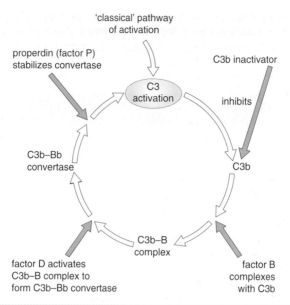

Fig. 10.15   Complement activation: the alternate pathway.

action of **certain proteins on C3b** and **factor B**, a molecule with a molecular weight of 100 000 which complexes with C3b produced by either the classical or alternate pathways. Factor B somewhat resembles C2 and, like C2, is coded for by the MHC. The C3bB complex is activated by an enzyme known as **factor D**, which cleaves factor B giving Ba and Bb. **The resulting complex C3bBb is the active convertase for C3** and is stabilized by factor P (properdin). If the convertase forms or is deposited on a foreign surface, amplification of the alternate pathway occurs. The stabilized convertase can now act on C3 to produce more C3b, which together with factors B and D leads to the production of more convertase and still more activation of C3. Thus there is a positive feedback loop with tremendous amplifying potential, kept under control in normal individuals by a C3b inactivator.

Normally, small amounts of C3bBb convertase are generated in plasma, but the inherent lability of this convertase together with the action of C3b inactivator prevents 'runaway' amplification leading to ultimate depletion of C3. Thus C3 activation via the alternate pathway is 'ticking over quietly'. The 'tickover' occurs because of the presence of an internal thioester bond in the C3 molecule. This becomes hydrolysed, leading to the formation of small amounts of C3b or its functional homologue C3i. The importance of C3b inactivation can be seen in patients lacking the inactivator. As C3b cannot be destroyed, there is continual activation of the alternate pathway through the feedback loop leading to very low plasma concentrations of C3 and factor B. Such patients suffer from repeated infections.

Once the amplification loop for alternate pathway activation has been triggered, **the C5 convertase C3bBb3b is formed**. Thereafter the events leading to the formation of the membrane attack complex are identical with those occurring in classical pathway activation.

THE IMMUNE RESPONSE IN DEFENCE AGAINST INFECTION

BACTERIA

In general terms bacteria are pathogenic because they:

- attach to host cell surface components
- proliferate within the host
- can, in some instances, avoid being phagocytosed
- may release toxins
- may invade tissues and cause tissue damage, in part only mediated by local toxin release.

These operational steps can all provide targets for host defence mechanisms. Some are based on the specific immune responses described in previous sections and some on triggering of the same defence mechanisms via **pathways that do not require lymphocyte-mediated recognition of specific bacterial antigens**. These pathways include:

- Triggering of the alternate pathway of complement activation (see pp. 172–173) by **C-reactive protein**, and **mannan-binding protein** (which somewhat resembles C1q). The release of the active fragments C3a and C5a activates mast cells which, in turn, release histamine, leukotriene B4, eosinophil chemotactic factor and IL-8. This results in:
  1) initiation of the vascular component of the inflammatory reaction
  2) chemotaxis of phagocytes
  3) activation of phagocytes.
- **Activation of NK cells, monocytes–macrophages and neutrophils by components of the bacterial cell wall**, such as lipopolysaccharide, peptidoglycan and lipoteichoic acid, **and by factors released from bacteria** such as f-Met-Leu-Phe. The activated cells release a range of cytokines which both activate phagocytes and upregulate endothelial adhesive properties, thus promoting defence mechanisms embodied in the cellular phase of acute inflammation.

Role of antibody in defence against bacterial infection

The ways in which antibody may counter infection have already been referred to (see p. 140). These mechanisms may be deployed against the pathogenic steps shown in *Table 10.3* (see also *Fig. 10.16*). The mechanisms involved in bacterial killing by **phagocytes** have already been described in the section on inflammation (see pp. 85–89).

Table 10.3   Antibodies may block bacterial pathogenicity at different stages

Pathogenic step	Antibody
Attachment	Antibodies directed against bacterial attachment molecules, fimbriae and some bacterial capsules
Proliferation of microorganisms	Antibody coating may initiate complement-mediated lysis of cell membranes Antibodies may block receptors and transport mechanisms needed for uptake of relevant substrates
Mechanisms for avoidance of phagocytosis	Antibodies can combine with bacterial M proteins and capsules, thus opsonizing the organisms. The opsonins bind to Fc and C3 receptors on phagocytes Antibodies can neutralize immunorepellant chemical species liberated by the organisms
Synthesis and release of bacterial toxins	Antibody can neutralize the toxins. Neutralization is accomplished either by binding to the biologically active site on the toxin molecule or by stereochemical blocking of a binding site on the substrate for the toxin. Some of the most successful immunization programmes are based on the eliciting of neutralizing antibody (e.g. immunization against diphtheria in which a modified form of the toxin (toxoid) is used as the immunogen)
Invasion mediated by the synthesis and release of spreading factors by the organisms (e.g. hyaluronidases)	Invasion is countered by neutralizing antibodies

Cell-mediated immunity in bacterial infections

The ways in which T cells cooperate with B cells so that the latter produce antibody are discussed in an earlier section (see pp. 151–152). In defence against infection, host cell-mediated immunity is very important, particularly in relation to bacterial species that grow *inside* cells and resist intracellular killing. Important examples in the context of human disease include:

* *Mycobacterium tuberculosis*
* *Mycobacterium leprae*
* *Salmonella typhi*
* *Brucella abortus*
* *Listeria monocytogenes.*

In defence against facultative intracellular parasites such as the bacteria named above, cell-mediated immunity is expressed in the form of cooperation between appropriately stimulated T lymphocytes and macrophages. *This is a process that is at once specific and non-specific.* Its **specificity** resides in the fact that T cells become activated after recognizing their

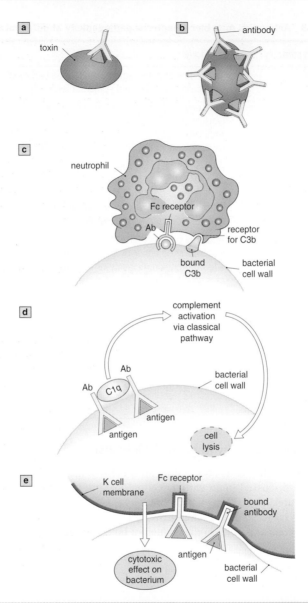

Fig. 10.16   Protective actions of antibody.

a The neutralization of bacterial toxins: antibody binds with toxin near its biologically active site and blocks the toxin's reaction with its substrate. **b** Antibody can block the entry of viruses and bacteria into cells by coating them and preventing their adherence to mucosal surfaces. **c** Bound immunoglobin acts as an opsonin and enhances phagocytosis. **d** Complement mediated lysis of a bacterial cell. **e** Antibody-dependent cell-mediated cytotoxicity (ADCC): the role of antibody in the binding of 'killer' lymphocytes (killer cells) to a bacterial cell.

homospecific antigen (in association with an appropriate MHC-coded antigen); this is supported by the fact that immunity against an organism such as *M. tuberculosis* can be transferred from one animal to another only through lymphocyte transfer.

The **non-specific** part of the process is mediated through the activation of macrophages by the cytokines (**lymphokines**) synthesized and released by activated T cells. Such soluble factors recruit macrophages to the site of infection, immobilize them at this site, and increase their ability to kill intracellular organisms (possibly by enhancing the oxygen-dependent bactericidal function). They can even increase the number of C5a receptors on the surface of blood monocytes. Once macrophages have been activated by the release of lymphokines by T cells responding to antigenic determinants on a specific organism, they acquire the ability to deal more effectively with the organisms that elicited the T-cell response, and also with other bacterial species.

VIRUSES

As with bacterial infections, some non-specific mechanisms exist to combat viral infection. These include:

- interferon production
- activation of NK cells.

Interferon production. There are three types of interferon, α, β and γ. IFN-α is encoded by a family of genes (about 20 of them) on chromosome 9, chiefly in leucocytes. IFN-β is coded for by a single gene on chromosome 9, chiefly in fibroblasts, and IFN-γ is coded for by a single gene on chromosome 12, chiefly in activated T lymphocytes.

Viral infection of a cell leads to the production of IFN-α and IFN-β; these activate mechanisms in adjacent cells enabling them to resist viral infection. The interferons are species-specific but not virus-specific. Interferons are discussed more fully in the sections dealing with viral infections (see pp. 305–308).

Activation of NK cells. Activated NK cells are important in the response to certain viral infections, most notably herpesvirus species with a special emphasis on cytomegalovirus. It is not clear which molecules the NK cells recognize on the surface of infected cells but their activity is certainly upregulated by increased local production of IFN-β. Interestingly, there is an *inverse* relationship between NK cell killing of infected cells and the expression of MHC class I-coded proteins on their surfaces.

Specific immune mechanisms in viral infection

Adaptive immune responses follow viral infections in the same way as bacterial infections. As in the latter, this response is characterized by:

- activation of T lymphocytes with expansion of clones of both helper and cytotoxic T cells
- activation and differentiation of B cells with antibody production.

Role of antibody in viral infections

Viruses are obligate intracellular parasites. When they are inside cells they are not exposed to antibody, but antibody can nevertheless play a significant role in combating viral infection, particularly when free virus is present in the bloodstream. This function is exercised in several different ways:

- **Antibody binds to free virus**. This may block **binding** of the virus to its target cell, inhibit **entry** of virus to that cell, or stop the **uncoating** of the virus once it has gained entry to the target cells (see p. 295).
- **Antibody and complement may bind to free virus** leading to lysis of the viral envelope.
- **Antibody may bind to cells infected by a virus** leading to ADCC.
- **Antibody and complement may bind to a virally infected cell** leading to lysis of the cell or to its opsonization and subsequent phagocytosis.

Cell-mediated mechanisms

Once viruses have entered their cell targets, cell-mediated immunity dominates the modulation of recovery from infection. Specifically sensitized T cells may counter the effects of invasion of cells by viruses:

Direct destruction of infected cells by cytotoxic T cells (Fig. 10.17). T-cell recognition of these infected cells involves alteration of the normal cell surface by the expression of virally encoded antigens. In addition, MHC class I surface antigens encoded by the HLA-A, -B or -C loci of the MHC are needed before T-cell recognition can occur. The importance of the MHC-coded part of the signal can be shown in vitro, where T cells that are cytotoxic for cells of a certain strain infected by a virus will not kill cells of another strain infected by the same virus.

While this system is clearly beneficial in terms of viral elimination, there are circumstances when cytotoxic T-cell activity damages host cells and tissues. In a very real sense, certain viral diseases, in both morphological and pathophysiological terms, are the expression of T cell-mediated attack on virally infected cells (e.g. hepatitis B).

Release of lymphokines from activated T cells. The lymphokines attract macrophages to the site of infection. These macrophages are activated by the lymphokines and may kill the infected cells, phagocytose free viral particles, or discourage the spread of virus from cell to cell.

Interferon release. T cells may release interferons which can block viral messenger RNA transcription and which render the cells adjacent to those infected unable to permit the replication of virus.

PROTOZOA AND HELMINTHS

Protozoa

Protozoal infections cause much disease and many deaths world-wide. This

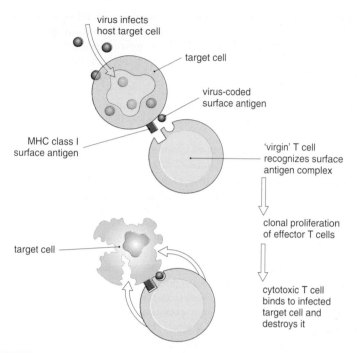

Fig. 10.17 Cytotoxic T cells in antiviral immunity.

is shown in *Table 10.4* which indicates the prevalence of four protozoal infections.

Both humoral and cell-mediated mechanisms may be involved in the immune reactions to protozoa. When the organisms are blood-borne, as in malaria and trypanosomiasis, antibody and complement appear to play a dominant role, whereas parasites that develop in tissues, such as *Leishmania*, usually elicit cell-mediated immunity.

In protozoal infections it is quite common for elimination of the parasites by the immune system to be incomplete. Thus, although able to resist a

Table 10.4 Protozoal infections

Disease	Protozoon	No. infected
Malaria	Plasmodium (*vivax, malariae, ovale* and *falciparum*)	100 million
Tropical sore	*Leishmania tropica*	
Kala-azar	*Leishmania donovani*	10 million
Espundia	*Leishmania braziliensis*	
Chagas' disease	*Trypanosoma cruzi*	no numbers
Sleeping sickness	*Trypanosoma gambiense* and *rhodesiense*	available

second infection, the host may still be harbouring a small number of living parasites. This state is known as **premunition (concomitant immunity)**.

Antibody-mediated defence is of greatest importance in **African trypanosomiasis** and **malaria**. In the former the parasites are free in the blood; in the latter red blood cells are parasitized. Antibody coating of trypanosomes leads either to complement-mediated cell lysis or to phagocytosis, the antibody functioning here as an opsonin. In malaria, antibody blocks invasion of the red cells or opsonizes them in the same way as trypanosomes.

In Chagas' disease, which causes chronic damage to heart muscle, and in the various forms of leishmaniasis, where the parasites reside within macrophages, T cells release cytokines such as IFN-γ which upregulate the killing power of the macrophages. Parasite killing is carried out by TNF-α, reactive oxygen species (free radicals) and nitric oxide.

Antigenic variation in evasion of the immune response

In the case of two important parasitic infections, **malaria** and **trypanosomiasis**, the effectiveness of antibody and complement in destroying the parasite may be overcome by the organisms varying their surface antigens into a form that cannot react with existing antibody. The trypanosome achieves this by expressing, in a **constant sequence**, alternative genes encoding surface glycoproteins. When sufficient antibody is present in the plasma to bring about complement-mediated lysis of organisms, the next gene in sequence is expressed and the surface antigens are altered. In due time, when new antibody has formed, the process is repeated; this can occur up to 20 times. Such a system clearly gives the trypanosome a great advantage in terms of survival.

Helminths

Helminth infestations are even more numerous than protozoal infections, schistosomiasis and hookworm infestations, affecting about 200 million individuals.

Two striking features of the immune reactions elicited by helminths are:

1) production of large amounts of IgE
2) a sharp rise in the number of circulating eosinophils.

Both these features suggest expression of the cytokines produced by T_H2 lymphocytes; indeed, antibodies to IL-4 reduce the IgE production in such infestations, and antibodies to IL-5 decrease the eosinophilia.

Degranulation of IgE-coated mast cells in the neighbourhood of the worm leads to release of histamine (which can affect vascular permeability) and of a factor chemotactic for eosinophils. In in vitro culture systems, eosinophils kill antibody-coated schistosomules, the cytotoxicity being associated with release of basic protein from the electron-dense core of the eosinophil granules.

THE IMMUNE SYSTEM

- Specific immunity involves **recognition** of foreign material and mounting a **specific response** to it.
- **Memory** also exists, as is shown by a quicker and greater response when foreign material is re-encountered.
- Molecules recognized as being 'foreign' are known as **antigens** and are protein, peptide or polysaccharide in nature.
- Antigens are 'introduced' to the immune system by antigen presenting cells of different types (e.g. macrophages).
- The response is a dual one – the production of immunoglobulins (antibodies) by B lymphocytes and the proliferation and activation of other types of lymphocytes with a wide range of functions. These lymphocytes are processed in the thymus and are termed T lymphocytes. T cells recognize antigens presented in association with Class II proteins encoded by the major histocompatibility complex and cooperate with B cells.
- Binding of antibodies to antigen may be followed by activation of complement, a protein cascade system, leading to generation of a lytic membrane attack complex, inflammatory mediators and opsonization of bacteria.

11 Disorders related to the immune system

All the mechanisms contributing to the immune response may go awry. Disorders arising from such defects are most easily understood when classified in relation to **individual defective functions** and, in **congenital immune deficiency**, in relation to the **ontogeny of the immune system**.

Defective or harmful immunological responses include:

- **Inadequate response to the introduction of an antigen** leading to the host being unable to mount an effective defence against infection. Such a defect may be **congenital** or **acquired** (sometimes deliberately induced) and is known as **immune deficiency**.
- **Excess and inappropriate response to antigen** leading to tissue damage by a variety of mechanisms. The term **hypersensitivity** is used for these, generally harmful reactions.
- **Loss of the ability to distinguish between self and non-self** leading to reactions against self antigens.This is known as **autoimmunity**.
- **Neoplastic proliferations** of elements of the immune system which involve either B- or T-cell populations.

IMMUNE DEFICIENCY

This can involve:

- **specific** afferent (antigen presentation and recognition) or efferent (T-cell activation and antibody production) pathways of the immune system
- **non-specific** effector mechanisms such as the complement system and bacterial killing by phagocytes.

Recognition that measurable defects in the immune system can cause reduced ability to combat infection dates back to 1952, when it was observed that a child suffering from repeated infections had no immunoglobulin (Ig) in his plasma. Since then a wide variety of immune deficient states has been described. Disorders of specific immunity may arise at any point in the differentiation of B and T cells. *The functional defect produced depends on the point in the differentiation process at which a block occurs:* the further back this point is, the broader the range of functions that is affected (*Fig. 11.1*).

PRIMARY IMMUNE DEFICIENCY

Stem cell deficiency: defects arising before lymphoid cells are processed by the thymus or bursa equivalent

If inadequate numbers of stem cells are produced, there is a deficiency or absence of the precursors of the B and T cells destined to undergo processing in the thymus or bursa equivalent. In its most severe form, known as **reticular dysgenesis**, there is complete failure of development of other bone

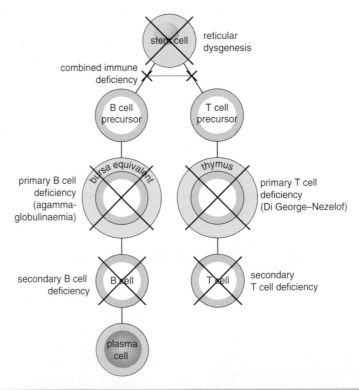

Fig 11.1   The cellular components of the immune system and the sites of immune deficiency.

marrow cells in addition to the obvious gross defects in B and T cells. Such infants may die within the first week of life, usually due to overwhelming sepsis.

Severe combined immune deficiency (SCID)

A more common type arising in the 'pre-thymus, pre-bursa' phase is severe combined immune deficiency (SCID). This may be inherited in either an X-linked or autosomal recessive pattern. In about half the sufferers the condition is due to lack of the enzyme **adenosine deaminase**. These patients may be helped by blood transfusions, as donor red cells contain this enzyme.

The thymus is usually very small or even absent. When present at post mortem examination, it shows a gross lack of thymic lymphocytes and complete absence of Hassall's corpuscles. Lymphoid tissue in the gut and other peripheral sites is also markedly atrophic.

The combined defect, which affects both the B- and T-cell systems, is expressed by low immunoglobulin levels and a low blood lymphocyte count (fewer than 1.0×10^9/l). Affected children can neither produce antibodies nor mount an effective cell-mediated reaction against intracellular bacteria or viruses. Normal immune function can be established by grafting bone marrow from a sibling with an identical or near-identical MHC. Blood transfusion and treatment with thymic extracts may also improve the situation, but many die within the first year or two of life, often as a result of pulmonary infections caused by agents that are normally not particularly virulent (**opportunistic infections**) as, for example, the protozoon *Pneumocystis carinii*. This organism proliferates within alveoli, filling them with material that appears foamy and eosinophilic in sections stained with haematoxylin and eosin. The use of silver staining methods shows the presence of many protozoa.

Other forms of combined immune deficiency

Two other forms of combined immune deficiency which are difficult to explain in terms of the development and maturation of the immune system are **ataxia telangiectasia** and **Wiskott–Aldrich syndrome**.

Ataxia telangiectasia
This syndrome, which is fortunately rare and inherited as an autosomal recessive trait, shows three basic features:

1) Cerebellar degeneration and spinocerebellar atrophy, leading to choreoathetoid (involuntary writhing and jerking) movements early in life.
2) Development at a somewhat later stage (5 and 8 years) of leashes of dilated blood vessels, especially in the skin on the flexor surfaces of the forearms, and in the conjunctiva (telangiectases).

3) Diminished resistance to infection. Plasma levels of IgE and IgA are lower than normal and there is also depression of cell-mediated immunity. Affected patients tend to have repeated infections of the sinuses and respiratory tract, which may lead to the development of bronchiectasis.

Ataxia telangiectasia is also one of a small number of syndromes associated with **chromosomal breakages** which include Bloom's syndrome and Fanconi's anaemia. In these there is an increased risk of developing malignant neoplasms, predominantly of lymphoid cells. This is the commonest cause of death in ataxia telangiectasia patients.

Wiskott–Aldrich syndrome
This is characterized clinically by:

- low platelet count
- eczema
- recurrent infection.

IgM concentrations are low; in keeping with this, there is a poor response to polysaccharide antigens. IgA and IgE concentrations are raised; IgG levels are usually normal. In addition, some depression of cell-mediated immunity is also present. T-cell numbers and effectiveness decline progressively over a few years. Both T cells and platelets lack certain surface glycoproteins (CD43, a ligand for intercellular adhesion molecule ICAM-1); it has been suggested that a defect of glycosylation, especially of sialidation of these cell surfaces, is present. As with ataxia telangiectasia, there is an increased risk of malignant neoplasms of the lymphoreticular system (5% of the patients die in this way).

The syndrome is inherited as an X-linked recessive trait; signs and symptoms of the disease usually appear in the first few months of life. Recently, it has been found that the disease is associated with abnormalities of a gene encoding the protein WASp. This protein has a role both in regulating signal transduction and in regulating the cytoskeleton.

Primary deficiencies of T-cell function

Di George's and Nezelof's Syndromes
Both of these show a selective T-cell deficiency because the thymus fails to develop normally as a result of defects in the development of the third and fourth pharyngeal pouches. Affected infants have grossly defective cell-mediated immunity and may succumb to viral infections such as measles. Bacterial infections elicit an antibody response but this is subnormal, presumably owing to lack of the normal cooperation between B and T cells.

In addition to thymic hypoplasia, infants with Di George's syndrome suffer from:

- cardiac defects
- cleft palate

- an abnormal facies
- hypocalcaemia due to absence of the parathyroids.

Most cases show a deletion on chromosome 22 but the disorder is inherited. Complete Di George's syndrome (i.e absence of the thymus) is rare; many of the sufferers have a very small but histologically normal thymus. In such cases the initially low number of T lymphocytes in the blood increases as the child grows and cell-mediated immunity may reach normality by the age of 5 years.

In Nezelof's syndrome, the same immune defects exist but only the thymus is affected. This disorder is inherited either in an autosomal or X-linked recessive fashion.

Infections with viruses and intracellular bacteria are particularly dangerous to these children, and even the bacille Calmette–Guérin (BCG) vaccine used against tuberculosis may have very serious results.

Primary deficiencies of B-cell function

Primary failure of normal B-cell function may result from:

- absence of B cells
- failure of B cells to differentiate into plasma cells
- inability of plasma cells to make one or other class of immunoglobulin.

Any of these will result in absent or very low plasma concentrations of immunoglobulin. Affected children develop repeated infections by pyogenic organisms (such as *Staphylococcus aureus*, *Streptococcus pyogenes* and *Streptococcus pneumoniae*) and also fall victim to opportunistic infections (e.g. *P. carinii*). Cell-mediated immunity is normal. Some cases are familial and sex-linked; others are sporadic.

Bruton's congenital agammaglobulinaemia

Bruton's congenital agammaglobulinaemia is one of the immune deficiency syndromes, including SCID and the Wiskott–Aldrich syndrome, associated with abnormalities on the X chromosome. The defect occurs at the pre-B-cell stage; B cells fail to mature and there is a lack of mature B cells in the circulating blood. The defect is associated in many cases with failure of rearrangement of the V_H genes. The affected gene on the X chromosome normally encodes a cytoplasmic tyrosine kinase belonging to the src family of proto-oncogenes (see pp. 485–486) which presumably mediates signal transduction. It is not yet known how a failure in this tyrosine kinase's function interferes with normal B-cell maturation.

Affected males have very low plasma immunoglobulin concentrations; the morphological correlate of this is a lack of lymphoid follicles and germinal centres in nodes and, not surprisingly, an absence of plasma cells in the tissues.

Repeated infections by pyogenic organisms such as *S. aureus*, *S. pyogenes*, *S. pneumoniae*, *Haemophilus influenzae* and *Neisseria meningitidis* occur in these children. There is also an increased risk of infection by the protozoon *P. carinii* (see p. 185) and by the intestinal parasite *Giardia lamblia*, which causes chronic diarrhoea. Purely cell-mediated responses to infection are normal.

IgA deficiency

IgA deficiency is common in Caucasians (1 in 700 population) but very rare in other ethnic groups. IgA-bearing lymphocytes fail to mature into plasma cells. In most cases there are no symptoms but there is an associated defect in IgG_2 and IgG_4 production in about 20% of individuals with IgA deficiency. The combined defect is associated with an increased risk of recurrent pyogenic infections.

Common variable immunodeficiency

This is an umbrella term for several different conditions which affect males and females equally and are all characterized by hypogammaglobulinaemia and a risk of recurrent infections. The defective immune response may be due to:

- failure of marrow pre-B cells to mature
- failure of circulating B cells to differentiate into plasma cells (possibly due to defective signalling from T cells)
- failure in about 30% of cases of T cells to respond to polyclonal activators
- the presence, in a small proportion of cases, of T cells with marked suppressor activity for B cells.

Transient hypogammaglobulinaemia of infancy

Neonates are protected against infections by maternal IgG that has crossed the placenta. By 3 months, when much of this IgG has been catabolized, infants start to synthesize their own. In some this immunoglobulin synthesis is long delayed and the infants are thus at risk, especially for respiratory tract infections. The deficiency situation usually rights itself by the age of 4 years.

X-linked hyper-IgM syndrome

These patients are deficient in IgA and IgG but synthesize large amounts of IgM. They are not only at increased risk of recurrent pyogenic infections but form IgM antibodies, which can be cytotoxic to various blood cells including neutrophils and platelets. The tissues show infiltration by large numbers of plasma cells containing IgM.

The functional defect is a failure to switch immunoglobulin class production from IgM to IgG and IgA. This appears to be due to failure of one of the ligand–receptor interactions necessary for class switching: the binding of a ligand on T_H cells to the CD40 protein on the surface of B cells. This results from a mutation in the gene encoding the CD40 ligand, located on the X chromosome.

Deficiencies related to non-specific immune functions

Phagocyte defects

These can be expressed as:

- failure to respond to chemotactic signals
- failure of lysosomal fusion
- failure of bacterial killing.

These defects are discussed in some detail in Chapter 5 (see pp. 87–89).

Defects in complement function

As each component of the complement sequence is separately encoded, it is theoretically possible for any one of them to be absent from the plasma. In some instances, instead of a component being absent, it is reduced in concentration; this suggests that the fault lies in a regulatory, rather than in a specific encoding gene.

Absence of certain inhibitors of complement activity may cause problems. For example, absence of C3b inhibitor results in continuous high-level activation of the alternate pathway, with depletion of C3 and thus an ultimate decline in the efficacy of the complement system. Absence of C1 inhibitor, inherited as an autosomal dominant trait, leads to unfettered production of C2 kinin activity, causing painful swollen patches in the skin and oedema in the gut and respiratory tract. This is known as **hereditary angio-oedema**. Sudden death from airway obstruction is a constant threat in these patients.

SECONDARY IMMUNE DEFICIENCY

Causes of acquired immune deficiency include:

Age

In both infancy and old age there is a relative lack of effectiveness of the immune response. The transfer of maternal IgG across the placenta tends to compensate for this in infants.

Malnutrition

This may be associated with defects in both B- and T-cell function and is, alas, very common. It may explain the relatively high mortality rate from diseases such as measles in underprivileged communities.

Neoplastic disorders of the immune system

Neoplastic B-cell proliferation, such as occurs in the majority of lymphomas, myelomatosis and chronic lymphocytic leukaemia, is associated with a decline in antibody responses. However, in Hodgkin's disease patients exhibit various manifestations of defective cell-mediated immunity and are more susceptible to infections caused by mycobacteria, viruses and fungi.

Iatrogenic immune deficiency

Suppression of immune reactions may be produced *deliberately* under two sets of circumstances:

1) where an attempt is made to reduce the reaction to allografts (see pp. 230–232).
2) in certain diseases, such as systemic lupus erythematosus, where tissue damage is caused by failure to distinguish between self and non-self antigens (autoimmune disorders), 'damping down' the immune response with appropriate drugs reduces the effects of the reaction and can improve the clinical state of the patient.

Iatrogenic immune suppression can also arise as a side-effect of treatments that are not aimed primarily at the components of the immune reaction. X-rays and cytotoxic drugs used in the treatment of malignant neoplasms may produce immune suppression, as may corticosteroids.

Infections

Certain viral infections can cause immune suppression. In some (e.g. measles), this effect is ascribed to a direct cytotoxic effect on certain lymphocyte subsets. Malaria and the lepromatous form of leprosy are also associated with a decreased ability to eliminate infecting microorganisms. In leprosy, macrophages are seen to contain very large numbers of apparently healthy mycobacteria.

Acquired immune deficiency syndrome (AIDS)

In recent years, increasing attention has been focused on a newly recognized form of acquired immune deficiency, known as the acquired immune deficiency syndrome (AIDS). *AIDS is the end-result of infection by a retrovirus known as human immunodeficiency virus (HIV).* Two strains of the virus, HIV-1 and HIV-2, are recognized. Most cases are caused by HIV-1, but HIV-2 infections are common in West Africa. HIV is an RNA virus closely related to the lentiviruses. Like other retroviruses, its single-stranded RNA genome is copied as double-stranded DNA via the viral reverse transcriptase system, and this DNA is then inserted into the genome of the host cell.

The consequences of HIV infection are due to the fact that the principal target cell is the **T helper lymphocyte**, as the **CD4 molecules** on the T cells bind with an envelope glycoprotein **gp120** on the surface of the virus. Other target cells are **macrophages, dendritic cells in lymphoid tissues, antigen-presenting Langerhans' cells in the skin** and **neuroglia**, all of which may express CD4 on their surfaces.

Infection of CD4+ cells leads ultimately to their destruction and a progressive fall in their numbers. This in turn exposes the affected individual to infection by a number of agents of low virulence, this situation being termed **opportunistic infection**. Agents commonly involved include *P. carinii* (causing pneumonia), *Mycobacterium tuberculosis*, *Mycobacterium avium intracellulare*, *Toxoplasma gondii*, *Cryptosporidium parvum* (causing chronic diarrhoea) and cytomegalovirus.

Infection with HIV may occur in several ways:

Sexual intercourse. In some parts of Africa where large proportions of the population have been infected, the common route is via heterosexual intercourse. In the West, risk appears to be associated chiefly with homosexual anal intercourse in males where infected lymphocytes may be present in the semen of one partner and enter the tissues of the other partner via abrasions in the anal or rectal mucosa.

Intravenous drug abuse.

Transfusion of infected blood or blood products (e.g. commercial factor VIII administered to haemophiliac patients). This risk is significantly diminished by testing donor blood for anti-HIV antibodies and by heat treatment of products such as factor VIII. However, seroconversion of an infected individual may take up to 3 months, during which time the blood will be infective despite the absence of antibodies.

Vertical transmission from infected mother to infant. This takes place via the placenta.

The HIV virus

Like all retroviruses, the single-stranded RNA genome of HIV contains *gag*, *pol* and *env* genes.

- *gag* encodes a protein that is cleaved into four nucleocapsid constituents known as p24, p17, p9 and p7. p24 elicits antibody formation in the infected host; these assist the diagnosis of HIV infection.
- *pol* encodes reverse transcriptase, an RNA-dependent DNA polymerase which uses RNA as its template for the formation of DNA.
- *env* encodes a glycoprotein with a molecular weight of 160; this becomes cleaved into two closely linked envelope glycoproteins, gp120 and gp41. Gp120 binds to CD4 and enters cells expressing this molecule on their surface (*Figs 11.2* and *11.3*).

In addition, the HIV genome contains other genes that are important in the natural history of infection:

- *tat*, a transactivator gene upregulating transcription of the viral genome
- *vpu* gene, required for efficient virion budding
- *vif*, controlling infectivity of free, rather than cell-bound, virus
- *rev* gene, which acts post-transcriptionally and promotes the transport of viral messenger RNA to the cytoplasm of the infected cell
- *nef* gene, the function of which is uncertain.

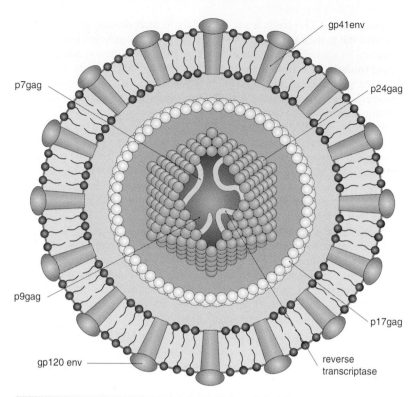

Fig 11.2 The structure of HIV-1 showing the genome and the outer glycoprotein coat.

Also important are long terminal repeats which, in addition to containing regions that bind products of *tat* and *nef*, contain core enhancer elements (NK-κB) activated when latently infected T cells or macrophages are stimulated.

Results of HIV infection

Once gp120 has bound to CD4, fusion occurs between the lipid bilayers of the viral and cell membranes, and the virus enters the cell. The viral genome becomes uncoated and the viral reverse transcriptase makes a single-stranded DNA copy of the virus's RNA genome. Complementary strands of DNA are synthesized, anneal and may then be inserted into the host cell's genome as a provirus. This provirus may be transcribed with the production of new HIV RNA, which may be translated in the endoplasmic reticulum of the host cells and result in the formation of new complete virions that bud from the host cell's plasma membrane and are released into the extracellular environment. This is termed a **productive** infection.

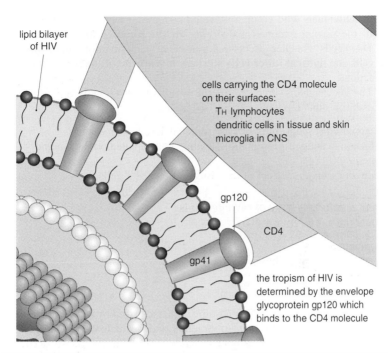

lipid bilayer
of HIV

cells carrying the CD4 molecule
on their surfaces:
TH lymphocytes
dendritic cells in tissue and skin
microglia in CNS

gp120

CD4

gp41

the tropism of HIV is
determined by the envelope
glycoprotein gp120 which
binds to the CD4 molecule

Fig. 11.3   The tropism of HIV is determined by the envelope glycoprotein gp120 which binds to the CD4 molecule.

Sometimes, the provirus is *not* transcribed and no new virus is made. This is described as **latency**. Latency is overcome if the infected T cells are stimulated either by other viruses or by increased concentrations of cytokines such as tumour necrosis factor α. *Latency is responsible for the often long, symptom-free intervals occurring in individuals infected by HIV.* During the latent period, some proviral transcription may be proceeding in the macrophage and follicular dendritic cell compartment.

HIV infection is followed by immune responses in which antibodies to p24 and the envelope glycoproteins are formed; this is accompanied by production of gp120-specific cytotoxic (CD8+) T cells which combat the viraemia. Virus plus antibody and complement are trapped in lymph nodes by follicular dendritic cells, which present viral antigens within germinal centres (see pp. 149–150) and cause hyperplasia of the B-cell zones, later followed by atrophy. Most of the antibodies formed during this phase fail to prevent infection of susceptible T cells. A major problem is the fact that the gp120 region of the viral genome is extremely variable and mutates readily and frequently. This has until now prevented active immunization against AIDS, as a vaccine prepared against one variant will have no effect against another.

In individuals who go on to develop serious consequences of HIV infection, the pivotal event is a **decrease in the number of circulating T$_H$ (CD4+) cells**. This has effects that transcend T-cell function: **macrophages**, **B cells** and **natural killer cells** all show impairment of the normal range of functions.

The mechanisms involved in the death of CD4+ cells are not clear. Possibilities that have been canvassed include:

- increased susceptibility of HIV-infected T cells to apoptosis
- failure in antigen presentation, leading to a depleted pool of memory T cells
- direct cytopathic effect of the virus on infected T cells.

Clinical natural history of HIV infections

Infection may be followed by:

- viraemia
- an asymptomatic phase
- AIDS-related complex
- full-blown AIDS.

Viraemia.   An acute early syndrome is characterized by fever, myalgia and joint pain. This is the correlate of viraemia, and the nucleocapsid antigen p24 can be identified in the patient's plasma. This clinical phase occurs in 50–70% of infected individuals.

Asymptomatic phase.   During the asymptomatic phase antiviral antibodies are present in the plasma. At this stage the affected individuals can transmit the disease to others despite their lack of symptoms. Hypergammaglobulinaemia is usually encountered at this stage and the B cells of affected individuals secrete immunoglobulin spontaneously in culture. The number of CD8+ cells specific for HIV antigens is increased in the blood. This phase may continue for years.

In a proportion of infected individuals, mild constitutional symptoms may develop, associated with **persistent generalized enlargement of lymph nodes**.

AIDS-related complex.   As the number of CD4+ cells in the circulating blood falls to below levels of 400 per mm^3, patients develop AIDS-related complex (ARC). This consists of:

- fever lasting longer than 3 months
- weight loss
- diarrhoea
- anaemia
- night sweats.

At this stage, the patient may develop superficial fungal infections, such as candidiasis, which are particularly likely to affect the mouth and oesophagus.

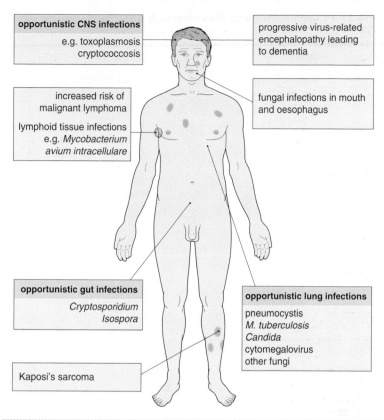

Fig. 11.4   Important clinical effects of AIDS.

Full-blown AIDS.   At the stage of full-blown AIDS the CD4+ cell count is likely to be 200 per mm^3 or less. Clinical manifestations (*Fig. 11.4*) are predicated on the basis of:

1) **immune deficiency**, laying the patient open to a wide range of opportunistic infections (see *Table 11.1*)
2) an increased risk of developing certain **malignant neoplasms**, most notably **Kaposi's sarcoma** and non-Hodgkin's lymphoma (including 'primary' lymphoma of the brain) and invasive squamous carcinoma of the uterine cervix
3) the **direct effects of HIV infection within the nervous system**; these include:
   • progressive encephalopathy associated with dementia
   • a range of opportunistic central nervous system infections, including toxoplasmosis and cryptococcal meningitis (caused by the fungus *Cryptococcus neoformans*)

Table 11.1 Opportunistic infections commonly occurring in patients with AIDS

Group	Agent	Target
Bacteria	Mycobacterium tuberculosis	Lungs and other organs
	Mycobacterium avium intracellulare	Lymphoid and other tissues
	Nocardia	Lungs, meninges
	Salmonella	All tissues
Viruses	Cytomegalovirus	Lung, gut, eye, brain
	Herpes simplex	Local or disseminated
	Varicella zoster	Local or disseminated
	Papova viruses	Brain causing progressive multifocal encephalopathy
Fungi	Candida	Mouth, oesophagus, trachea and lung
	Cryptococcus	Brain and meninges
	Coccidioides	Disseminated
	Histoplasma	Disseminated
Protozoa and helminths	Toxoplasma gondii	Brain and lung
	Pneumocystis carinii	Lung and other tissues
	Cryptosporidium parvum	Gut
	Isospora belli	Gut

- peripheral neuropathies
- vacuolar changes in the spinal cord.

HYPERSENSITIVITY

Foreign antigen in an immunologically normal host induces a state of **altered reactivity**, expressed by antibody production and/or the proliferation of sensitized T cells. In such a **primed** host, a second encounter with the same antigen produces a reaction that is greater both in degree and in speed of response. Sometimes this second reaction may be excessive in degree and cause tissue damage. Such injurious reactions are subsumed within the term **hypersensitivity**.

Hypersensitivity reactions are best classified on the basis of the **mechanisms** involved in their production. This approach is embodied in the classification proposed by Gell and Coombs, in which four major types of immunologically mediated tissue injury are recognized.

Type I hypersensitivity (immediate hypersensitivity, anaphylactic sensitivity, reagin-mediated allergy)

In type I hypersensitivity foreign antigen reacts with IgE bound to mast cells via the Fc portion. The bridging of the Fab portions of two adjacent IgE molecules by antigen initiates a complex series of reactions resulting in:

- release of preformed contents from the mast cell granules into the surrounding micro-environment
- synthesis of arachidonic acid metabolites, which have powerful pharmacological effects, notably in relation to smooth muscle tone which is greatly increased.

Excessive IgE response to the introduction of, for the most part, harmless antigens lies at the heart of type I hypersensitivity. In affected individuals there is presumably a failure to inhibit responses of B cells to certain antigens. Such people, who are spoken of as being **atopic**, make large amounts of IgE which is specific for some normally innocuous protein. This antibody then binds to the tissue mast cells, which are widely distributed in the skin, membranes of the nose, mouth, trachea, bronchi and bronchioles, gut and lymphoid tissues.

The surface of a mast cell is studded with between 100 000 and 500 000 receptors (FcεRI); the inappropriately large amounts of IgE synthesized by allergic patients bind to these via the Fc fragment. At this point there is no functional disturbance. Disturbance occurs only on a second or subsequent exposure to divalent homospecific antigen, which reacts with the adjacent bound IgE molecules to cause 'bridging' between the Fab portions and resulting cross-linking of the Fc receptors on the mast cell (*Fig. 10.7*). This cross-linking leads to degranulation of the mast cells. The sequence of events that follows binding of antigen to IgE is similar in many respects to that which occurs in the course of reception and transduction of chemotactic signals. Serine proesterase is activated and the resulting serine esterase causes changes in the fluidity of the cell membranes through methylation of phospholipids. The result is an influx of calcium ions through the membrane; this has two quite separate effects.

The **intracellular cyclic nucleotide concentration increases** leading to microtubule and microfilament assembly. Microfilament contraction causes granules containing histamine, heparin, 5-hydroxytryptamine, platelet-activating factor and eosinophil chemotactic factor to move towards and then fuse with the plasma membrane of the mast cell, and to discharge their contents.

The influx of calcium leads to the **activation of phospholipase A_2 and release of arachidonic acid**. With arachidonic acid as a starting point, a two-branched cascade occurs (*Fig. 11.5*). One (the **cyclo-oxygenase pathway**) leads to the formation of prostaglandins via the endoperoxides prostaglandin (PG) G_2 and PGH_2. The second, catalysed by the enzyme **lipo-oxygenase**, leads to the formation of powerful inflammatory mediators known as the **leukotrienes** by converting arachidonic acid via 5-hydroperoxy-eicosotetraenoic acid (5-HPTE). A number of such leukotrienes is formed. These include B_4 (see pp. 73–74), C_4, D_4 and E_4. The mixture of C_4, D_4 and E_4 constitutes what was formerly known as **slow-reacting substance A (SRS-A)**, a powerful and long-acting agent for the contraction of smooth muscle.

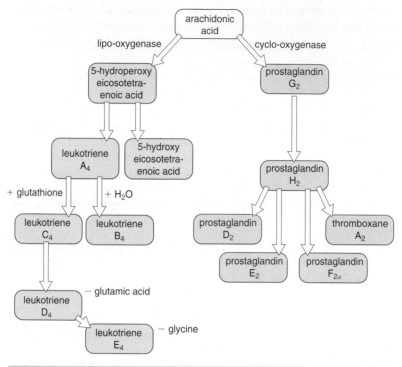

Fig. 11.5 Arachidonic acid metabolism in the activated mast cell membrane.

The release of these powerful agents leads to a number of different clinical expressions mediated, at least in part, by the **route of exposure** to the offending antigen and thus the location of the affected mast cells. These include:

- Allergic rhinitis (hay fever).
- Extrinsic allergic asthma, dominated by bronchospasm. The small airways in asthma show evidence of inflammation in the form of infiltration by T cells, macrophages and, especially, eosinophils. Migration of eosinophils is determined largely by the local release from T cells of interleukin (IL) 3, IL-5 and granulocyte–macrophage colony-stimulating factor (GM-CSF). IL-5 is particularly powerful in this context, promoting eosinophil migration in a number of different ways. Eosinophils contain a protein known as **major basic protein** which upregulates bronchial responsiveness to allergens and is also toxic for bronchiolar and bronchial epithelium. The presence of large amounts of IL-5 in the affected airways suggests a T_H2 type of response to antigen, which seems to be associated with the atopic state.
- Atopic conjunctivitis, caused by spores, danders, pollens and faeces from the house dust mite *Dermatophagoides pteronyssinus*.

- Atopic dermatitis resulting from a variety of allergens (penicillin, heavy metals, local anaesthetics, etc.).
- Urticarial angio-oedema, characterized by intensely itchy skin papules and often related to insect bites or food allergies.
- Gastrointestinal disturbances such as pain, vomiting and diarrhoea, usually related to food allergies. Mucosal mast cells which are presumably involved in this syndrome, differ from the more widely distributed connective tissue mast cells in that they are induced to proliferate by IL-3, release less histamine and release relatively more leukotriene C_4 and less prostaglandin D_2.

Type 1 hypersensitivity can be transferred passively via serum

The relationship of hypersensitivity to a plasma component (IgE) can be demonstrated by **transfer of serum from an allergic to a non-allergic subject**. If such serum is injected into the skin of the non-allergic person and this is followed by intradermal injection of the allergen at the same site, a characteristic wheal and flare reaction develops very quickly (the Prausnitz–Kustner reaction).

Treatment

Treatment is based on a number of factors relating fairly logically to the steps involved in the development of the specific hypersensitivity:

- The specific allergen should be avoided if possible.
- The allergic reaction can be reduced by giving repeated injections of small amounts of allergen. This is known as desensitization.
- Calcium entry into the mast cell can be blocked by the administration of disodium cromoglycate. This is ineffective in the case of mucosal mast cells found in the gut and lung.
- The contraction of microfilaments, which is an essential precursor of mast cell degranulation, can be inhibited by the use of corticosteroids.
- The effects of histamine can be blocked by administration of antihistamines.
- Smooth muscle contraction can be inhibited by isoprenaline or adrenaline.
- The adenosine 5′-cyclic monophosphate (cAMP) to guanosine 5′-cyclic monophosphate (cGMP) ratio can be increased by the use of theophylline or compounds that inhibit the enzyme phosphodiesterase and thus raise intracellular cAMP concentrations. As cAMP increases, the intracellular events described above are damped down.

Type II hypersensitivity (cytotoxic hypersensitivity)

Here tissue damage arises primarily from the presence of circulating antibody directed against some tissue component and the binding of that antibody to its specific epitope. Once such binding has occurred, damage to and

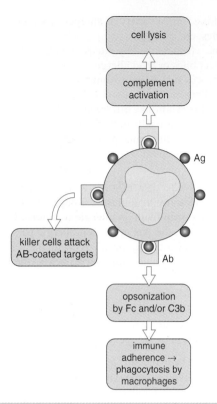

Fig. 11.6   Effector mechanisms in type II hypersensitivity.

death of the affected cells can come about through the operation of a number
of effector mechanisms (*Fig. 11.6*) (see also Chapter 10).

- Lysis of the cell membrane may occur as a result of activation of the
  complement system.
- The cell to which antibody has bound may be phagocytosed by
  macrophages via the adherence mechanisms mediated through C3b or
  the Fc portion of immunoglobulin.
- The antibody-coated cells may be killed by killer cells (antibody-
  dependent cytotoxicity).

*Cytotoxic hypersensitivity is of particular clinical importance in relation
to the cells of the blood.* **Immune haemolysis** is an archetypal type II
reaction. It may occur under three different sets of circumstances: incompatible blood transfusion, haemolytic disease of the newborn (*Fig. 11.7*), and
autoimmune haemolytic disease.

Other examples of autoimmune type II hypersensitivity are considered in
Chapter 12.

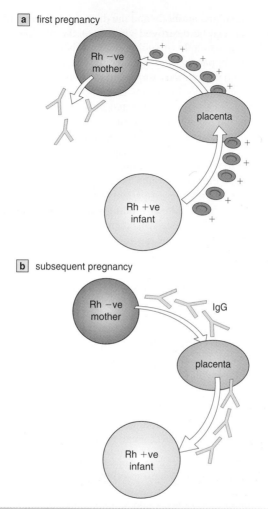

Fig. 11.7   Haemolytic disease of the newborn.

a Rhesus (Rh)-positive red cells from the fetus leak into the maternal circulation at parturition and cause the mother to produce antibodies directed at the Rh antigens. **b** In subsequent pregnancies, if the infant is Rh positive, the IgG antibodies against Rh antigens cross the placenta and cause haemolysis of the fetal red blood cells.

Drug-induced type II hypersensitivity

All varieties of hypersensitivity can be elicited by drugs, but only those operating through type II mechanisms are considered here. Even in this restricted frame of reference, diverse mechanisms may be involved.

In one form, the drug or part of it binds to a carrier (which may be a cell such as the red cell or platelet) and thus acts as a hapten. When binding takes place between the resulting antibody and the drug-related antigenic determinant, the carrier cell can be destroyed via one of the mechanisms already described. A classical example of such a reaction is the purpura caused in some people by the hypnotic drug Sedormid. The drug acts as a hapten bound to platelets, and the antibody formed in response binds to the drug and destroys the innocent platelet by means of complement-mediated lysis. In vitro, the platelet lysis can be demonstrated only if the drug is added to a mixture of platelets and the patient's serum.

A totally different mechanism appears to operate in the case of some other drugs. Antibodies are formed, which, instead of binding with the drug, react with **self antigenic determinants** and thus, by implication, are elicited by them. An example of this is the once very widely used antihypertensive agent α-methyldopa. In a number of patients taking this compound, the red cells become coated with an antibody binding with one of the antigens of the **rhesus system** (e). The suggested mechanism is that the interaction of the drug with the red cell membrane has revealed antigenic determinants that are normally masked.

Type III hypersensitivity (immune complex-mediated hypersensitivity)

The union of antibody and antigen in very finely dispersed or soluble form is known as an **immune complex**. Such complexes are capable of causing inflammation, usually by complement activation and the consequent attraction of neutrophils and platelets (*Fig. 11.8*). The tissue injury itself is largely due to:

- release of lysosomal enzymes from the neutrophils
- release of vasoactive amines from aggregated platelets
- formation of platelet aggregates that can occlude vessels of the microcirculation.

The role of the complement system in bringing about these events is thus a key one.

The effect of immune complexes can be reduced greatly if the actions of C3 and later components of the complement sequence are inhibited. The *size* of the complexes is important in determining the type of reaction.

- **Large complexes** are usually phagocytosed, although phagocytosis may be preceded by an inflammatory reaction if the complex is localized within tissues.
- **Very small complexes** may circulate in the plasma and pass harmlessly through the glomerular filter into the urine.

The nature of the complex is partly governed by the relative proportions of antigen and antibody. If there is **antibody excess** or **mild antigen excess**, the complexes are rapidly precipitated and tend to be localized to the site of antigen introduction, thus giving **local tissue reactions**. If there is **moderate**

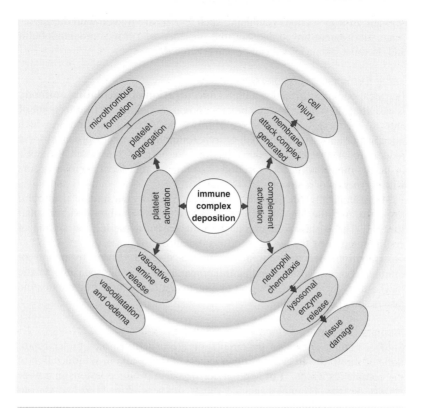

Fig. 11.8   Type III hypersensitivity: results of immune complex deposition.

to gross antigen excess, the complexes formed are **soluble**. They can thus circulate widely and become deposited in relation to the basement membranes of small blood vessels (e.g. the glomerular capillaries), in the joints and in the skin.

Immune complex localization in such sites can produce a spectrum of lesions, those affecting small blood vessels showing characteristic features. Tissue reactions in response to immune complexes are influenced by whether the complexes are formed **locally** or are **within the circulation**.

Microscopic features of small blood vessel lesions caused by immune complex deposition

There may be extensive necrosis of smooth muscle cells associated with deposition of fibrin and immunoglobulin. This type of reaction is called **fibrinoid necrosis**. Microscopically, in sections stained with haematoxylin and eosin, the necrotic portions of the blood vessel walls show a great affinity for the eosin and stain bright red with a curious 'smudged' appearance. These changes may involve the whole circumference of the vessel wall or only a segment of it. If sections containing such lesions are treated with the appropriate fluorescein-linked antisera, the presence of fibrin, immunoglobulin and, in most instances, C3 can be demonstrated.

Local formation of complexes

For local complex formation a **high concentration of circulating antibody** is essential. This leads to rapid precipitation of antigen at or near its point of entry to the tissues. The archetype of this is the **Arthus reaction**, in which injection of antigen into the skin of hyperimmunized rabbits produces local reddening and oedema at the injection site within 3–8 hours. In some instances the inflammatory reaction is so intense that local necrosis occurs with formation of a slough.

Microscopically such a lesion is characterized by an intense neutrophil response, and the antigen is often precipitated by antibody within small venules. The Arthus reaction can be blocked by depleting the animal of complement or by the use of specific antineutrophil sera.

Arthus-type reactions occur in human disease. Local formation of immune complex with a resulting inflammatory response is the pathogenetic mechanism operating in a number of human disorders, including rheumatoid disease and farmer's lung .

Immune complexes formed in the circulation

Soluble complexes within the circulation are usually formed under conditions of **moderate to gross antigen excess**. This results in solubilization of the complexes which, if of appropriate size, can produce lesions in a wide variety of sites. Examples include serum sickness (*Fig. 11.9*) and various forms of glomerulonephritis.

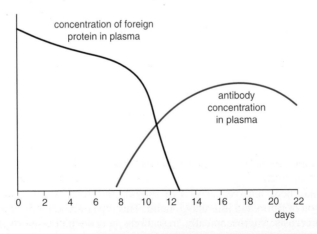

Fig. 11.9   Antigen and antibody concentrations in serum sickness.

Pathogenic immune complexes are formed during the period of antigen excess.

Type IV hypersensitivity (cell-mediated reactions)

Tissue injury resulting from the activity of sensitized T cells is common and includes some of the most widespread and serious disorders, such as tuberculosis and leprosy (see pp. 251–276). Such injury occurs under three main sets of circumstances:

1) **Hypersensitivity reactions elicited by a number of microbial agents**. These include **bacteria** (tuberculosis and leprosy), **viruses** (smallpox, measles and herpes) and **fungi** (candidiasis, histoplasmosis). The delayed skin reactions induced by the injection of tuberculoprotein into the dermis of persons previously exposed to *Mycobacterium tuberculosis*, and hence having some degree of cell-mediated immunity, are highly characteristic. The tissue reactions characteristic of some of the pathological expressions of cell-mediated reactions are considered in more detail in the section dealing with granulomatous inflammation (see pp. 241, 247, 255–257).
2) **Rejection of tissue or organ grafts**.
3) **Contact dermatitis**, as seen after exposure to certain chemicals, plant products and metals (e.g. watchstrap dermatitis). Contact dermatitis is induced by complex antigens which are formed as the result of binding between the foreign substance and a carrier protein derived from the host's skin.

Stimulatory reactions caused by antibody (called type V by some writers)

Some types of cell hyperfunction may be brought about as a result of immune reactions. The example most often cited is that of **thyrotoxicosis** (Graves' disease). This condition is characterized by:

- an enlarged thyroid gland
- increased plasma concentrations of the hormones produced by the thyroid
- the clinical features that arise from such an increase in hormone concentration (e.g. weight loss, tremor, anxiety, increased basal metabolic rate).

A significant proportion of patients show in their plasma an immunoglobulin with a stimulatory effect on mammalian thyroid epithelium.

Antibodies that **block** thyroid function bind to the **glycoprotein** component of the receptor; those that **stimulate** thyroid activity bind to the **ganglioside** portion. Other models of antibody-mediated 'switching on' of cell functions have been described, but their relevance in clinical practice has yet to be established.

DISORDERS RELATED TO THE IMMUNE SYSTEM

- Inadequate responses to antigens constitute **immune deficiency**.
- An excessive response is termed **hypersensitivity**.
- Immune deficiency leads to increased susceptibility to infections which may be life threatening.
- Primary immune deficiency is inborn, due either to a failure at some point in the ontogeny of the cells of the immune system (e.g. severe combined immune deficiency) or to a single gene defect (e.g. Wiskott–Aldrich syndrome).
- Secondary immune deficiency may be due to cytotoxic drugs, certain neoplasms and, most notably, HIV infection leading to AIDS.
- Hypersensitivity is of four main types:
  — the effects being mediated by release of histamine and leukotrienes from mast cells (I) as in asthma
  — membrane damage directly mediated by antibody and complement (II) as in certain haemolytic anaemias
  — immune complex-mediated damage (III) such as occurs in certain forms of glomerulonephritis and vasculitis
  — cell-mediated reactions (IV) such as are seen in tuberculosis and leprosy.

12 Autoimmune disease

It is fundamental that the immune system be able to distinguish between **self** and **non-self**. Not only does this protect against invasion by foreign species, but it prevents immune injury to the host's own tissues. Loss of the immune system's normal unresponsiveness (**tolerance**) to self components is known as **autoimmunity**.

Tolerance is normally induced in the perinatal period

Tolerance is normally induced during fetal development and in very early neonatal life. Introduction of potential antigens during the perinatal period, when the immune system is developing rapidly, leads to failure to respond to those antigens when the animal becomes immunologically mature. For instance, the injection of cells from one strain of mouse into newborn of another strain suppresses the ability of the recipient strain, in adult life, to reject a skin graft from the donor strain.

It is possible that exposure of immature lymphoid cells to a specific antigen might lead to the **deletion** of that particular clone and thus account for the immunological unresponsiveness in later life. Such tolerance is just as highly specific as any other aspect of immunological reactivity. If, for example, the pituitary is removed from a tree frog larva while its immune system is developing, and the excised tissue is kept alive by transplanting it into another tree frog larva, the animal from which the organ was removed will be found to regard its own pituitary as foreign after the neonatal period.

Tolerance can be induced in adult animals as well as in neonates. This can occur under two sets of circumstances which, one might have imagined, would be mutually exclusive. The first of these, known as **low zone tolerance**, is induced when repeated **low** doses of certain antigens are used. Such tolerance is induced most easily by antigens that are **weakly immunogenic**, but can occur with strongly immunogenic antigens provided that antibody synthesis is inhibited during antigen dosage by an immunosuppressive drug such as cyclophosphamide.

Tolerance can also be induced by the use of repeated **high** doses of antigen (**high zone tolerance**). The **state** of the antigen is also of some importance in experimental induction of tolerance. Proteins that are soluble, rather than in macromolecular or aggregated form, can more easily induce tolerance. Avoidance of antigen processing by macrophages before presentation to lymphocytes is also more likely to lead to tolerance of that antigen than to an immune response.

In low zone tolerance, only T cells are unresponsive; in high zone tolerance both B and T cells are involved. High zone tolerance is much more likely to maintain immunological unresponsiveness to self antigens than the low zone variety, because tolerant T cells could be bypassed by a change in one or more of the determinants in an antigen complex to which they had been made tolerant.

Another possible way of maintaining tolerance is via the operation of **suppressor T-cell activity**. Any reduction in the population of suppressor cells is associated with a tendency to form antibodies against self components. Neonatal thymectomy, which greatly reduces the population of suppressor T cells, exacerbates the autoimmune haemolytic anaemia characteristic of the New Zealand Black mouse. Similarly, the injection of thymocytes from young unaffected members of the same strain delays the appearance of the anaemia.

There are some self components to which tolerance does not normally develop but which do not elicit the formation of autoantibodies. It is possible that there is a small number of self components to which the immune system has never been exposed and to which, therefore, tolerance never develops. Such antigens are spoken of as being **secluded** and probably include lens protein and the antigens of sperm and the myocardium. Damage to tissues containing these antigens and their subsequent release elicits autoantibody formation and this may be associated with immune-mediated injury to the parent tissue.

AUTOIMMUNITY

The concept that some diseases could be autoimmune stems from three very important sets of observations:

1) recognition that certain haemolytic anaemias were associated with the presence of antibodies that were cytotoxic to the patient's red cells
2) the discovery, in 1956, that the serum of patients suffering from a disorder of the thyroid known as Hashimoto's thyroiditis contained antibodies binding to thyroglobulin and also to certain components of thyroid epithelium
3) the production of experimental thyroiditis in rabbits by injecting extracts of thyroid tissue.

Since then, autoimmunity has been invoked as the pathogenetic mechanism in a large number of diseases. It is not always easy to prove that a specific disease has an autoimmune origin. Factors suggesting that this may be the case include:

- **indirect evidence** of immunological disturbance, such as increased plasma levels of immunoglobulins
- **direct evidence** of autoimmune reactivity as shown by autoantibodies in the plasma and blast transformation in vitro of lymphocytes exposed to self antigen
- tissue changes characterized by infiltration by lymphocytes, mononuclear phagocytes and plasma cells, all of which mediate immune reactions
- clinical and serological associations with other autoimmune diseases in either the patient or his or her family
- the occurrence of a similar disease in animals that can be shown to be mediated by immune mechanisms.

Do autoantibodies change tissue function and structure?

Effector mechanisms for producing tissue damage in autoimmune disorders are essentially the same as those operating in hypersensitivity. Many autoimmune diseases are associated with either circulating autoantibody or soluble immune complexes; these can be grouped roughly into two categories: **organ specific** or **multisystem**.

Organ-specific diseases can be still further subdivided:

- those with specific lesions in target organs and where the accompanying autoantibodies are directed against specific organ components.
- those where the lesions tend to be restricted to a single organ but the autoantibodies are not organ specific and, indeed, sometimes not species specific (e.g. primary biliary cirrhosis, where the in vivo target is intrahepatic bile duct epithelium but the antibody reacts in vitro with all mitochondria); the pattern of autoantibody production in such organ-specific diseases shows a considerable degree of overlap.

Thyrotoxicosis and autoimmune haemolytic anaemia are clearly diseases that are due directly to the binding of autoantibody to a tissue target (*Table 12.1*). Another striking example of this is **myasthenia gravis**, in which muscle contraction is impaired either by blocking of the acetylcholine receptors on the voluntary muscle or by actual destruction of the receptor, which can be shown to be stripped from the membrane of the muscle cells after they have been cross-linked by autoantibodies (*Fig. 12.2*).

Some of the autoantibodies directed against acetylcholine receptors are produced by the thymus. Thymocytes obtained at thymectomy from patients suffering from myasthenia gravis produce antibodies against acetylcholine receptors when cultured, and such antibodies lead to the muscle changes of

Table 12.1 Organ-specific autoimmune disorders with autoantibodies that react only with antigens in the affected organ (*Fig. 12.1*)

Disease	Antigen
Hashimoto's thyroiditis	Thyroglobulin
Primary myxoedema	Thyroid peroxidase
Thyrotoxicosis	TSH receptors on cell surface
Addison's disease	Hydroxylases in adrenal cortical cells
Pernicious anaemia	Intrinsic factor
Insulin-dependent diabetes mellitus	Islet cell cytoplasmic antigen; insulin
Goodpasture's syndrome	Basement membranes of glomeruli and lung
Myasthenia gravis	Acetylcholine receptors on muscle
Idiopathic thrombocytopenic purpura	Platelet antigens
Pemphigus vulgaris	Desmosomes between prickle cells
Pemphigoid	Epidermal–dermal basement membrane
Autoimmune haemolytic anaemia	Red cell membrane antigens
Phacogenic uveitis	Lens
Sympathetic ophthalmia	Uveal tract antigens

myasthenia when injected into rats. The thymus contains a substance on some of its cells that resembles the acetylcholine receptor, and this substance is immunogenic in cell culture systems.

Autoantibodies in the plasma do not necessarily signify autoimmune disease. Such antibodies are found in a number of healthy people and may have no pathogenetic significance. In addition, autoantibodies may occur as a result, rather than being the cause, of tissue damage. For instance, antibodies that react with human heart muscle are often found in the serum of patients who have undergone open heart surgery.

Many autoimmune diseases exist in which there are autoantibodies in the plasma for which no pathogenic role has as yet been identified. If autoantibodies are not responsible for the tissue damage occurring in some autoimmune diseases, it is necessary to invoke some other mechanism. It seems likely that the guilty party here is either the T or the K cell. In Hashimoto's thyroiditis, where antibodies reacting with thyroglobulin and thyroid microsomes can cross the placenta, there is no evidence of damage to the thyroid in infants born to patients with this disease. In the experimental form, caused by injected thyroid extracts in complete Freund's adjuvant, the disease can be reproduced in non-immunized animals **only by the transfer of lymphoid cells** from affected animals, **not by transfer of plasma**.

Possible mechanisms for the production of autoimmunity

Loss of tolerance leading to autoimmunity could, theoretically, occur in several ways.

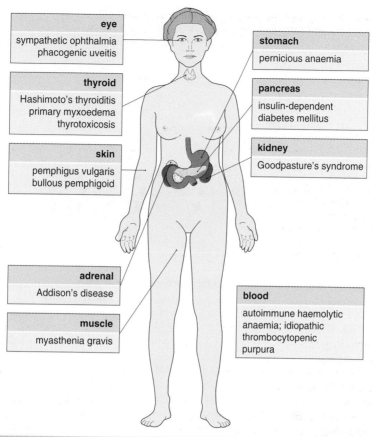

Fig. 12.1 Organ-specific autoimmune disorder with autoantibodies reacting with the affected organ.

Exposure of previously secluded antigens

The possibility that tissue components exist that normally are not encountered by the immune system, such as sperm and lens proteins, has already been mentioned. Certainly some cases of open trauma to one eye may be followed 2–3 weeks later by a severe inflammatory reaction in the other eye. This has been termed **phacogenic ophthalmitis**. Similarly, some cases of male infertility are associated with the presence of antibodies directed against sperm, which are not normally encountered by the developing immune system. At one time it was thought that this secluded antigen situation existed in relation to thyroglobulin. This is incorrect; a small amount of thyroglobulin can be found in lymph draining from the normal thyroid.

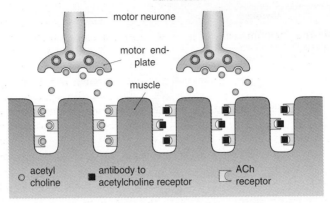

normal: acetylcholine from motor end-plate binds to receptors on muscle

myasthenia: antibodies to acetylcholine receptors block binding of ACh and thus interfere with neuromuscular transmission

motor neurone

motor end-plate

muscle

○ acetyl choline

■ antibody to acetylcholine receptor

⊏ ACh receptor

Fig. 12.2   Blocking of acetylcholine receptors in myasthenia gravis.

At the motor end-plate, acetylcholine normally binds to receptors on muscle cells. If antibodies to these receptors are present in sufficiently high titres, the binding is blocked and muscle stimulation to contract does not occur.

Alteration of self antigens so as to bypass tolerant T cells

Tolerance is due in many cases to the failure of T cells to respond to a certain antigenic determinant and thus to help appropriate B cells produce antibody. This unresponsiveness can be overcome by changes in the **carrier** molecule, accomplished either by alteration of determinants on the carrier or by addition of new ones.

In experimental conditions, extracts of unaltered tissue components do not usually elicit an autoimmune response. When such extracts are altered, either by treating them with certain chemicals or by incorporating them in Freund's adjuvant, autoantibodies are formed and tissue damage occurs. However, there is no evidence that such alteration of self antigens plays a role in spontaneous autoimmune disease, although low density lipoprotein molecules within the arterial intima which have undergone oxidative modification elicit the formation of autoantibodies. Such autoantibodies are found in many 'normal' individuals.

'Self' antigens can be altered by certain drugs and probably by some viral infections. One of the best known of the drug reactions is the autoimmune haemolytic anaemia that occurs in some patients treated with the anti-hypertensive agent α-methyldopa. In affected patients, autoantibodies are produced against the e antigen of the rhesus system, presumably as a result of changes in the red cell surface produced by the drug or one of its metabolites.

Cross-reactions in bypassing tolerance

There is no doubt that the immune system encounters certain exogenous antigens that share antigenic determinants with native tissue antigens. Normally tolerance for these determinants would be expected. In just the same way as T-cell tolerance can be overcome by a modification in the carrier molecule associated with an autoantigen, the presentation of one of these '**shared**' determinants on a totally different carrier brings normal immunological unresponsiveness for that antigen to an end.

Rheumatic fever, a multisystem inflammatory disease which affects the heart most severely, follows an infection by certain strains of **β-haemolytic streptococci**. The antibodies produced as a result of such an infection bind *inter alia* to antigenic components of heart muscle. Some patients with this disease develop a neurological syndrome characterized by abnormal, jerky, involuntary movements (**Sydenham's chorea**). Their serum contains antibodies that bind to neurones, and this binding can be inhibited by prior absorption of the serum by streptococcal cell membranes. A similar mechanism is believed to operate in the encephalitis that sometimes followed the use of rabies vaccine containing heterologous brain tissue.

Idiotype bypass

T helper cells with specificity for the idiotype on a certain B-cell receptor play a role in the stimulation of that B-cell clone. If, perhaps as a result of an infection, an antibody was formed with an idiotype that cross-reacted with the receptor of a potentially autoreactive T or B cell, then an autoimmune response might occur. Cross-reacting idiotypes have been found in certain autoimmune diseases such as rheumatoid arthritis and systemic lupus erythematosus (SLE).

Inappropriate Ia expression

Most organ-specific antigens appear on the surface of the cells as class I but not as class II major histocompatibility complex (MHC)-coded molecules. As a result they cannot communicate with T helper cells and cannot act as immunogens. It has been suggested that if class II genes could become derepressed, MHC class II-coded proteins would be synthesized and appear on the surface of cells, thus rendering them able to present antigen to T helper cells. Thyroid epithelial cells in culture can be persuaded to express Ia molecules (HLA-DR) on their surfaces after stimulation by phytohaemagglutinin, and the epithelial cells from thyroid glands of patients suffering from Graves' disease bind anti-HLA-DR antibodies, suggesting that such inappropriate expression of MHC class II proteins can take place in 'real life' as well as in cell culture systems.

Impaired regulation of T cells

B cells from normal individuals have the potential to produce autoantibodies. It has been shown, for example, that *normal lymphocytes in culture will produce immunoglobulin (Ig) M antibodies of the type* seen in rheumatoid disease when stimulated with non-specific mitogens, and normal mice will also produce autoantibodies when injected with non-specific lymphocyte activators. In these situations the autoantibodies formed combine with widely distributed antigens. These include DNA, IgG phospholipids, red blood cells and lymphocytes themselves. It has been suggested that these antibodies form a group whose production is an inherent property of the immune system.

Regulation of these potentially autoreactive B cells is probably one of the functions of the T-cell population. The normal dormancy of autoreactive B cells could be regarded as being the result either of the **action** of T suppressor cells, **lack of activity** on the part of appropriate T helper inducer cells, or both.

Certainly there is a reduction in the number of suppressor T cells in some autoimmune diseases. In one such disease, **multiple sclerosis**, clinical exacerbations and remissions parallel changes in the suppressor T-cell population. We cannot be absolutely sure, however, that the decrease in the number of suppressor T cells is responsible for the activation of autoreactive B cells. Indeed, it is possible that the reduction in the T-cell subpopulation may be caused by the autoantibody; soluble immune complexes, for example, can impair both the function of suppressor cells and the expression of their markers.

An **excess of T helper cells** has been recorded in a strain of mouse prone to develop a disorder resembling human lupus erythematosus. Such excesses have not yet been described in human autoimmune disease. However, **increased T helper cell activity** has been noted in procainamide-induced lupus erythematosus. This may be due to an inhibition of adenosine 5'-cyclic monophosphate (cAMP) formation by the drug or its metabolites. A decline in intracellular cAMP concentration stimulates helper cells.

On the other hand, α-methyldopa, which can cause autoimmune haemolysis, stimulates cAMP formation, an effect that inhibits suppressor cells. Thus autoimmunity could arise from either stimulatory or inhibitory effects on T-cell subpopulations.

Possible role for anti-idiotype antibodies

Possible mechanisms for the activation of dormant, potentially autoreactive, B lymphocytes are discussed above. These cells tend to produce autoantibodies that react with widely distributed antigens. In autoimmune states associated with the presence of highly specific autoantibodies, a normally regulated immune network seems essential. Examples include **myasthenia gravis**, in which there are antibodies directed against the insulin subunit of the acetylcholine receptor, antibodies against the insulin receptor in type I **diabetes mellitus**, and the thyroid-stimulating antibody found in primary **thyrotoxicosis**.

It has been suggested that the autoantibody binding to the acetylcholine receptor in myasthenia gravis may be an anti-idiotype antibody. An **idiotype** is a serologically identifiable configuration in the antigen-binding region of

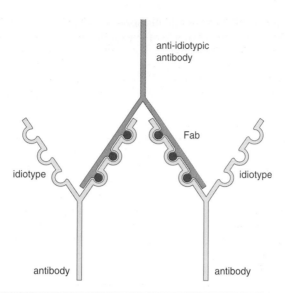

Fig. 12.3   Binding between idiotypes and an anti-idiotype antibody.

an antibody. An anti-idiotype reacts specifically with this site (*Fig. 12.3*). Binding between idiotype and anti-idiotype can be inhibited by the antigen that originally elicited the formation of the first antibody. In a similar fashion the anti-idiotype can inhibit binding between the antigen and the specific combining site on the first antibody.

In myasthenia gravis, acetylcholine plays the role of a ligand that binds both to its normal receptor and to its corresponding antibody. Thus both the receptor and the antibody must have similar ligand-binding structures. An anti-idiotype that combines with the ligand-binding structure in the variable region of the antibody can also bind to the corresponding structure in the receptor. Such an antibody has been described as 'a key that fits two similar but not identical locks'.

The validity of this view has been shown in experimental models in which the eliciting of anti-idiotype antibodies leads to a myasthenia-like syndrome.

SOME EXAMPLES OF AUTOIMMUNE DISEASE

The clinical and pathological features of autoimmune diseases encompass a wide spectrum:

- **organ-specific disease associated with organ-specific antibodies** (as seen in Hashimoto's thyroiditis)
- **disorders limited to one organ or tissue but where the antibodies are not organ specific** (such as primary biliary cirrhosis)

- **non-organ-specific or systemic diseases**, where lesions may be found in many organs and a wide range of autoantibodies may be encountered (e.g. SLE, rheumatoid arthritis).

The range of these disorders is illustrated in *Tables 12.1–12.3*. These disorders are considered in other chapters, and only one example is discussed briefly here.

SYSTEMIC LUPUS ERYTHEMATOSUS (SLE)

SLE is a multisystem autoimmune disease in which the lesions are caused by immune complex deposition, and which is characterized by a generalized excessive autoantibody production. There is a strong predilection for the disease to occur in females (female:male ratio 9:1), and Negro females in the USA are particularly at risk. An increased risk also seems to be conferred by the HLA antigens DR2, DR3 and BW15. Additional evidence of a genetic component comes from family clustering of cases and from a high degree of concordance in monozygotic twins.

Table 12.2   Organ-specific autoimmune disorders without organ-specific autoantibodies (*Fig. 12.4*)

Disease	Antigen
Primary biliary cirrhosis	Mitochondria
Chronic active hepatitis	Smooth muscle, nuclear lamins
Ulcerative colitis	A lipopolysaccharide

Table 12.3   Multisystem autoimmune disorders (*Fig 12.5*)

Disease	Antigen
Sjögren's syndrome	Single-stranded RNA (Ro), duct epithelium, mitochondria
Rheumatoid arthritis	IgG
Scleroderma	DNA topoisomerase, centromeres
SLE	Double-stranded DNA, single-stranded DNA, histones, Sm (Smith) antigen (an extractable nuclear antigen), ribonucleoprotein, Ro (another small ribonucleoprotein), cardiolipin
Discoid lupus erythematosus	Nuclear antigens
Mixed connective tissue disease	DNA
Wegener's granulomatosis	Antigen in neutrophil cytoplasm (ANCA anti-neutrophilic cytoplasmic antigen)
Dermatomyositis	Extractable nuclear antigens

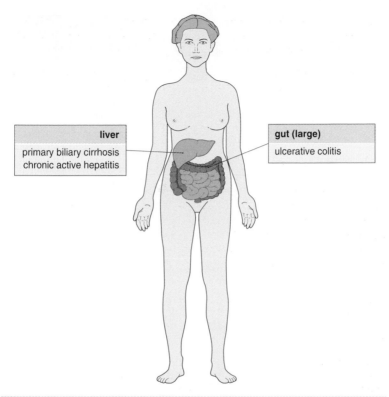

Fig. 12.4 Organ-specific autoimmune disorders with no organ-specific autoantibodies.

The tissues most frequently involved are the **skin**, where there is a highly characteristic erythematous rash in the 'butterfly area' of the face, the **joints** (with the production of a polyarthritis), and the **kidney**, where a life-threatening glomerulonephritis may occur (*Fig. 12.5*). Other tissues such as the pleura and pericardium are not infrequently involved, and increasing attention has recently been paid to the effects of the disease on the central nervous system. In about half the cases, small warty excrescences may be seen on the heart valves (Libman–Sacks endocarditis).

Two views have been put forward to explain the hyperactivity of the B cells in SLE.

1) The first of these postulates a decline in suppressor T-cell activity, thus allowing B cells an unfettered opportunity to produce large amounts of autoantibodies. Certainly a good number of patients with SLE show evidence of decreased T-cell activity, but this is by no means a universal phenomenon.

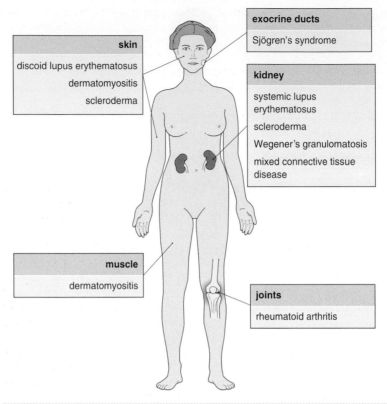

Fig. 12.5   Non-organ-specific autoimmune disorders.

2) The second suggests some direct polyclonal activation of B cells, thus bypassing the need for a non-specific signal from T helper cells. Such activation can occur when B cells are exposed to lipopolysaccharides such as bacterial endotoxins, and it has been suggested that similar lipopolysaccharides can be derived from cell membranes.

The LE cell phenomenon

In 1948, long before autoimmunity had been recognized, Hargreaves found that when blood was taken from patients with SLE, heparinized and allowed to incubate for between 40 and 60 minutes at 37°C, smears made from the buffy layer showed the presence of phagocytic cells containing large basophilic masses composed of nuclear material.

It is now known that these phagocytosed nuclear masses arise as the result of interaction between nucleated blood cells and antibodies against deoxyribonucleoprotein. Healthy cells are not damaged by this antibody, but cells damaged during the taking of blood allow entry of the antibody and consequently binding to its nuclear homospecific antigen. The damaged nucleus swells, is extruded from the cells and is then phagocytosed by a phagocyte, usually a polymorphonuclear leucocyte. There is no good evidence of significant damage being produced in vivo as the result of cytotoxic antibody, but occasionally the homologue of the nuclear material within the LE cell may be seen in the tissue in the form of amorphous masses that stain a purplish blue with haematoxylin and are found in relation to the necrotic lesions characteristic of SLE.

Animal models of SLE

Our understanding of the processes involved in SLE has been improved by the finding of a number of animal models of the disease. Three of these exist in different strains of mouse (NZB/W, BXSB and MRL/1) and one in the dog.

The hybrid strain produced by mating New Zealand Black (NZB) with New Zealand White (NZW) mice has for many years been the classical model for SLE. The NZW parent produces large amounts of antibody when immunized with DNA, but does not develop the disease, and the NZB parent is similarly free from SLE, although it tends to develop autoimmune haemolytic anaemia. Thus at least two genes must be involved in producing the greatly increased degree of susceptibility of the hybrid.

This hybrid shows a decline in suppressor T-cell activity fairly early in life. This is followed by the appearance of antinuclear antibodies and the onset of autoimmune disease. The picture is complicated by the fact that both parent strains are infected with leukaemia virus and there is similar evidence of viral infection in canine lupus and in some human patients. In the NZB/W hybrid, the predilection for females noted in humans is also present and 50% of the female mice are dead by the age of 9 months. Males, on the other hand, usually live for 14–15 months before death on this scale occurs. Early castration and treatment with sex hormones can alter this state of affairs; an ovariectomized female given androgens will survive much longer than her untreated counterpart. In other murine SLE models, sex hormones do not appear to influence the situation. The MRL/1 mouse has a recessive gene which, when homozygous, codes for a tremendous degree of lymphocyte proliferation. In the BXSB mouse, the factor that accelerates the development of the lupus syndrome appears to be associated with the Y chromosome. Thus, even in the mouse, SLE appears to be a destination that can be reached by a variety of paths, some of which may involve infection.

Drug-induced SLE

A lupus-like syndrome, although usually without significant renal involvement, has been described following administration of a number of drugs, including the antihypertensive agent hydralazine, procainamide and isoniazid. Withdrawal of the drug is usually followed by significant regression of clinical and pathological features. Antibodies reacting with double-stranded DNA are not present, antibodies to nucleoprotein (which fix complement rather poorly) being most prominent. The risk of developing drug-induced SLE appears to be associated with the HLA antigen DR4; it has been suggested that the basic defect in these patients is an inability to acetylate hydralazine or amine groups, thus leading to an accumulation of metabolites that might alter the antigenic properties of certain cell constituents as a result of covalent binding.

AUTOIMMUNE DISEASE

- **Autoimmunity** is the loss of the ability to distinguish between 'self' and 'non-self' antigens, i.e. **loss of tolerance for self**.
- There are several putative mechanisms by which tolerance is overcome.
- Autoimmunity is expressed by the presence of autoantibodies in the blood, 'blast' transformation of host lymphocytes exposed to self antigen, infiltration of affected tissue by lymphocytes, plasma cells and macrophages and, in some cases, clinical and serological associations with other autoimmune diseases.
- Autoimmune disorders may be **organ-specific** when autoantibodies react only with antigen in the affected tissue (e.g. Hashimoto's thyroiditis), or **multisystem** in which the antigen is widely distributed (e.g. DNA or nuclear antigens as seen in systemic lupus erythematosus).

13 Transplantation and the major histocompatibility complex

There are situations where prolongation and an adequate quality of life can be obtained only by replacement of a defective organ (**transplantation**). Examples include chronic renal failure due to a variety of disorders, intractable cardiac failure secondary to ischaemia or to one of the primary disorders of heart muscle, chronic respiratory failure due to widespread pulmonary fibrosis or widespread disease in the small pulmonary vessels, bone marrow failure and chronic liver failure. Transfer of a 'spare part' from one individual to another is not simple; unless the donor and the recipient are genetically identical or, at least, very similar, the graft undergoes a series of changes resulting in its destruction as a functioning entity. This sequence of events is known as **rejection**.

Like every other branch of science, transplantation has its own jargon. Thus a graft:

- taken from the patient him/herself is an **autograft**.
- where both donor and recipient are genetically identical (syngeneic), as in the case of identical twins, is an **isograft**.
- where donor and recipient are of the same species but not identical in genetic make-up (allogeneic) is an **allograft**
- where donor and recipient are *not* of the same species (xenogeneic) is a **xenograft**, e.g. monkey to human.

REJECTION

Allograft rejection can be studied easily in models where skin from one strain of mouse is grafted on to a mouse of another strain. The graft becomes normally vascularized in a few days, but shortly after this it becomes infiltrated by lymphocytes and macrophages, and the blood flow through the part begins to diminish. By 10 days or so after transplantation, the graft is necrotic and is sloughed off leaving a bare area of exposed dermis.

What is the evidence that rejection is immunological in nature?

First and second set reactions
In granuloma formation, the **second contact with the responsible antigen** (such as **schistosome ova**) **leads to an accelerated and increased tissue response**; this is a universal pattern in immune reactions. If graft rejection is mediated by immunological mechanisms, rejection of a second graft from a given donor to a given recipient should be accelerated and this is indeed the case. In the case of mouse skin, adequate vascularization of the graft may never occur and necrosis may be obvious within a few days. This very rapid rejection is known as a **second set reaction**.

Its specificity is shown by the fact that, if a graft from a donor of genetic make-up different from that of the first donor is transplanted into a previously skin-grafted mouse, a second set reaction does not occur and the graft is rejected at the same speed as the first graft (**first set reaction**).

Cell-mediated reaction
Again, as in the case of granuloma, transfer of lymphoid cells from an animal that has had an allograft to an animal that has not, results in the second animal showing accelerated rejection of a graft from the original donor animal. In animals that have been thymectomized during the neonatal period, allografts survive for prolonged periods. The ability to reject such grafts at a 'normal' speed is restored by the injection of lymphocytes from a genetically identical normal animal.

Antibody production
Humoral antibodies reacting with donor cells can be found in the blood of the recipient after rejection.

All these data indicate that **rejection is immunologically mediated**. The success of isografts between animals with an identical genetic constitution suggests that the antigens responsible for rejection are genetically determined.

THE MAJOR HISTOCOMPATIBILITY COMPLEX (*Fig. 13.1*)

The basis of rejection is the recognition by the recipient's immune system of a group of glycoprotein antigens on the surface of the donor cells known as histocompatibility antigens. In some ways, this is a misleading name

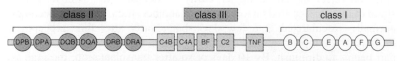

Fig. 13.1 Principal genes of the MHC on chromosome 6.

because it obscures the vital role these antigens play in regulating immune responses in general.

The major histocompatibility complex (MHC) has been studied extensively in the mouse and in humans; in the latter it is made up of a group of genes on the short arm of chromosome 6. In the mouse there are at least 20 transplantation loci, the most important being the H-2 locus. This provokes intense allograft rejections, which are difficult to suppress. The H-2 locus consists of at least three loci, two of which code for the very 'strong' transplantation antigens H-2K and H-2D. The third locus codes for H-2L.

All lymphoid cells contain large amounts of the H-2K/D antigens; liver, lung and kidneys have moderate amounts; and brain and voluntary muscle have rather little.

Antigens of this group have been termed **class I molecules** (see p. 159) and can be identified on lymphoid cells by the cytotoxicity of antibodies that react with them. The mouse histocompatibility complex, however, also codes for another group of antigens, called **class II molecules** or **Ia antigens**. These antigens are recognized by T helper cells and are thus the signals that stimulate a variety of T-cell functions. They cannot be identified by means of a panel of antibodies. However, when lymphocytes from animals that have different genes determining Ia antigens are mixed together they undergo 'blast' transformation and mitosis.

The MHC in humans and transplantation

As stated above, the MHC in humans is located on the short arm of chromosome 6. The dominant group of antigens governing rejection reactions is spoken of as the HLA system. HLA stands for **human leucocyte antigen**, as the class I molecules have been delineated through the effect of their homospecific antibodies against human leucocytes, which, of course, constitute an abundant source of nucleated cells. The combination of genes coding for transplantation antigens which is inherited from each parent is known as the **haplotype**.

Class I molecules

Class I molecules are encoded at three major loci: A, B and C. HLA-A and -B are probably homologues of the 'strong' mouse transplantation antigens H-2D and H-2K and readily induce formation of complement-fixing cytotoxic antibodies, which are used for tissue typing. These antibodies are found in the plasma of patients after blood transfusions, and in multiparous women, immunized against fetal antigens defined by paternally derived genes.

A and B gene products act as cell surface recognition markers for cytotoxic T cells. They usually present viral antigen on infected cell surfaces, thus enabling the cytotoxic T cells (CD8) to eliminate the virus by destroying infected cells. In kidney grafts, class I antigens are present on vascular endothelium, tubular epithelium and interstitial and mesangial cells.

HLA typing

HLA typing in respect of class I antigens is done by setting up an individual's lymphocytes against a panel of known antibodies in the presence of complement. Binding of antibody to its homospecific antigen on the surface of the lymphocyte leads to cell membrane damage; this is monitored by testing the cells' ability to exclude dyes such as trypan blue or eosin. A marked degree of polymorphism exists in respect of the MHC loci. There are 24 alleles for HLA-A, 42 for HLA-B and 11 for HLA-C.

Class II molecules

Class II molecules were originally defined by the HLA-D locus. This is not a single locus; it is split into DR, DQ and DP, each encoding class II molecules. There are six DP alleles, 20 DR and nine DQ. Class II antigens are expressed on the surfaces of B lymphocytes, monocytes and macrophages, and other antigen-presenting cells.

The antigens encoded by D genes are recognized by performing the **mixed lymphocyte reaction test**. In this test, lymphocytes (for example, those from a patient awaiting a renal transplant) are mixed with an equal number of lymphocytes drawn from a potential donor. The donor cells are pretreated, either by irradiation or with mitomycin, which prevents them undergoing blast formation in response to the D antigens on the surface of the recipient's lymphocytes, should these be different from the donor's. Blast transformation of the potential recipient's cells is detected by measuring the uptake of tritiated thymidine, which is greatly increased if blast transformation occurs. Unfortunately this test takes 5 days to perform and thus is of no practical use if transplantation of a cadaver kidney is being contemplated. Newer serological methods are now available, however, for the detection of D and DR antigens.

MHC complex products show a marked degree of polymorphism and it is virtually impossible, other than in the identical twin donor–recipient situation, to obtain a complete match of the MHC-encoded antigens. Nevertheless, the closer the match, the greater are the chances of long-term graft survival.

The most important factor in predicting success in transplantation is the degree of matching between the class II antigens, especially DR, of the potential donor and the recipient. When the donor is a sibling of the recipient with good HLA matching, the chance of 10-year survival in the presence of appropriate immunosuppression is now about 90%. However, if the donor and recipient are not siblings, the same degree of HLA-A and -B matching gives a success rate over a 10-year period of only 60–70%. The explanation given for this discrepancy is that, when brothers and sisters share a common heritage of HLA-A and -B antigens from one of their parents, they are likely to have inherited most or all of the genes that lie between these two loci.

Individuals who are not related may seem to be identical at their A and B loci but they may well have many genes in between that are not identical.

MECHANISMS INVOLVED IN ALLOGRAFT REJECTION

In humans, renal allografts have been most extensively studied. Here, rejection can be seen to occur at different times after transplantation; the events at these different stages probably mirror different mechanisms (*Fig. 13.2*).
   Thus rejection may be:

- hyperacute – the graft being rejected within minutes or hours
- acute – usually occurring within the first few weeks after transplantation

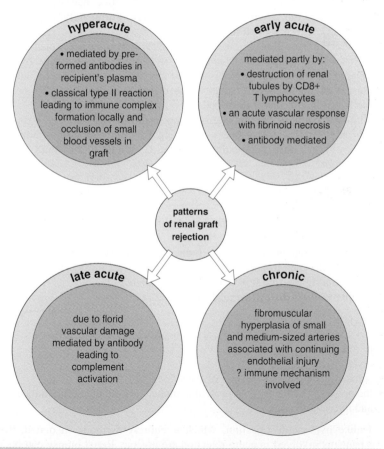

hyperacute

- mediated by pre-formed antibodies in recipient's plasma
- classical type II reaction leading to immune complex formation locally and occlusion of small blood vessels in graft

early acute

mediated partly by:
- destruction of renal tubules by CD8+ T lymphocytes
- an acute vascular response with fibrinoid necrosis
- antibody mediated

patterns of renal graft rejection

late acute

due to florid vascular damage mediated by antibody leading to complement activation

chronic

fibromuscular hyperplasia of small and medium-sized arteries associated with continuing endothelial injury
? immune mechanism involved

Fig. 13.2 Patterns of renal graft rejection.

- chronic – usually manifesting some months or even years after transplantation; it may follow several episodes of acute rejection or may appear as an insidious decline in the function of the transplanted kidney with no history of acute rejection episodes.

Hyperacute rejection

This occurs within minutes of the graft being inserted. It is characterized by small thrombi and sludged red cells in the glomeruli. *It is a classical example of a type II immunological reaction*. Preformed antibodies, present either as a result of ABO incompatibility between donor and recipient or because the recipient has formed antibodies after previous blood transfusions, bind to small vessel endothelial cells in the donor kidney and activate complement. Complement then activates platelets and the clotting system, leading to blood vessel occlusion in the graft and to ischaemic necrosis. This is irreversible and the failed graft must be removed. Fortunately, hyperacute rejection is rare (0.5% of all rejections).

Hyperacute rejection is, in morphological terms, quite spectacular. The donor kidney, instead of being pink and firm as it is perfused by the recipient's blood, becomes blue, mottled and flabby. Angiography shows occlusion of the intrarenal small vessels, and over the next day or so complete cortical necrosis develops.

Biopsy specimens shows extensive occlusion of the small vessels by fibrin and platelets, this process extending into the glomeruli. Immunohistology shows immunoglobulin (Ig)G and C3 bound to the small vessel endothelium.

Early acute rejection

This occurs 7–10 days after transplantation. The affected kidney is densely infiltrated by cytotoxic T cells.

Acute rejection is common. A kidney showing acute rejection is not necessarily doomed to fail; many patients have one or more acute rejection episodes during the first few weeks after transplantation.

Acute rejection shows several clinical features:

- oliguria
- a rise in serum creatinine concentration (which may be the only evidence of rejection)
- fever
- some swelling and tenderness of the kidney
- the presence in the urine of protein, lymphocytes, tubular epithelial cells and interleukin (IL)-2.

Unlike hyperacute rejection, which is entirely antibody mediated, the mechanisms involved in acute rejection are diverse. Renal biopsy can be a helpful guide to the pathogenesis and progress of the kidney following treatment for the rejection. Thus acute rejection can be the result of a cellular response mediated by T cells or a vascular response mediated by antibody.

Cellular response mediated via recipient T cells

The principal targets for such a reaction are the tubules and interstitial tissues. Renal biopsies show severe interstitial tissue oedema, associated with a dense mononuclear cell infiltrate. Many grafts not undergoing rejection show some interstitial cells, but the infiltrate in rejection is much more extensive and severe. The T lymphocytes and macrophages constituting the infiltrate often invade the walls of the tubules, and evidence of tubular necrosis is frequent. Immunohistological examination shows the T cells to be activated and to be producing IL-2 as well as other activation and proliferation markers.

The response is due to a reaction by the recipient's T cells to antigens present on donor vascular endothelium and on dendritic cells present in the donor kidney interstitium. There is no evidence of binding of either IgG or C3. Recognition of donor antigens by recipient T helper cells is followed by the release of lymphokines including IL-2. IL-2 is not synthesized by cytotoxic T cells and, therefore, a cytotoxic T-cell response in acute rejection depends on IL-2 synthesis by the helper cells (*Fig. 13.3*). In this connection, it is not without interest that the most effective immunosuppressive drug in common use, cyclosporin A, inhibits the synthesis of IL-2 and the expression of HLA class II antigens (see *Fig. 13.4*).

Acute vascular response mediated by antibody

The clinical and laboratory findings are, for the most part, identical with those of acute cellular rejection but an additional feature, seen in some cases, is platelet sequestration within the transplanted kidney.

Cell infiltration is concentrated on and between the vascular endothelial cells of the donor kidney. In severe cases, small blood vessels show fibrinoid necrosis extending into glomerular capillary tufts with resulting thrombosis.

IgG and IgM antibodies are often bound to the donor endothelium, as are C1q and C3 components of complement. The presence of C1q suggests classical pathway activation of the complement system.

While it is clear that an antibody-mediated reaction with subsequent complement activation occurs, it is likely that T cells are also involved (CD8 cells are found in relation to the damaged endothelium). Once there is evidence of fibrinoid necrosis and/or thrombosis in the small blood vessels and glomerular capillaries, the outlook for long-term survival of the graft is bleak.

Acute late rejection

This occurs in patients immunosuppressed with prednisolone and azathioprine. This regimen damps down the T-cell response but is not completely effective in stopping antibody production. Rejection occurs 11 days to 6

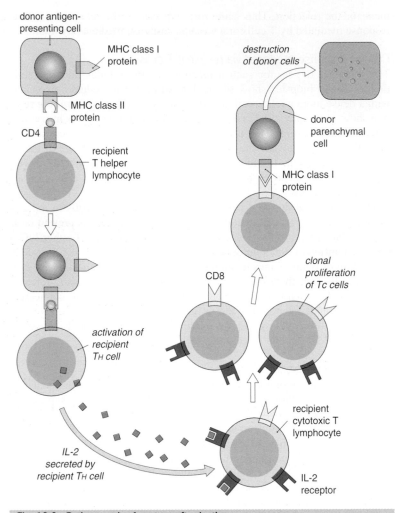

Fig. 13.3   Pathogenesis of acute graft rejection.

weeks after operation and is characterized by florid vascular damage, mediated by antibody and complement. Immunoglobulins and complement can be identified within the vessel walls.

Acute transplant glomerulopathy

About 4–10% of allogeneic kidney transplants develop a rather characteristic glomerular lesion. Clinically, the patient presents with an acute rejection episode, no different from any other. Affected glomeruli show occlusion of the capillary lumina by swollen endothelial and mononuclear inflammatory cells. Glomerular lesions are often accompanied either by tubulointerstitial rejection or, in a minority of cases, by vascular rejection. The pathogenesis is not known.

Chronic rejection

Chronic rejection causes about 8% of the renal graft rejection in the first year after transplantation and the vast majority of those rejected after this time. Because chronic rejection is basically ischaemic in nature, most of the affected patients become hypertensive.

Chronic rejection may occur years after transplantation. The most prominent histological feature is fibromuscular hyperplasia of the intimal lining of small and medium-sized renal vessels, with eventual occlusion leading to ischaemic necrosis of glomeruli. Chronic rejection is thought to be mediated via the reaction of antibodies binding to HLA antigens on the endothelium of vessels in the donor kidney. Antibody and complement may also be seen to be deposited within the glomeruli.

Arterial changes in chronic vascular rejection
The arcuate and interlobular arteries are most commonly affected. The intima is grossly thickened, the whole circumference of the vessel wall being involved. This is due partly to the presence of cells and partly to mucin-rich, connective tissue. Lipid-laden macrophages are also present.

As the lesion ages, so the amount of intimal collagen increases and the vessels become stiff and non-compliant. The pathogenesis of this arterial lesion is unclear. There is no direct evidence for the involvement of immune mechanisms but, equally, there is no doubt that the closer the match between donor and recipient in terms of histocompatibility antigens, the lower the risk of chronic vascular rejection.

Serial renal biopsies show that the intimal thickening of chronic vascular rejection is associated with mural thrombi on the endothelial surface of affected vessels. This tells us two things:

1) Chronic vascular changes are likely to be due to continuing or recurrent endothelial injury leading to thrombus formation in the affected vessels.
2) The intimal thickening itself is likely to be mediated by growth factors released from the thrombi.

Glomerular changes in chronic rejection
Glomerular damage as part of chronic rejection occurs in about 4% of all grafted kidneys. Clinically, it is expressed in the form of a moderately heavy proteinuria (> 1 g per day); the loss of protein may be so great as to lead to the nephrotic syndrome.

Renal biopsy material shows thickening of glomerular capillary walls, due in part to widening of the subendothelial region with interposition of mesangial cell cytoplasm. This results in a double-contour basement membrane similar to that of mesangiocapillary glomerulonephritis. In addition there is some increase in the mesangial matrix and mesangial cell population.

AVOIDING REJECTION

The chances of rejection may be reduced in two ways:

1) **Good matching between donor and recipient**. The perfect match would be one in which the haplotypes of both donor and recipient were identical as, for example, in the case of monozygotic twins. This situation is rare.
2) **Suppression of the immune responses of the recipient**.

Immunosuppression by drugs

Azathioprine
Azathioprine, broken down in the body to 6-mercaptopurine, is particularly helpful in inhibiting T cell-mediated rejection. It interferes with enzyme systems involved in nucleic acid synthesis and is thus most likely to affect actively replicating cells. In the first days after transplantation, the cells most likely to be undergoing clonal expansion are T cells, and the drug thus inhibits lymphocyte proliferation. However, it is by no means specific for these cells and affects other cell systems in which replication is a prominent feature.

Cyclosporin A
Cyclosporin A is a fungal product which, unlike azathioprine, has no effects on the replicating cells of the bone marrow. It selectively penetrates antigen-sensitive T cells in the G0 and G1 phase and inhibits an RNA polymerase, leading to blocking of the IL-2 production by T_H cells that is required for clonal expansion of cytotoxic T cells (*Fig. 13.4*). It is now regarded as the first-line drug in the prevention of rejection. At certain doses it is nephrotoxic and thus its blood concentration must be monitored carefully.

Tacrolimus (FK506)
Tacrolimus is another fungal product which also suppresses lymphokine production by recipient T_H cells.

Rapamycin
The fungal macrolide rapamycin differs from the previously mentioned compounds by interfering with the intracellular signalling pathways of the IL-2 receptor.

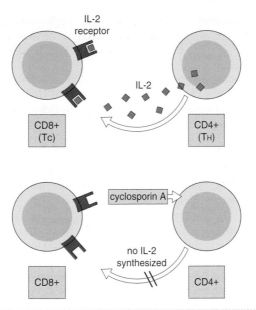

Fig. 13.4   The action of cyclosporin A in preventing graft rejection.

Biological immunosuppression

Increasing attention is being paid to the potential for **selective immuno-suppression by biological methods** that might lack the toxicity of drugs. Such approaches include the use of:

- monoclonal antibodies against T_H (anti-CD4) cells or activated T cells (anti-CD25, the IL-2 receptor)
- monoclonal antibody conjugated with a toxin, such as ricin; the complex is targeted against CD5, a molecule expressed on activated T cells
- a lymphokine complexed with toxin (e.g. diphtheria toxin); for example, IL-2 plus toxin would lock on to the IL-2 receptors on activated T cells and kill the cells.

Effects of immunosuppressive treatment

The survival of renal allografts depends, in most cases, on adequate immunosuppression. This is not without problems, which may be caused in a number of ways and have a number of effects.

Nephrotoxicity
There may be a direct nephrotoxic effect of the immunosuppressive agent.
Cyclosporin A, for example, can cause acute nephrotoxicity at high dosages. In such cases there may be vacuole formation in the cells of the proximal

tubules and hyalinization of arterioles. Chronic nephrotoxicity can also occur as a result of cyclosporin treatment. This takes the form of interstitial fibrosis and tubular atrophy. The fibrosis shows a peculiar 'striped' pattern, being focal in distribution.

The use of antilymphocyte globulin to combat rejection occasionally leads to serum sickness. This is associated with a diffuse endocapillary proliferative glomerulonephritis similar to that which can occur after streptococcal infections.

Infection
Immunosuppression must increase the risk of infection. Any variety of infectious agent may be involved. Viral inclusions may be seen, commonly as a result of cytomegalovirus infection.

Hypertension
Hypertension is quite common following renal transplant, being seen in about 50% of patients. It has been suggested that cyclosporin may contribute to this. The vasoconstriction associated with cyclosporin does not appear to be due to action by the renin–angiotensin system and is very responsive to restriction of the patient's sodium intake.

Hyperlipidaemia
Hyperlipidaemia occurs in about 60% of post-transplant patients. The hyper-lipidaemia is of the combined type, both cholesterol and triglyceride being increased. As patients have both hyperlipidaemia and high blood pressure following transplantation, it is not surprising that they show an increased risk of cardiovascular events, such events being responsible for 30% of the deaths that occur in these patients.

Post-transplant neoplasia
The concept that immunosurveillance may play a role in inhibiting the development of malignant neoplasms gains some support from the fact that post-transplant patients have an increased incidence of such tumours. In order of frequency, the tumours that complicate renal transplantation are:

1) squamous carcinoma of the skin
2) B-cell lymphomas, especially those associated with infection by the Epstein–Barr virus
3) Kaposi's sarcoma
4) cancer of the cervix uteri.

BONE MARROW TRANSPLANTATION AND GRAFT VERSUS HOST REACTIONS

Another aspect of the transplantation problem is what has been termed graft versus host (GvH) reaction. This is a major factor in bone marrow transplantation, which is used in patients with aplastic anaemia or immunological deficiencies and in those whose bone marrow has been ablated by therapy, for example for acute leukaemia.

The basis of a GvH reaction is the transfer of competent lymphoid cells from a donor to a recipient who is unable to reject them. If the donor cells survive long enough to recognize the recipient's cells as 'foreign', the former mount immunological reactions against the recipient's cells, hence the term 'graft versus host'. In mice there is inhibition of growth (so-called 'runting'), haemolytic anaemia and splenomegaly. In humans, GvH reaction is characterized by fever, weight loss, rashes, splenomegaly, anaemia and diarrhoea. Cyclosporin A reduces the frequency of GvH reaction. Recently some success has been obtained by treating the bone marrow sample that is to be transplanted with monoclonal anti-T cell antibodies so that cells capable of responding to recipient antigens are removed.

HLA RELATIONSHIPS WITH DISEASE

Why do some people get certain diseases and others not? For many years geneticists have tried to answer this question. Apart from various familial disorders for which the inheritance patterns have been worked out, some associations, although rather weak, have been noted; an example is the relationship between ABO blood groups and gastric carcinoma. In 1963 an association was noted between susceptibility to spontaneous murine leukaemia and certain antigens of the H-2 system, and in 1967 an association was described between certain HLA antigens in humans and the risk of developing Hodgkin's disease. These early reports have led to exploration of the relationships between human haplotypes and various diseases.

In considering this question it must be remembered that a number of genes not directly concerned with transplantation reactions are closely linked to the HLA complex on the short arm of chromosome 6. These include:

- the gene determining factor B (involved in the alternate pathway of complement activation)
- genes for controlling production of the second and fourth components of complement (failure to produce these proteins increases the risk of immune complex-mediated disease)
- a gene controlling production of the enzyme 21-hydroxylase
- a gene encoding the heat shock protein hsp70
- genes encoding tumour necrosis factors α and β.

The distribution of HLA genes is non-uniform on a world-wide basis

The prevalence of various HLA-determined antigens varies between populations. For instance, A30 is found in 28% of black-skinned people, in only

5% of Caucasians and not at all in Japanese people. Aw24 occurs in 58.5% of Japanese, in 18% of Caucasians and in only 6% of black-skinned people. HLA-B8 occurs in 16% of Caucasians, but in less than 0.5% of Japanese.

Linkage disequilibrium

Sometimes the alleles of two or more loci, for instance A1 and B8 or A1, B8 and DR3, occur together more frequently than would be expected if their association was only random. This is known as linkage disequilibrium.

Several explanations have been offered for this phenomenon.

1) At some point during evolution, a particular combination of alleles may have conferred some selective advantage. This, while not provable, gains a little support from the fact that the frequency of certain alleles and haplotypes differs between populations living under different environmental conditions. Thus the haplotypes showing linkage disequilibrium in European Caucasians are quite different from those occurring in West African Negros.

2) Some haplotypes have arisen relatively recently (in evolutionary terms) and there has been insufficient time for equilibration to occur by random recombination.

3) As a result of migration, some 'foreign' haplotype or gene has been introduced into a population, leading to linkage disequilibrium in the genetic pool of that population. Many generations of random breeding may be required before this effect vanishes.

Linkage and association in human disease

The appropriate distinction between linkage and association should be made in considering genetic relationships in human disease. The term **linkage**, strictly speaking, applies to a situation where gene loci are close to each other on a particular chromosome. The presence of such linkage can be recognized only by carrying out family studies on more than one generation to see whether certain characteristics are transmitted together. Not many human diseases have been shown to be linked to the HLA system in this way. Those that have been found include:

- 21-hydroxylase deficiency, which leads to congenital adrenal hyperplasia (see pp. 423–424).
- deficiencies of the second and fourth components of complement.
- some cases of haemochromatosis in which regulation of iron absorption is defective; large amounts of iron are deposited in parenchymal cells in various tissues, most notably, from the functional point of view, the liver and heart.

The term **association** refers to a relationship between two separate characteristics. This can be recognized by examining a sufficiently large number of cases of a certain disease and an equal number of controls. For example, HLA-B27 occurs more frequently in patients with ankylosing spondylitis (95%) than in a randomly selected control population (5%).

The most striking association with HLA-determined antigens is to be found in disorders in which immune mechanisms are implicated. These are the rheumatic diseases and a group of diseases characterized by chronic inflammation and abnormal immunological reactions.

Family studies in autoimmune diseases suggest a genetic influence

Two striking family studies reported in 1982 can be quoted as strong support for the operation of genetic factors in autoimmune disease. The two families between them contained 70 relatives and 23 spouses. In one family the patient originally identified had autoimmune haemolytic anaemia and hypothyroidism. Five relatives had hyperthyroidism and three others had ulcerative colitis. In the second family, the proband had autoimmune thrombocytopenia. Four of her relatives had rheumatoid arthritis, SLE, autoimmune thrombocytopenia and asthma. There was no evidence of autoimmune disease in the spouses. Other studies also show evidence of this type of familial clustering. Even more suggestive is evidence obtained from studying identical twins. The concordance of SLE in identical twins ranges from 50 to 60%. In type I diabetes, the concordance is also about 50% with respect to insulin requirement.

Ankylosing spondylitis

The most convincing of all HLA associations with disease is that between HLA-B27 and ankylosing spondylitis. It might be better here to use the term 'the spondyloarthropathies', because, although ankylosing spondylitis is the archetype, a number of other arthritides involving the spine, sacroiliac and axial joints have this association. This group of disorders includes:

- ankylosing spondylitis
- Reiter's disease
- psoriatic arthritis
- post-*Shigella*, post-*Salmonella* and post-*Yersinia* arthritis
- spondylitis associated with inflammatory bowel disease.

The B27 antigen is found in more than 90% of Caucasian patients with ankylosing spondylitis and in only 5% of Caucasian controls. Possession of the antigen confers a risk of developing the disease that is 80–90 times greater than that in the control population. Even so, individuals with the B27 gene stand a chance of only 5–20% of developing ankylosing spondylitis. 50% of first-degree relatives of spondylitics with B27 also have the antigen, and 30% of them develop either ankylosing spondylitis or some other spondyloarthropathy. The relative risks of developing one of these diseases in association with HLA-B27 are shown in *Table 13.1*.

The prevalence of B27 in different populations correlates quite well with the risk of developing the disease. B27 is virtually absent in Japan and

Table 13.1   Relative risk of HLA-B27 associated spondyloarthropathies

Disease	Relative risk
Ankylosing spondylitis	87.4
Reiter's disease	37.0
Post-*Salmonella* arthritis	29.7
Post-*Shigella* arthritis	20.7
Post-gonococcal arthritis	14.0

ankylosing spondylitis is very rare among the Japanese. Conversely, there is a tribe of native Canadians in British Columbia (the Haidas) in whom the prevalence of B27 is more than 50%. This tribe also has a very high prevalence of ankylosing spondylitis. B27 is associated with a lesser degree of increase of risk in other spondyloarthropathies (*Table 13.1*).

One problem in relation to the association between B27 and ankylosing spondylitis is the different prevalence of the disease between the sexes. Males are affected five times as frequently as females, but the distribution of B27 is the same in both sexes.

Rheumatoid arthritis

Classic rheumatoid arthritis is associated with the class II antigens Dw4 and DR4. These are present in 25% of the control population and in 45% of those with the disease. The DR4 association is strongest for patients with severe erosive changes in the articular cartilage and underlying bone, and who have rheumatoid factors in the plasma. Patients with rheumatoid arthritis treated with gold or D-penicillamine, who develop an immune complex nephritis as a result, have an association with HLA-B8 and -DR3.

A group of other diseases, in all of which immune mechanisms appear to be implicated, have associations with antigens of both the class I and class II variety.

Coeliac disease

Coeliac disease is characterized by malabsorption associated with subtotal or total atrophy of the villi in the duodenum and jejunum. Patients are sensitive to the gliadin fraction of gluten; when this is withheld from the diet, both their symptoms and the appearance of the gut mucosa improve markedly. Such patients show a strong association with HLA-B8 (this being present in 60–81% of the patients and in only 16–22% of controls). DR3 is found in 79% of the patients, and D7 in 45%.

Myasthenia gravis

Myasthenia gravis, which has already been discussed in relation to anti-idiotype antibodies, appears to exist in two forms with respect to its genetic associations. The early-onset type, associated with thymic hyperplasia, has an association with B8 and DR3. The adult-onset type, usually associated with a tumour of the thymus (thymoma), does not show any strong HLA association.

Juvenile diabetes

So-called 'juvenile' diabetes, usually early in onset and associated with a need for insulin, shows associations either for B8 and DR3 or for B15 and DR4. The presence of DR3 increases the relative risk to 3.3 and that of DR4 to 6.4. Being homozygous for either of these antigens increases the relative risk to 10 and 16 respectively, and if both DR3 and DR4 are present the relative risk rises to 33. The presence of an antigen encoded by an allelic variant of the factor B gene (BF1) is eight times more common in patients with juvenile diabetes than in the general population. It is not known whether DR3 and DR4 *per se* confer increased susceptibility to diabetes mellitus or whether they may be linked with some, as yet unknown, susceptibility gene.

Genes other than those coding for HLA antigens may show associations with certain autoimmune diseases

Correlations exist between genes specifying certain phenotypic markers of immunoglobulins and some autoimmune diseases. One of these phenotypes (Gm) is a polymorphic marker on the Fc portion of immunoglobulin. Its variants are associated with thyrotoxicosis (Graves' disease), myasthenia gravis and type I diabetes mellitus. The use of these markers, and of certain others, in association with HLA typing may greatly strengthen our recognition of a genetic component to certain diseases. For example, there is a recognized association between Graves' disease and HLA-B8/DR3. When Gm typing is added to the study of these patients, much stronger associations are found.

Possible mechanisms underlying the association with HLA type and disease susceptibility

Various explanations have been proposed for the associations between certain diseases and HLA type.

* According to the 'molecular mimicry' hypothesis, histocompatibility antigens might show partial homology with some of the determinants of certain microorganisms and this might lead to cross-reaction phenomena. For instance, cross-reactions have been shown between certain

Klebsiella pneumoniae antigens (the bacterial nitrogenase) and B27, and the urease produced by *Proteus mirabilis* and DR4.
- Certain HLA antigens might be susceptible to alterations as a result of events such as viral infection, exposure to toxins and neoplastic transformation, and this alteration might lead to a loss of tolerance of the HLA surface antigens.
- Genes, associated with the HLA complex and determining the degree of immune reactivity, are involved in HLA-associated diseases and determine the immune over-reaction that is a feature of many of the disorders.

It may be that the undoubted complexities in this area could be simplified if the genes associated with increased susceptibility to certain diseases were divided into two classes:

- those related to the regulation of the immune response
- those related to the effector arm of the immune system.

In this scheme the former would determine whether or not autoantibodies were formed, and the latter would determine the development of lesions. The two varieties of gene would be unlinked, to explain the **presence of auto-antibodies but the absence of disease** (such as may be seen in the relatives of some patients with autoimmune diseases). Only when **both classes of gene** are inherited does the disease develop.

Regulation of immune responses

An example that is cited to support this view is the frequent association between the HLA antigens B8 and DR3 and autoimmune disease. Both of these have independently been associated with abnormalities of immune regulation in individuals without any evidence of autoimmune disorder.

Lymphocytes from normal individuals who have the HLA-B8 antigen respond less well to T-cell mitogens such as phytohaemagglutinin than do the cells of those without this HLA antigen. Not all HLA-B8 subjects show this defect, which suggests that HLA-B8, by itself, may be insufficient to produce it. HLA-B8 is the commonest phenotype in the 'healthy' autoantibody-producing relatives of patients with autoimmune diseases.

Normal individuals with HLA-DR3 have lymphocytes showing some impairment of suppressor cell function when tested in vitro, and the number of immunoglobulin-secreting B cells is increased relative to that in DR3-negative persons. In vitro, possession of the DR3 allele is associated with abnormalities of phagocytosis by macrophages, and defects in Fc receptor function have been reported in normal individuals with the HLA-B8/DR3 haplotype. DR4, the allele associated with classical rheumatoid arthritis, is said to correlate with the ability of lymphocytes from normal persons to mount an immunological response in vitro when exposed to collagen.

In connection with some autoimmune disorders (SLE, primary biliary cirrhosis and type I diabetes), clinically healthy first-degree relatives show impaired function of T suppressor cells, another indication of the influence of the genetic constitution of an individual on immune regulation.

The effector arm of the immune response in autoimmune disease

The elimination of immune complexes may well be mediated by the binding of C3b to its appropriate cell surface receptor, this being followed by binding and phagocytosis of the complex. The number of these receptors for C3b is genetically determined, and is reduced both in patients suffering from SLE and in their clinically healthy first-degree relatives. Thus one might possibly view systemic lupus as a disorder characterized by a genetically determined propensity to form autoantibodies in large amounts and a genetically determined inability to eliminate the immune complexes formed as a result of the presence of autoantibodies at appropriate concentrations.

It is also not without interest that some relatives of patients with autoimmune diseases show mild changes in their tissues of a type characteristic of the disease process; for example, a moderate degree of villous atrophy of the small intestinal mucosa is found in about 10% of the asymptomatic first-degree relatives of patients with dermatitis herpetiformis.

TRANSPLANTATION AND THE MHC

- It is now technically possible to replace certain defective organs, e.g. kidney, liver, heart, bone marrow, lung and pancreas (**transplantation**).
- Most transplanted organs (grafts) come from individuals of the same species but not of identical genetic make up (**allografts**).
- Some allografts fail to function over different periods of time and show characteristic pathological features. This is known as **rejection.**
- Rejection is immunologically mediated; the chances of it occurring are affected by the degree of homology in donor and recipient of certain antigens encoded by a group of genes on chromosome 6 known as the **major histocompatibility complex** (MHC).
- Rejection occurs at different times after transplantation and shows several microscopic patterns. Both reflect the different immunological mechanisms operating.
- The combination of alleles in the MHC of an individual (the **haplotype**) may have significant implications for the risk of developing certain diseases such as insulin-dependent diabetes mellitus and ankylosing spondylitis.

14 Granulomatous inflammation

Granulomatous inflammation is a special type of chronic inflammatory reaction characterized by the local accumulation of large numbers of activated macrophages. It occurs when either a living pathogen or some foreign material (e.g. beryllium) cannot be eliminated from the host by phagocytosis and killing or digestion.

The cell biology of the macrophage dictates many of the features of this type of inflammation, which is the expression of some of the most widespread, common and serious infections. At any given moment, just three – tuberculosis, leprosy and schistosomiasis (bilharziasis) – affect more than 200 million people.

Viewed superficially there are marked differences between many of the granulomatous disorders in their tissue and clinical manifestations. Some, such as tuberculosis, may cause extensive tissue destruction if local, whereas others show only focal or more diffuse infiltration by macrophages. The common factor, however, is the macrophage with:

- its role in antigen presentation
- its reactions to T cell-derived lymphokines
- its capacity to function as both phagocyte and secretory cell.

CELL BIOLOGY OF THE MACROPHAGE

Macrophages are derived from bone marrow. A marrow precursor, the **promonocyte**, is released into the circulation as a **monocyte**. After 12–32 hours, this cell migrates into the tissues where it matures to form the **macrophage**. The term macrophage was coined by Metchnikoff in the late nineteenth century and literally means '**big eater**', a term applicable equally to its large size, its ability to engulf large particles, and its great reserve capacity for phagocytosis. Macrophages possess certain inbuilt advantages over the neutrophils in that they:

241

- have a longer natural lifespan
- can resynthesize membranes and intracellular enzymes lost during phagocytosis (which the neutrophil cannot)
- can ingest particles far larger than those that can be coped with by the neutrophil
- can undergo mitotic division.

PHAGOCYTOSIS AND ENDOCYTOSIS

The macrophage can ingest many substances; these then exist intracyto-plasmically in membrane-bound vesicles (phagosomes). Large particles are engulfed in phagocytosis. This process is triggered by close contact between the plasma membrane of the macrophage and the object to be engulfed, and this is aided by the process of **opsonization**. Like neutrophils, macrophages have surface receptors for the common opsonins immunoglobulin (Ig)G and C3b. Binding to these starts a series of membrane and intracytoplasmic events leading to pseudopod formation; these surround the target particle. Other receptors exist for activators of the alternate complement pathway and for **lectins**, proteins binding with exquisite specificity to different sugars on the cell surface.

Receptor expression can be influenced profoundly by factors external to the macrophage. Monocytes have hardly any receptors for the chemotactic C5a component of complement. However, if they are incubated in a medium containing lymphokines, expression of this receptor soon starts and eventu-ally some 40 000 receptors are found on the plasma membrane.

BACTERIAL KILLING

Just as with neutrophils, ingestion of particles by macrophages is associated with a respiratory burst and phagosome/lysosome fusion. If the ingested particle is a microorganism it may be killed, the most important mechanism being the oxygen-dependent one described earlier (see pp. 85–86). It seems likely that an additional microbicidal mechanism exists in the inducible pathway for nitric oxide (NO) synthesis.

NO is synthesized in a wide variety of cells from the amino acid L-arginine via operation of a NO synthase. In vascular endothelium, NO synthesis is constitutive (i.e. it proceeds constantly), and its synthesis and local release constitute an important mechanism for regulating vascular tone. NO can, however, be synthesized in other cells, including macrophages, via an inducible rather than a constitutive pathway. Triggering of this inducible pathway is not only important in the killing of certain pathogens but is one of the pathogenetic factors involved in septic shock.

However, for some organisms, engulfment by macrophages does not inevitably result in bacterial killing. *Mycobacteria* (including those respon-sible for tuberculosis and leprosy), *Brucella*, *Listeria*, *Salmonella*, *Toxo-plasma*, *Leishmania*, *Chlamydia*, *Rickettsia* and *Legionella pneumoniae* are among those that maintain a symbiotic relationship with the macrophage unless the latter becomes activated, usually by soluble **lymphokines** released from activated T cells, most notably interferon γ.

FATE OF MACROPHAGES IN GRANULOMATOUS INFLAMMATION

After migration to a site of infection or tissue injury a macrophage may undergo a number of possible fates (*Fig. 14.1*):

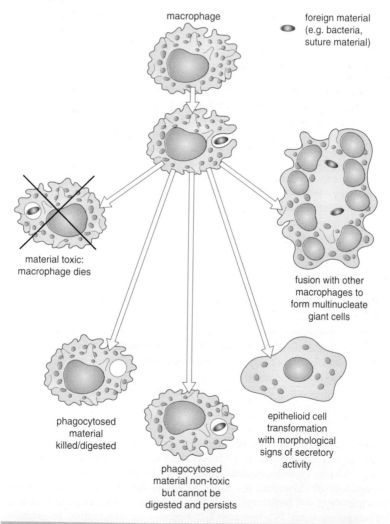

Fig. 14.1 The possible results of encounters between macrophages and foreign material (living or dead).

- The material phagocytosed may be toxic and kill the macrophage, releasing its intralysosomal contents into the surrounding extracellular milieu.
- If the inflammatory stimulus disappears, the macrophage infiltrate may resolve.
- Ingestion of non-toxic but undegradable material leads to conversion of the macrophage into a very long-lived form which persists in the tissue together with its intracytoplasmic load.
- Macrophages can undergo either conversion into so-called '**epithelioid cells**' or fusion to form multinucleate giant cells or **macrophage polykaryons**.

Epithelioid cell transformation

In many granulomas (most notably in those occurring in tuberculosis and sarcoidosis) some of the aggregated macrophages undergo a series of morphological changes which have led to them being called epithelioid cells. This is a rather inaccurate term, coined by nineteenth century pathologists who thought, wrongly, that these cells resembled squamous epithelium.

The morphological changes include elongation of the cells. They appear to be in close contact, the cell boundaries being indistinct on light microscopy. When examined with the electron microscope, the plasma membranes of adjacent cells are seen to be closely applied to one another and often interdigitate. *The epithelioid cell has much more rough endoplasmic reticulum, much more plasma membrane and a much more developed Golgi apparatus than the untransformed macrophage, features suggesting that the cell has become differentiated towards the secretory rather than the phagocytic end of the spectrum of macrophage activity.* Indeed:

- Epithelioid cells are only one-tenth as effective in phagocytosis as non-activated macrophages.
- There is less expression of surface receptors such as those for Fc and C5a.
- Phagocytosed material is seldom, if ever, seen in the cytoplasm. By differentiating in this way, the epithelioid cells appear to have lost the normal ability of the macrophage to react with extracellular particles, although they retain the ability to express HLA-DR-coded antigens on their surface receptors and thus still have the potential to interact with T lymphocytes.

Activation of human macrophages by exposure to interferon γ leads to the expression of the enzyme 1α-hydroxylase. This causes conversion of circulating 25-hydroxycholecalciferol to the active form of vitamin D, $1,25(OH)_2$ cholecalciferol. Macrophages have receptors for this metabolite, which activates them still further but tends also to shift responses in granulomatous inflammation from T_H1 towards T_H2 lymphocyte expression. In granulomatous disorders such as sarcoidosis and tuberculosis active vitamin D production may be so great as to cause hypercalcaemia.

Functions of the activated macrophage

The macrophage has a wide range of secretory products (see pp. 76–79). This, apart from its phagocytic powers, gives the cell a central role in inflammation, healing and immunity (*Fig. 14.2*), its functions encompassing:

- production of fever
- expression of mediators of acute and chronic inflammation
- microbicidal activity
- a role in the preferential selection of T_H1 or T_H2 responses
- a role in lymphocyte activation via antigen processing and presentation and interleukin 1 production
- tissue breakdown through secretion of metalloproteinases, tumour necrosis factor α and oxygen free radicals
- a role in connective tissue matrix formation and remodelling.

Multinucleate giant cell formation (macrophage polykaryons)

Persistence of any foreign material in tissues, whether living or non-living, elicits a response dominated by the macrophage in one or other of its functional and morphological forms

The simplest example of this is the presence within the dermis of unabsorbed suture material. Here, as in many other types of granulomatous inflammation, some of the infiltrating macrophages fuse to form multinucleate giant cells. Classic morphological pathology teaches us (wrongly) that there are two distinct forms of the multinucleate giant cell: the **foreign body giant cell** and the **Langhans' giant cell**. The former has its many

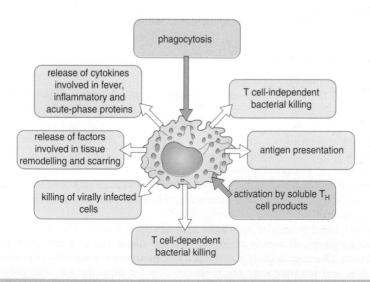

Fig. 14.2 Roles of the macrophage.

nuclei dispersed more or less evenly through the cytoplasm. It commonly appears in response to the presence of **exogenous** foreign material such as sutures or of misplaced **endogenous** material such as hair, cholesterol crystals or keratin.

The so-called Langhans' giant cell has multiple nuclei, which tend to lie peripherally in a horseshoe pattern, leaving a clear zone of cytoplasm in the cell centre. Langhans' cells are found archetypally in chronic infective granulomas such as tuberculosis. In fact the Langhans' cell merely represents a later stage in the development of the macrophage polykaryon; it has a greater content of lysosomal enzymes and a more highly developed Golgi apparatus than the foreign body giant cell. If microtubule function in the latter is interfered with by adding colchicine, transformation into the Langhans' variant is blocked.

How do multinucleate giant cells form?

In certain experimentally induced chronic inflammatory lesions, macrophage fusion forming multinucleate giant cells occurs only when the initial macrophage infiltrate is reinforced by the arrival of new macrophages. If a glass coverslip is placed in the subcutaneous tissues of a mouse, within a very short time the glass becomes covered with macrophages. If the coverslip is removed at this time and placed within a diffusion chamber into which no further cell migration can occur and the whole apparatus is returned to the subcutaneous tissue, no fusion of macrophages takes place, despite the fact that mitotic division occurs. If holes are made in such a diffusion chamber so that cells can gain access to it, macrophage fusion can be seen to occur.

An additional factor stimulating macrophage fusion, and thus giant cell formation, is the attempt by two or more cells to endocytose the same material. Once such fusion has occurred, the resulting cell can fuse with other macrophages and hence acquire the impressive number of nuclei commonly seen in some granulomas.

Role of the multinucleate giant cell

Giant cells in chronic inflammatory lesions behave like other multinucleate cells in that their nuclei enter the mitotic cycle in a near-synchronous fashion. This is likely to lead to pooling of genetic material, and some of the resulting chromosomes are defective. Polyploidy is present in some nuclei and this appears to shorten the lifespan of the cell. It has been suggested that formation of the polykaryon, with the implication that its lifespan will inevitably be shorter than that of the unfused macrophage, is one of the ways in which the multiplication of macrophages in a chronic inflammatory focus can be controlled.

It is probably unwise to accept uncritically the thesis that the multinucleate giant cell merely constitutes a stage of the macrophage's path to oblivion. One recent study compares the bone resorptive activity of mononuclear and multinucleate macrophages derived from the rat. The polykaryon variants bound and degraded significantly more bone than the mononuclear cells. This suggests that, at least in the frame of reference provided by osteoclast formation, existence in a multinucleate form confers some advantage.

CLASSIFICATION OF THE GRANULOMATOUS RESPONSE

In terms of process, the question of how to classify granulomatous reactions has been considered in two ways.

CELL KINETICS

One type of classification is based on the cell kinetics of the lesion, granulomas being classified as either **low** or **high turnover** in type.

An aggregate of macrophages whose presence has been elicited by some persistent irritant will remain until the irritant is cleared (which may, of course, be never). The cell population is maintained, firstly, by continuing migration of macrophages to the site of the irritant. If this migration is balanced by death of macrophages, either within the lesion or by emigration to draining nodes, then the lesion will remain more or less **constant in size**.

Another mechanism for maintaining the cell population within the lesion is mitotic division of the aggregated macrophages. The number of successful mitoses is usually restricted to two or three, so that in the long term this mechanism cannot be very effective.

Lastly, the macrophages that have aggregated at the site of the irritant may become immobilized and remain *in situ* for prolonged periods, with few changes in the cell number due to either death or division.

In the **low turnover** type of granuloma, aggregated macrophages remain for a long time within the lesion and there is little new migration of macrophages and little cell death or mitotic division. The irritant, which is typically non-toxic to the macrophage but poorly degradable by it (e.g. barium sulphate, carageenan), persists within the cells in relatively large amounts. Epithelioid cells are usually not present in such granulomas. The presence of lymphoid cells, which might suggest the involvement of immune mechanisms, is distinctly unusual.

In contrast, the macrophage population in the **high turnover** type of granuloma needs constant replenishment to compensate for the high death rate and the relatively short lifespan of the cells originally forming the lesion. The causative agents are usually highly toxic for the macrophages (e.g. mycobacteria, silica) and can be identified in only a small proportion of these cells. Such granulomas show evidence of functional heterogeneity within the macrophage population, and epithelioid cell transformation is a common phenomenon. Some of the most important disorders affecting humans are characterized by this high turnover type of granulomatous inflammation, amongst them tuberculosis and leprosy.

IMMUNOLOGICAL MECHANISMS IN GRANULOMA FORMATION

As most granulomas of clinical significance are of the high turnover variety, additional methods of classification would be useful in understanding the pathogenesis. Recently some writers have attempted to classify granulomas on the basis of whether or not immune mechanisms are involved in their formation.

Granulomas without evidence of immunological mechanisms

The major feature of such granulomas is the lack of specific recognition of the irritant by the immune system and, therefore, the lack of an enhanced response on a second exposure to that irritant. Thus, no matter how great the frequency of exposure, the lesions always appear at the same time after the irritant has entered the host, and the size of the lesions is the same on each occasion. It is impossible to transfer reactivity from one animal to another with either serum or cells, and immunosuppressive measures do not affect the development of the lesion.

An experimental model of this type of reaction which has been studied extensively is the granuloma that follows the injection of small plastic beads into the tissue. In vitro the beads activate Hageman factor and generate kinin activity in normal human and mouse plasma. When such beads are injected into pigeons, which lack Hageman factor, no granulomas are formed. Agents such as talc and silica, which cause granulomas of this type, are believed to operate via similar mechanisms.

Granulomas in which immunological mechanisms are involved

The fundamental difference between granulomas in which immune mechanisms play a part and those described above is that, in the former case, the **first exposure to an irritant induces an altered state of reactivity**. *This expresses itself in the form of an accelerated and more severe reaction on second and subsequent exposures to the irritant.* Formation of the granuloma can be inhibited by measures designed to suppress immunity and the altered reactivity can be transferred from animal to animal by either cells, serum or both.

Mechanisms underlying the induction of 'immunologically mediated' granulomas

Much of the basic knowledge relating to immunologically mediated granulomas has been derived from studies of the tissue reactions to infestation by the helminth *Schistosoma* (bilharzia), a parasite affecting more than 100 000 000 people. The worms themselves induce no lasting tissue response, but many of the eggs they lay do not escape from the body of the host and it is these eggs that induce granuloma formation. When eggs of *Schistosoma mansoni* are injected into the tissues of a mouse, no inflammatory response is seen for 48 hours (a fact possibly related to the presence of anti-Hageman factor activity in the eggs).

Macrophages and eosinophils start to accumulate around the eggs about 60 hours after injection; this occurs at much the same time as delayed hypersensitivity can be demonstrated in the mouse foot pad following injection of soluble schistosomal egg antigens. Priming of the mouse host by prior intraperitoneal injection of *S. mansoni* leads to faster and more severe granuloma formation. A similar enhancement of the reaction can be seen on first exposure to *Schistosoma* in mice who have received injections of spleen or lymph node cells from an animal with schistosomal granulomas (**passive transfer**).

It is possible to culture living granulomas isolated from the livers of infected mice. These studies have demonstrated the secretion of two lymphokines from the cells of the granuloma: **macrophage migration inhibiting factor** and a factor that promotes the activity of eosinophils. In addition, lysosomal enzymes and a factor that stimulates fibroblast proliferation and the synthesis of collagen can be identified in the culture fluid. Very little antibody globulin can be isolated from these lesions. These data indicate the importance of cell-mediated immunity, at least in this model, and also show that such a granuloma carries within itself the means by which both necrosis and scarring can be brought about.

Scar tissue formation in granulomas

The formation of scar tissue in and around granulomas is probably controlled largely by the secretion of cells making up the lesion. The degree of such scarring is determined by the balance between factors that stimulate fibroblasts and hence collagen formation, and those that work in a contrary way causing collagen breakdown. Both these sets of factors are governed, at least in part, by the macrophage. The macrophage can secrete substances that stimulate fibroblast division (e.g. IL-1); fibronectin and platelet-derived growth factor, which it also secretes, are also chemotactic for fibroblasts. On the other hand, macrophages can secrete enzymes that break down collagen, and fluid in which macrophages have been cultured has been described as able to inhibit collagen synthesis.

This brief general account of the nature of immunologically modulated granulomatous reactions sets the stage for consideration of some of the serious human disorders in which the development of such lesions is a dominant feature.

GRANULOMATOUS INFLAMMATION

- Granulomatous inflammation is characterized by focal aggregates of macrophages showing evidence of both functional and structural changes.
- It occurs when foreign material (living or non-living) cannot be eliminated from the tissue and is expressed in some common and serious disorders (e.g. tuberculosis, leprosy and schistosomiasis).
- Its features are dictated by the cell biology of the macrophage and the interactions between macrophages and T helper cells.
- Many changes follow the encounters between macrophages and certain antigens, the most noteworthy being a decline in the phagocytic ability of the cell and activation of its secretory properties.
- This activation follows the release of soluble products from the T helper lymphocytes, which have themselves been activated by encounters with certain antigens.

15 Some specific granulomatous disorders

Tuberculosis is a disease of great antiquity, diagnosable lesions having been found in Egyptian mummies dating back as far as 3400 BC. Its infective nature was confirmed in 1882 by the great Robert Koch who at this time put forward three essential postulates for ascribing the origin of a disease to an infective cause. **Koch's postulates** are:

1) The suspected organisms must be present in the lesions in all cases of the disease.
2) It must be possible to isolate the suspected organisms in pure culture from the lesions.
3) It must be possible to reproduce the disease by injecting or otherwise introducing the organisms into a healthy animal.

Epidemiology

In the affluent West, mortality and morbidity due to tuberculosis have decreased so sharply that it is difficult now to conceive of its dominant position as a cause of death and misery even as recently as 50 years ago. In the USA between 1900 and 1965, deaths from tuberculosis dropped from 200 per 100 000 of the population annually to 4.1 per 100 000. However, in deprived areas, the prevalence of tuberculosis remains much as it was half a century ago, and it has been estimated that three to five million people world-wide die each year from this disease.

Unfortunately tuberculosis is showing signs of resurgence in the West, largely because of the emergence of multidrug-resistant strains of the responsible organism. In addition, the appearance of **acquired immune deficiency syndrome** (**AIDS**) has greatly increased the toll exacted by tuberculosis in economically underprivileged populations. In some parts of

Africa almost 40% of deaths in individuals suffering from AIDS are due to tuberculosis.

The decline in tuberculosis in the West is due as much to socio-economic factors as to medical advances. They include:

- improved housing with less overcrowding
- improved nutrition
- improved sanitation
- effective chemotherapy for sufferers of the disease
- early detection by mass miniature radiography and hence early treatment
- pasteurization of milk and tuberculin testing of dairy cattle leading to the virtual elimination of primary intestinal tuberculosis.

Those members of the population at highest risk include:

- uncontrolled **diabetics**
- patients on **immunosuppressive treatment**
- individuals suffering from **AIDS**
- patients with **silicosis**
- in Britain, Asian immigrants, who are many times more likely to develop the disease than indigenous Britons.

The organism and its identification

Tuberculosis is caused by *Mycobacterium tuberculosis*, a slender, slightly curved, rod-shaped organism which is difficult to stain. Once stained, it has the remarkable property of resisting decolourization by acid and alcohol. This '**acid fastness**' is related to the presence of large amounts of complex lipid substances (neutral fats, phosphatides and various long-chain fatty acids) in the capsule of the bacillus.

The organism is most commonly stained by the **Ziehl–Neelsen** method (hot carbolfuchsin with methylene blue or malachite green). The organisms stain red with the carbolfuchsin and this red colour is *not* removed by treatment with acid and alcohol. Mycobacteria may also be stained with auramine which fluoresces yellow in ultraviolet light; it is often easier to identify mycobacteria in material treated in this way than by conventional light microscopy.

Mycobacteria are aerobic and grow slowly in culture. The media used are the egg-based Lowenstein–Jensen medium and the agar-based Middlebrook 7H10 and 7H11. A positive culture is regarded as the 'gold standard' for the diagnosis of tuberculosis. More than 85% of the confirmed cases of tuberculosis in the USA are culture positive. The major disadvantage of culture methods for diagnosing tuberculosis is that the organisms grow slowly and colonies may not be visible for 4 weeks or more.

The sensitivity and specificity of direct examination of smeared material are much lower and are influenced by the amount of time and trouble put into doing the test and the population from which the samples derive. Sensitivity ranges from 22 to 80% (mean approximately 55%).

Recently molecular probes for mycobacterial DNA have been used in diagnosis. With chemical amplification of small amounts of DNA present in samples, the time taken to make a diagnosis can be reduced to a few hours; both sensitivity and specificity are greater than with conventional staining techniques. A positive result with DNA probing in an individal with a positive smear test result gives a positive predictive value of close to 100% for culture. The combination of negative smear and negative probe results indicates that, in 94% of cases, mycobacteria will *not* be identified on culture of clinical samples.

How does infection occur?

Mycobacteria are very resistant to drying; this means that infection can follow inhalation of dust in which infected dried sputum is present. At least five strains of the organisms exist:

1) human
2) bovine
3) murine
4) avian
5) reptilian.

In humans the infection may be acquired in three ways:

1) inhalation
2) ingestion
3) inoculation.

In communities where dairy herds are free from mycobacterial infection, only the first of these is at all common or important.

Pathogenesis

The lesions of tuberculosis are the result of the interaction between the organisms and the host's immune system. Unlike organisms such as *Clostridium perfringens* or *Staphylococcus aureus*, which produce toxins that directly damage the tissues, the mycobacterium has not yet been shown to have any direct cytotoxic effect. Indeed, it survives and multiplies within macrophages in cell culture without any harm to the cultured cells.

The tissue damage effects of tuberculosis are largely, if not entirely, mediated by the **specific altered reactivity of the immune system**, following introduction of mycobacteria into the host. This altered state of reactivity expresses itself in two ways:

- by enhanced resistance to infection and more effective **clearing** of the mycobacteria from the tissues of the host
- by the appearance of **hypersensitivity** through which tissue damage is caused, the likely mechanisms being locally released cytokines and direct action of cytotoxic T cells (*Fig. 15.1*).

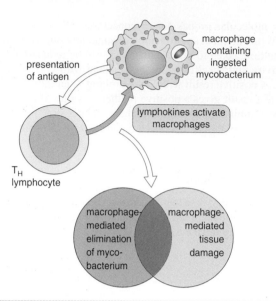

Fig. 15.1   The pathogenesis of tuberculosis.

Mycobacterial antigens are presented to T_H lymphocytes by antigen-presenting cells which have ingested the organisms. The subsequent release of lymphokines activates the macrophages to eliminate the bacteria from the host tissues and to cause some degree of tissue damage. The relative severity of these two macrophage responses determines the outcome of the infection in each case.

While it is true that *M. tuberculosis* does not synthesize or secrete exotoxins, it is clear that different strains exhibit differences in their ability to cause extensive disease. This increased 'virulence' is associated with the presence in the organisms of certain **components that protect the organisms from intracellular killing**:

- **'cord' factor**, a surface glycolipid (trehalose-6-6'-dimycolate) which, when present, causes the bacteria to grow in 'cords' in media; it is associated with the ability to induce granuloma formation and it inhibits neutrophil chemotaxis
- **sulphatides**, also surface glycolipids which inhibit fusion between phagosomes and lysosomes within macrophages that have ingested the organisms; this is likely to decrease antigen processing
- **lipoarabinomannan**, a lipopolysaccharide resembling endotoxin; it inhibits the upregulation of macrophage killing power by interferon γ, increases output of tumour necrosis factor (TNF) α, associated with fever, weight loss and tissue destruction, and increases interleukin (IL) 10 secretion, which inhibits mycobacteria-induced T-cell proliferation.

TUBERCULOUS GRANULOMAS

The essential lesion of tuberculosis is the tuberculous granuloma. The granuloma, or follicle as it is sometimes called, is the archetypal response of all tissues to *M. tuberculosis*. The extensive tissue destruction that can occur in this disease depends on the number of such granulomas, their growth and confluence, the degree of the characteristic **caseation necrosis** that occurs, and the attempts at repair which the long-continued presence of the lesions ultimately stimulates.

Evolution of a tuberculous granuloma (*Fig. 15.2*)

Following the entry of bacilli into the tissues, there is a very mild, transient, acute inflammatory reaction. The organisms are engulfed by local macro-

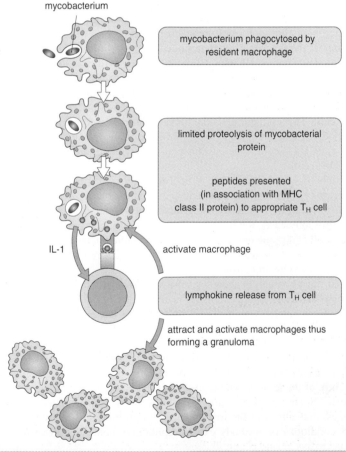

Fig. 15.2 **Genesis of an immune-mediated granuloma.**

phages and, in association with major histocompatibility complex (MHC) class II-coded membrane proteins, mycobacterial antigens are presented to appropriate T helper (T_H) cells. Interaction between these two groups of cells leads to proliferation of specifically coded T cells and to lymphokine release from them. This is followed by infiltration by macrophages, which group together to form focal accumulations and then become immobilized at the site of infection.

The whole process is subtly modulated by the immune system. One lymphokine is **chemotactic** for the macrophages, while another migration-inhibition factor (MIF) renders them relatively **immobile**. The fact that, in an **unprimed host**, bacillus-bearing macrophages travel from the site of infection in the tissue to the draining lymph nodes suggests that the full action of MIF takes some time to express itself *in vivo*. In addition, the stimulated T cells secrete **interferon γ**, which increases the expression of MHC class II-coded proteins on the macrophage membrane; thus it can increase the ability of local macrophages to present antigen and upregulate the microbicidal properties of the macrophage.

Many of the macrophages then undergo **epithelioid cell** transformation. This, as described in Chapter 14, is associated with loss of the ability to phagocytose foreign particles. Some of the macrophages fuse, with the formation of multinucleate giant cells which mature and acquire the characteristic 'horseshoe' arrangement of nuclei found in the Langhans' giant cell. The epithelioid cells become surrounded by a mantle of T lymphocytes. In granulomas the lymphocytes in the lesion centres are likely to be T_H (CD4+) cells, whereas those at the periphery are more likely to be T_C (CD8+) cells.

Within 10–14 days, evidence of necrosis begins to appear in the centre of the lesion. The necrosis is coagulative and is characterized by the appearance of firm, allegedly cheesy, material (hence the name caseation necrosis). On microscopy caseation necrosis shows virtually complete obliteration of normal cell and tissue outlines, all the tissue elements being merged into an amorphous mass of material which appears bright red in sections stained with haematoxylin and eosin.

What causes caseation necrosis is not well understood. Presumably one of the important effector mechanisms is release of lysosomal enzymes from dying macrophages, which disappear from the lesion centres as necrosis develops. Some believe that caseation necrosis is the structural expression of a marked degree of delayed hypersensitivity, although evidence gained from experimental mycobacterial infections in rats suggests that humoral factors also play a part. It is suggested that local formation of immune complexes in the centre of the lesions, where antigen is in excess, modulate the degree of necrosis. Such complexes are said to form if cell-mediated immunity declines, thus allowing the mycobacteria to proliferate. If complexes form under conditions of antibody excess, epithelioid cell transformation rather than necrosis tends to occur.

The type of T_H cell response probably plays an important part in determining whether extensive necrosis occurs or not. This is discussed in a later section (see pp. 259–260).

The sum of all these events constitutes the basic tissue response in tuberculosis.

Natural history of the tissue response

Different tissues and different individuals react very differently to the presence of *M. tuberculosis*. Some lesions are small and heal readily; some may cause extensive local tissue destruction; and others may release organisms that can spread throughout the body. These differences are probably accounted for by interactions between:

- the virulence of the organisms
- the size of the dose of mycobacteria
- the degree of local and general resistance, which may be innate or acquired
- the type and degree of hypersensitivity which, as already stated, may correlate with the type of T_H cell response.

Some of these factors are discussed below.

Innate immunity
This is difficult to disentangle from factors related to exposure to the organism and to unfavourable socio-economic circumstances. Certain groups are inherently more susceptible to tuberculosis, notably North American Indians and the Negro races.

Experimentally, where conditions are much easier to control, strains of certain species of animal can be bred that differ markedly in their degree of resistance to infection by *M. tuberculosis*.

Age
In communities where tuberculosis is very prevalent, the very young (under 5 years) and the elderly appear to be more at risk for developing overt tuberculosis. In the UK, the increased risk in young children appears to have been eliminated. Those at greatest risk are socially and economically deprived middle-aged and elderly men, many of whom are poorly nourished and unsatisfactorily housed.

Immunosuppression
Immunosuppression associated either with certain disorders (such as AIDS) or with certain treatments (such as prolonged administration of high doses of corticosteroids) increases the risk of tuberculosis.

Effects of previous exposure to mycobacteria
Previous exposure to mycobacteria is one of the most important factors in modulating the natural history of a tuberculous infection. A second infection

produces tissue reactions differing markedly from those of primary infection. Robert Koch's exploration of this in the guinea-pig has a significant bearing, not only on the natural history of tuberculosis, but also on the evolution of the basic pathological unit – the tuberculous granuloma.

The Koch phenomenon

If *M. tuberculosis* is injected subcutaneously into a guinea-pig not previously exposed to the organism, no reaction is seen at the injection site for the first 10–14 days. Then a nodule develops; if this is excised and examined microscopically, tuberculous granulomas are seen. Meanwhile mycobacteria have been transported by macrophages to the regional draining nodes and in due time produce caseous lesions within them. In time, infected macrophages escape from the nodes and the animals usually die from disseminated disease.

If the size of the initial dose was such that the animal survived at least 4 weeks and a second subcutaneous injection of *M. tuberculosis* is given at that time and at a different site, a nodule forms rapidly (within a few days), ulcerates and then heals. *No regional lymph node involvement occurs.*

These observations indicate that:

- The local tissue response to the second infection is much more rapid than that to the first.
- Local clearance of organisms by activated macrophages following a second infection is much more effective than after a first infection since the inflammatory process resolves quite rapidly.
- Macrophages containing viable organisms are immobilized at the site of the local infection: there is no evidence of spread to the draining lymph nodes in the second infection.
- Local hypersensitivity is increased after a second infection; rapid central necrosis leading to ulceration may occur.

These events have been interpreted as being due to the development of altered reactivity on the part of the host immune system. This leads to an increased ability to clear the infecting organisms from the tissue and thus to an enhanced resistance to the infection (immunity). There is also an increased tendency for tissue damage, probably also mediated by immune mechanisms, to occur (hypersensitivity). However, in the light of the failure of certain large-scale trials of the efficacy of vaccination using attenuated strains of *M. tuberculosis*, some workers have challenged this view of the Koch phenomenon.

Favourable aspects of the altered reactivity of the immune system

The altered reactivity occurring after infection with *M. tuberculosis* is largely, but not entirely, expressed in the form of cell-mediated reactions (delayed hypersensitivity). T_H cells with appropriate receptors encounter bacterial antigens expressed on the surface of macrophages or other antigen-presenting cells and proliferate. T_H cells release lymphokines (see pp. 260–261), including factors chemotactic to the macrophage and factors that tend to immobilize them at the site of bacterial lodgement (MIF). The macrophages become better able to kill intracellular organisms, and the symbiotic relationship that can exist between mycobacteria and virgin macrophages is largely ended. This aspect of the altered immune state is obviously favourable for the survival of the infected host, although the enhanced resistance to the mycobacteria is not nearly as effective as that seen, for example, after smallpox or diphtheria.

Hypersensitivity to components of the mycobacterium

Most agree that the chief factor modulating the degree of tissue destruction in tuberculosis is hypersensitivity to some antigenic components of the bacillus. In addition to its role in causing caseation necrosis, hypersensitivity is probably also associated with the very severe constitutional effects that accompany the lodgement of large numbers of the bacillus. It is most likely that these effects are mediated by release of large quantities of **TNF-α**. The liquefactive necrosis that tends to occur when there is active local proliferation of mycobacteria may be associated with the same phenomenon.

Such liquefied tissue debris usually contains very large numbers of mycobacteria and tends to rupture into adjacent tissue planes or into bronchi, lymphatics and blood vessels. Sometimes the debris tracks down through a tissue plane and may present as a soft mass at a point some distance away. Such a lesion is called a '**cold abscess**' because it consists of a localized mass of what looks like pus but lacks the heat and redness normally associated with abscess formation.

Relationship between immunity and hypersensitivity

The relationship in tuberculosis between enhanced resistance to infection and tissue-damaging hypersensitivity is one of the most difficult questions to answer satisfactorily. *Is the difference between these two expressions of altered reactivity (allergy) merely a quantitative one or is the 'protective face' of altered reactivity distinct from the 'tissue-damaging' hypersensitivity?* At present there is no definite answer but there is evidence that the latter is correct.

- The degree of **protection** produced by vaccination with an attenuated strain of the organism (bacille Calmette–Guérin (BCG) vaccination) is not related to the degree of **hypersensitivity** produced. For example, an immunized guinea-pig reacting to a skin dose of tuberculin (mycobacterial protein) at a titre of 1/10 000 is likely to survive an intramuscular challenge with live mycobacteria for about 99 days, whereas one reacting to tuberculin at a titre of only 1/10 is likely to survive a subsequent challenge for 250 days.
- It is possible to protect against live bacilli by injecting a guinea-pig with bacilli extracted using methyl alcohol, without hypersensitivity developing.

- Hypersensitivity can be induced without any protection against live bacilli being conferred at the same time, by injecting mycobacterial protein together with some of the bacillary lipids.

In both mice and humans, two types of response can follow exposure to mycobacteria. In the first of these responses, the injection of tuberculo-protein is followed by a fairly rapid reaction which peaks at 48 hours, resolves rapidly, itches but is not painful, and is often seen in recipients of BCG vaccine in the UK. The other response develops a little more slowly, peaks at 72–96 hours, lasts for 2–3 weeks, often shows evidence of necrosis and is often seen in those with a history of previous tuberculosis. The first is believed to be associated with a higher degree of resistance to infection, the second with a greater degree of hypersensitivity. Individuals may develop one or other of these responses because of previous exposure to mycobacteria other than the major pathogens *M. tuberculosis* and *M. leprae*. There are some 30 species of mycobacteria. The two major pathogens are usually encountered only following contact with patients who have open tuberculosis or leprosy. Many of the other species may be encountered frequently in the environment. It has been suggested that when there has been a 'moderate' exposure to such more or less harmless mycobacteria via the oral route, the first type of skin response is likely to develop. Where there has been 'excessive' exposure to these mycobacterial species a high degree of hypersensitivity is found and BCG vaccination confers little protection.

KEY POINTS: CASEATION NECROSIS

The balance between cell-mediated immunity (as manifested by an enhanced ability to clear mycobacteria from host tissues) and the tissue damage related to hypersensitivity determines the natural history of tuberculous infections. The tissue damaging component is the major contributor to the clinical expressions of tuberculosis.

The effect of TNF-α differs depending on whether infection causes a pure T_H1 response or a mixed T_H1 and T_H2 response

In animal models of tuberculosis, necrosis of granulomatous lesions is accompanied by the release of large amounts of TNF-α. Similarly, direct injection of TNF-α into tuberculous granulomas also causes necrosis. At the same time, secretion by macrophages of TNF-α is a vital component in defence against *M. tuberculosis*, shown by the fact that mice in whom the gene encoding TNF-α has been 'knocked out' in the embryo show greatly increased suceptibility for tuberculosis.

Thus TNF-α has a double role and can be either helpful or harmful in the context of tuberculosis. The factor determining which of these operates in a given case appears to be the type and degree of priming of the host by

Table 15.1 Secretion patterns of T_H1 and T_H2 lymphocytes

T_H1	T_H2
Interferon γ	IL-3
IL-2	Met-encephalin
TNF-α	IL-4
TNF-β	IL-5
Granulocyte–macrophage colony-stimulating factor	IL-6
IL-3	IL-10

mycobacteria, and, in particular, what type of TH cell response occurs in the course of such priming. Two types of T_H cells exist: T_H1 and T_H2; their secretion patterns are shown in *Table 15.1*.

A **pure T_H1 response** is characterized by increased resistance to *M. tuberculosis*. A **mixed T_H1 and T_H2 response**, in which a much broader range of cytokines is expressed, is characterized by extensive necrosis occurring in tuberculous granulomas.

PATTERNS OF TUBERCULOSIS

First infection-type pulmonary tuberculosis (childhood tuberculosis)

Lodgement of *M. tuberculosis* in a child's lung is usually followed by the development of a small lesion, often measuring not more than 1 cm along its longest axis. This lesion, known as the **Ghon focus**, is almost always situated just beneath the pleura, either in the basal segment of the upper lobe of the lung or in the apical segment of the lower lobe. As might be expected in a primary infection, macrophages laden with organisms travel to the draining hilar lymph nodes and, as in the guinea-pig, these nodes become enlarged and show caseation necrosis. It is characteristic of childhood infection that, irrespective of the lodgement site of the organisms, there is a relatively inconspicuous local tissue response which tends to be overshadowed by involvement of the draining lymph nodes. The combination of this inconspicuous parenchymal lesion and the prominent lymphadenopathy is known as the **primary complex** or **Ghon complex** (*Fig. 15.3*).

Natural history of the primary complex

Healing. Most lesions, in both the lung parenchyma and hilar nodes, will heal. This may be brought about by one of the following:

- complete replacement of any areas of caseation necrosis by fibrous tissue
- more often, by the local walling off of the necrotic area by scar tissue followed by deposition of calcium salts in the caseous material (**dystrophic calcification**); organisms may survive in these calcified foci

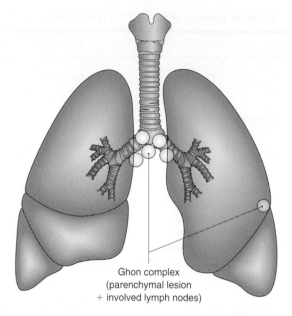

Ghon complex
(parenchymal lesion
+ involved lymph nodes)

Fig. 15.3　Primary infection with *Mycobacterium tuberculosis*.

and, even years later, if immune regulatory mechanisms become less efficient may start to proliferate.

Exudative responses. High-grade hypersensitivity following infection causes a severe exudative response, characterized by outpouring of fibrin-rich exudate containing scanty epithelioid and giant cells. This type of reaction may also manifest as a large pleural effusion with massive accumulation of serous fluid with a scanty cell population; the number of organisms that can be isolated is very small.

Spread. If the primary reaction is dominated by caseation and softening of the necrotic material, then spread via the bronchi or bloodstream (**haematogenous spread**) may occur. This is most frequent in relation to softening of the caseous lymph node component of the primary complex. Organisms may reach the blood either by direct involvement of small blood vessels or via thoracic duct lymph.

Miliary tuberculosis. If many organisms are released into the circulation and host resistance is low, the systemic spread of the mycobacteria is expressed by the development of very large numbers of small granulomatous lesions. These are more or less equal in size and stud the **lungs**, **kidneys**, **spleen**, **brain**, **meninges**, **adrenals** and, to a lesser extent, the liver. The rather distressing habit of pathologists of an earlier day to describe lesions in terms of food led to these lesions being compared with millet seeds, hence the term miliary tuberculosis.

Classically miliary tuberculosis was associated with childhood infection, but it is far from uncommon in the elderly receiving immunosuppressive therapy and in patients suffering from AIDS. These patients show both diminished resistance to the infection and diminished hypersensitivity, the latter in the form of negative skin reactions to intradermal injections of tuberculoprotein. Bone marrow or liver biopsy may be useful diagnostic procedures in such cases, as lesions are so widespread that the chances of obtaining a positive result on biopsy are quite high.

'Organ' tuberculosis.   If the dose of mycobacteria reaching the bloodstream is small, disseminated organisms may cause lesions in only one organ or tissue; the clinical picture will be determined by the site of such lesions. For example, a patient with tuberculous granulomas in the brain may present with the clinical features of a space-occupying lesion. Many tissues can be involved in this way, some of the most commonly affected being the **kidneys**, **adrenals**, **fallopian tubes**, **bones**, **joints** and **tendon sheaths**.

Adult-type pulmonary tuberculosis

In adult pulmonary tuberculosis the parenchymal lesions usually start in the subapical region of the upper lobe, where they are known as **Assmann foci** (*Fig. 15.4*). Apart from the possibly irrelevant fact that the bacilli are

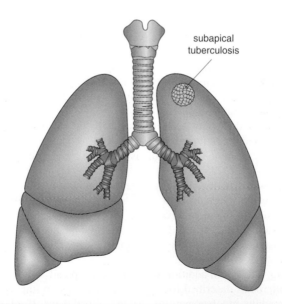

subapical
tuberculosis

Fig. 15.4   The typical 'adult' or secondary type of infection in the lung.

This is usually expressed in the form of a subapical lesion associated with much tissue destruction.

obligate aerobes and that the ventilation in this part of the lung is said to be greater than in other segments, the reason for this localization is not known. The prominent lymph node involvement seen in primary infections is not present, although microscopic lesions may be seen.

The origin of adult-type infections is still poorly understood and controversial. The lesions might arise from:

- a primary infection which, for unknown reasons, has elicited a tissue response differing from that seen in childhood
- a second infection in someone previously exposed to *M. tuberculosis* and who has, as a result, developed some degree of both immunity and hypersensitivity
- reactivation of a previous infection owing to a decline in the efficiency of cell-mediated immunity as a result of malnutrition, overindulgence in alcohol, immunosuppression, etc.

Natural history of adult-type pulmonary tuberculosis

Healing.   As with childhood lung lesions, if the host has a high degree of immunity the lesions may heal with some scarring and calcification. Appropriate antimicrobial therapy reduces the amount of scar tissue formed and if there has been cavitation (see below) the end-result may be a smooth-walled cavity with very little peripheral fibrosis.

Softening and cavitation.   Softening of caseous material may occur; if this is associated with erosion into a bronchus, a **cavity** develops. Apart from the resulting destruction of lung tissue, cavitation is an extremely unfavourable development. Direct communication of lesions with major airways increases oxygen tension and thus favours multiplication of the aerobic bacilli. The patient coughs up infected material and thus is a danger to his/her contacts. Also, a natural pathway is created for spread within the patient's own lung via the bronchial tree.

Blood vessels in the cavity walls are frequently involved in the inflammatory process. Sometimes they become blocked by small thrombi but not infrequently they become eroded; this is followed by bleeding, which may be massive.

Caseating lesions within the lung parenchyma may involve the **pleura**, leading to a **serous effusion** or a persistent **fibrinous exudate**: this may cause obliteration of the pleural cavity by the processes of organization and repair. Occasionally the affected pleural cavity contains abundant, partly liquefied, caseous material; this situation is known as a **tuberculous empyema**.

Spread (Fig. 15.5).   In addition to bloodstream spread, which can follow the same patterns as described for childhood infection, an important aspect of spread in adults involves natural anatomical pathways. If a bronchus is eroded, spread of infected material may occur by inhalation, with distal extension of the inflammatory process within the lung. This usually leads to a patchy tuberculous bronchopneumonia, but if the number of bacilli is very

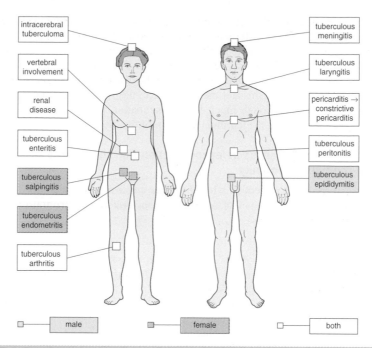

Fig. 15.5   The patterns of organ involvement seen in tuberculous infections that spread.

large and there is high-grade local tissue hypersensitivity, a massive degree of caseation may occur involving several segments of lung tissue or even a whole lobe.

Spread of infected caseous material can also occur proximally with involvement of the larynx. The patient may swallow some of the infected material and tuberculous involvement of the bowel may follow.

LEPROSY

Leprosy is a chronic infectious disease of humans caused by **Mycobacterium leprae**. It affects principally the skin, the nasal mucosa, the peripheral nerves and the testes, the organisms having a predilection for tissues that are relatively cool.

The organism is similar morphologically to other mycobacteria, but is more easily decolourized by acid than *M. tuberculosis*. Thus a modified Ziehl–Neelsen method is used to take account of this (the Wade–Fite stain). Unlike *M. tuberculosis*, *M. leprae* is an obligate intracellular parasite and cannot be cultured in any known medium. However, it does survive and proliferate in the footpad of the mouse and in the nine-banded armadillo.

Leprosy is rare in Western communities but it is estimated that there are more than 11 million sufferers world-wide, 60% of these in Asia. In India alone there are 3.5 million lepers.

Transmission occurs from person to person. The infectivity rate is low, only 5–10% of contacts actually developing the disease. The period between exposure to the organisms and the first appearance of tuberculoid lesions is about 3–6 years, although much longer incubation periods (10–20 years) have been reported in the lepromatous form of the disease.

Local tissue responses in leprosy depend on the degree of cell-mediated immunity

Tissue responses to infection with *M. leprae* cover a wide spectrum. At the two extremes are the types of response characterized as **lepromatous** and **tuberculoid** leprosy.

Lepromatous leprosy
In this form there are widespread lesions in the **skin and mucous membrane**. The lesions consist of poorly organized infiltrates comprising very large numbers of macrophages, which look foamy, and smaller numbers of lymphocytes, plasma cells and mast cells. In appropriately stained sections, acid- and alcohol-fast bacilli can be seen in enormous numbers within the macrophages, being arranged either in compact masses or in bundles, somewhat similar to cigarettes in a pack. Ultrastructural studies also show organisms within Schwann cells ensheathing cutaneous nerves. One gram of tissue from a lepromatous area may contain as many as 10^7 bacilli.

Tuberculoid leprosy
Here lesions are far scantier and involvement of peripheral nerves is quite common. On histological examination, in contrast to the lepromatous form, there are tightly packed and well-organized macrophage granulomas without caseation. Lymphocytes are numerous, the macrophages have often undergone epithelioid cell transformation, and occasional multinucleate giant cells may be seen. Mycobacteria are extremely difficult to find in these lesions; it may be impossible to see any on light microscopic examination, although electron microscopy may reveal some bacterial remnants.

Intermediate forms
A large number of intermediate forms of tissue response exist. The more closely they resemble the lepromatous type, the more bacilli can be identified in sections; the more closely they resemble the tuberculoid type, the smaller the number of bacilli found.

Lepromatous and tuberculoid leprosy represent two extremes of the cell-mediated response

In tuberculoid leprosy, the type of lesion and the presence of demonstrable cutaneous hypersensitivity to antigen extracted from leprous tissue suggests that some cell-mediated immunity is present which is not sufficient to eliminate all the mycobacteria. In lepromatous leprosy, the absence of well-formed epithelioid cell granulomas, the absence of skin hypersensitivity, and the absence of effective microbicidal function on the part of the infiltrating macrophages all suggest the opposite: poor or absent cell-mediated immunity.

This impression is strengthened by the observation that lymphocytes from patients with lepromatous leprosy fail to respond by undergoing blast transformation in the presence of *M. leprae* in vitro, whereas those from patients suffering from the tuberculoid form of the disease respond strongly. The relative failure of T cell-directed microbial elimination in lepromatous leprosy may be due to a local change in the relative proportion of T-cell subsets in the lesions themselves. The T cells in lepromatous lesions consist almost entirely of **suppressor cells** while, in contrast, those in tuberculoid lesions are mainly **helper cells**. No marked differences are noted in the blood of these two groups of patients in respect of the T-cell subsets.

Interestingly, whereas patients with lepromatous leprosy exhibit impaired cell-mediated immunity, at least in relation to *M. leprae*, they are capable of making large amounts of antibody directed against determinants of the leprosy bacillus; autoantibodies may be formed as well, however, suggesting some fault in B-cell regulation. Immune complexes are formed in some patients; these occasionally deposit in small subcutaneous blood vessels giving rise to slightly tender nodules (**erythema nodosum leprosum**). The killing of organisms in patients with lepromatous leprosy by appropriate antimicrobial agents can lead to an increase in cell-mediated immunity, and there may be a change in the character of the lesions with some progression towards the tuberculoid type. This suggests that the local T-cell deficiency may be related in some way to the antigen load.

SARCOIDOSIS

Winston Churchill once wrote of Russia that it was a 'riddle, wrapped in a mystery, inside an enigma'. The same might be said of sarcoidosis.

Sarcoidosis is a disease of unknown aetiology which is fairly common in northern Europe and has its highest incidence in Sweden. It is characterized morphologically by well-formed epithelioid granulomas showing little or no central necrosis. These may be present in any organ or tissue. Multinucleate giant cells in the granulomas often show calcified bodies within the cytoplasm. These are sometimes star-shaped (hence the name **asteroid bodies**) or rounded and basophilic. Their presence is not diagnostic of sarcoidosis. The granulomas are often very sharply demarcated from the surrounding tissue and are cuffed by a mantle of lymphocytes much less conspicuous than that seen in relation to tuberculous lesions.

Distribution of the lesions

Sarcoidosis is a systemic disease in that most organs and tissues may be affected. The lung is the most frequently and prominently involved target. Chest radiography shows widespread, miliary mottling associated with hilar lymph node enlargement. The pulmonary symptoms are usually much milder than radiological appearances would suggest.

Other lymph nodes, liver and spleen are also frequently involved. In the skeleton the small bones of the fingers are most conspicuously affected; radiological examination shows the presence of small cyst-like lesions.

A variety of skin lesions may be seen. The uveal tract in the eye, the lacrimal gland and the salivary glands may also be involved; when all three are involved at the same time, the triad is spoken of as Heerfordt's syndrome. On rare occasions sarcoidosis has been reported as affecting the neurohypophysis, with the production of diabetes insipidus. Hypercalcaemia is not uncommon in these patients due to the activation of 1α-hydroxylase in epithelioid cells.

Aetiology and pathogenesis

Both the aetiology and the pathogenesis of sarcoidosis are poorly understood. A major difficulty is the fact that the basic pathological unit, the epithelioid granuloma, is a non-specific tissue reaction found after exposure to a large number of irritants, both living and non-living. While it is likely that the tissue response in sarcoidosis is an expression of cell-mediated immunity, we cannot be sure of this. In this connection it is not without interest that patients usually show diminished skin hypersensitivity as judged by their lack of response to tuberculoprotein.

Suggestions have been made that sarcoidosis may be the result of:

- A mycobacterial infection in a patient with altered cell-mediated immune reactions.
- A non-specific reaction to a wide variety of irritants. This would account for the histological features but would not explain the peculiar clustering of lesions that constitutes the clinical syndromes of sarcoidosis.
- Infection by an agent not as yet identified. Evidence that might be interpreted as supporting this view is derived from experiments in immunologically deficient mice. If such animals are injected with material from the lesions of a patient with sarcoidosis, they will develop large numbers of epithelioid cell granulomas. Material from these can then be transferred to another immunologically deficient mouse, with the same results.

SYPHILIS

Syphilis is still an important sexually transmitted disease. It is alleged that the disease was unknown in Europe until the last decade of the fifteenth century when Columbus's sailors were said to have introduced it on their return from the first voyage to the Americas. A large-scale outbreak was recorded after the siege and capture of Naples by Charles VIII of France in 1495–1496. The French called syphilis 'the Italian disease' and the Neapolitans dubbed it the 'French pox'. This episode tells us more about people than it does about syphilis.

The name 'syphilis' is derived from a poem by Girolamo Fracastoro, who died in 1533, in which a presumptuous shepherd boy named Syphilus was afflicted as a punishment for having taken his pleasure with the goddess Aphrodite. The poem, now entitled *Syphilis or a Poetical History of the French Pox*, was translated into English in about 1680 by Nahum Tate, the poet laureate of the day, who is perhaps better known for having provided Shakespeare's King Lear with a happy ending in which Cordelia marries Edgar and lives 'happily ever after'.

The organism

Syphilis is caused by a spirochaete, *Treponema pallidum*. This is a corkscrew-shaped bacillus, resistant to ordinary staining methods. As yet the bacillus cannot be cultured in artificial media or in tissue culture systems and can be maintained only in the tissues of living animals; the rabbit testis is most frequently used for this purpose. The spirochaetes can be seen in fluid taken from ulcerated lesions in the early stages of the disease either by using dark-field microscopy or by silver staining methods. The organism is very sensitive to heat and drying; stories of syphilis having been acquired via the medium of 'cracked tea cups' and the like are thus inherently improbable. Other than in congenital syphilis, where the infection is transplacental, direct contact is required.

T. pallidum spreads widely throughout the body aided by its invasive properties. These probably derive, in part, from the mucopolysaccharide capsule, which is antiphagocytic and may also downregulate the T-cell response. In addition, the treponema possesses enzymes that attack the constituents of the intercellular ground substance. *T. pallidum* shows considerable ability to **adhere** to the surface of a number of cell types. Only the tapered end of the organism adheres to subjacent plasma membranes, suggesting the presence of a receptor in this part of the bacterial cell wall.

The immune response to infection

An antibody response can be demonstrated within 1–3 weeks of the appearance of the first lesions of syphilis. Two interesting groups of antibodies have been identified. The first of these forms the basis for widely used diagnostic tests: the VDRL (Venereal Disease Research Laboratory) and Wassermann reactions.

Wassermann antibodies (anticardiolipin)
The Wassermann antibody is an immunoglobulin M molecule which reacts with a constituent of the lipid membranes of many cell organelles, notably

mitochondria. The antigen is diphosphatidylglycerol, often called **cardio-lipin** because a common source is an alcoholic extract of beef heart. The presence of this antibody in serum is not an absolutely reliable indicator of syphilis as biological false-positive reactions may occur in association with a number of non-treponemal and non-venereal diseases, including:

- malaria
- leprosy
- glandular fever
- trypanosomiasis
- some other treponemal disorders (e.g. yaws, pinta and bejel)
- mycoplasmal pneumonia
- some autoimmune haemolytic anaemias
- systemic lupus erythematosus
- some Coxsackie B virus infections.

Initially the wide range of disorders capable of eliciting the presence of the anticardiolipin antibody and the wide distribution within tissues of cardiolipin suggested that antibody formation was secondary to tissue damage and was not related to any specific antigen associated with *T. pallidum* itself. Cardiolipin has, however, now been shown to be present in *Treponema*, and it may be that this bacterium-associated cardiolipin acts as the antigen. Anticardiolipin antibodies do not react with intact organisms, and the case must still be regarded as not proven.

Antibodies binding specifically with intact T. pallidum
These antibodies can be detected in two ways:

1) by the **immobilization** of organisms in suspension
2) by the **fluorescent antibody** technique; in this group there are antibodies that react with all treponemas and others that react only with *T. pallidum*.

NATURAL HISTORY OF SYPHILIS

Apart from the congenital form of the disease, syphilis is contracted as a result of direct sexual contact with an infected person. Minute abrasions of the skin and mucous membranes in areas making such contact facilitate entry of the organisms into the tissues. After a 3–4-week incubation period, the **primary lesions** appear at the site of infection. Such a lesion is usually situated in the genital region, but in those preferring more recherché forms of sexual congress, they may occur on the lips, tongue, fingers or anus. In at least half the patients, the disease will follow a course lasting many years if untreated. The natural history in these cases appears to fall into three clearly defined and separable stages, which have been termed **primary**, **secondary** and **tertiary**.

Primary syphilis

The primary lesion usually occurs within 1 month of infection; occasionally the incubation period may be longer. The lesion, an indurated papule which is usually painless but often ulcerated, is known as a **chancre**.

In microscopic terms the tissue response is that of a localized inflammatory reaction characterized by a dense cellular infiltrate in which plasma cells, lymphocytes (both T and B cells) and macrophages are prominent. The endothelial linings of small blood vessels in affected areas show marked swelling. If extreme, the swelling can lead to virtual obliteration of the vessel lumina and to patchy local ischaemia, which may contribute to ulceration. The draining lymph nodes are usually enlarged.

Organisms are usually plentiful in the tissues at this stage and can be found in the fluid that oozes from ulcerated chancres. Local clearance of organisms appears to be effective, as the chancre heals spontaneously. In about half the patients the disease progresses no further, but in the others widespread dissemination of the treponema occurs and within a few weeks to a few months the next stage of the disease appears.

Secondary syphilis

This stage commonly occurs within 2–3 months after exposure to infection. A generalized skin rash appears; the face, palms and soles are particularly likely to be involved. The rash usually consists of many reddish or copper-coloured papules, but other types of lesion have been described.

The mucous membranes of the mouth and pharynx show the presence of whitish patches, some of which break down to give the lesions known as 'snail track' ulcers. In the moist cutaneous and mucocutaneous areas of the anus, vulva and perineum, flat papules develop known as **condylomata lata**. These contain large numbers of organisms and are very infectious. Generalized slight enlargement of lymph nodes is common, those in the epitrochlear region and those related to the posterior border of the sterno-mastoid being involved most frequently. Immune complexes may be formed; these can give rise to lesions in a number of different places, the most noteworthy being the kidney where glomerulonephritis may occur. Fever, muscle pains and a general malaise occur quite commonly.

These symptoms and the various lesions disappear spontaneously after a few months, and such patients no longer constitute a hazard to their sexual partners. A fairly high grade of immunity has now been established, but complete clearance of organisms usually does not occur. The treponemas appear to enter a latent phase, which may last for many years. Presumably this latent period is brought to an end when some diminution in cell-mediated immunity occurs, although it is not known how this comes about.

Tertiary syphilis

Unlike the tissue responses seen in the primary and secondary stages of syphilis, the lesions occurring when the latent period ends are destructive and may lead to crippling or life-threatening situations. Two basic tissue responses are seen in the tertiary stage of syphilis:

1) A special type of coagulative necrosis known as **gummatous necrosis**.
2) Inflammatory damage to small blood vessels in a wide variety of sites. This may lead to necrosis of the areas of tissue that they perfuse. Affected vessels show a severe degree of endothelial thickening with reduction of the lumina, and are cuffed by plasma cells and lymphocytes.

Gummatous necrosis

Gummas may occur anywhere in the body, producing clinical features that depend on their localization. The gumma is an area of rubbery coagulative necrosis somewhat resembling caseation necrosis. However, the centre of a gumma does not show the complete obliteration of cell and tissue outlines characteristic of caseation. The borders of the gumma are surrounded by plump fibroblasts, macrophages and lymphocytes. Blood vessels at the periphery show narrowing of their lumina and this may contribute to the necrosis. Treponemas are very scanty and difficult to demonstrate in lesions. Healing differs from the healing seen in tuberculosis in that fibrous bands criss-cross the necrotic area producing coarse scarring. Sites of predilection for gummatous necrosis include the liver, testis, subcutaneous tissue and bone (especially the tibia, ulna, clavicle, skull, nasal and palatal bones).

The pathogenesis of gummatous necrosis is still unknown. It has been suggested that it is a hypersensitivity phenomenon.

Small blood vessel disease

Small blood vessels in many sites show periadventitial cuffing by lymphocytes and plasma cells. Endothelial cells swell and may proliferate leading to obliteration of the lumina.

Such changes in the small blood vessels have a particularly baneful effect on the cardiovascular system. The ascending and thoracic parts of the aorta are the chief targets. The vasa vasorum in the adventitia and their extensions into the outer tunica media become cuffed by inflammatory cells. This is followed by destruction of both the elastic laminae and the smooth muscle cells in the media, inevitably leading to loss of the normal recoil of the aortic wall. The weakening of the aortic wall can lead to local dilatation of the vessel or **aneurysm** formation. The intimal surface of a vessel affected in this way often shows a curious wrinkled pattern, which has been likened to the appearance of tree bark. Any destructive process associated with scarring of the media of large elastic arteries shows this feature, which is therefore not diagnostic of tertiary syphilis.

Not infrequently the weakening process in the aortic media extends proximally to involve the aortic root, which becomes dilated as a result. This will give rise to incompetence of the aortic valve with consequent regurgitation of blood during diastole. Apart from the obvious dilatation of the aortic ring, the commissures between the valve cusps are widened and the cusps themselves show a characteristic cord-like thickening along their free edges, presumably due to the alteration in haemodynamics. As with the wrinkling of the intimal surface mentioned above, these appearances of the aortic valve can occur in any condition that gives rise to dilatation of the aortic root (e.g. ankylosing spondylitis) and are not diagnostic of syphilis. Before the introduction of penicillin treatment for syphilis, aortic valve disease of this type was a common cause of both left ventricular failure and sudden death. Its frequency in Western countries has declined very steeply.

Syphilis and the central nervous system

The lesions of tertiary syphilis occurring in the central nervous system fall into two distinct groups:

1) Lesions that involve the meninges and their small blood vessels lead to a chronic meningitis, patchy gummatous necrosis and severe narrowing of arterial lumina as a result of swelling of endothelial cells. These tend to occur early in the tertiary stage and have even been recorded in the secondary stage of the disease.
2) So-called **parenchymatous neurosyphilis** occurs late in the tertiary stage and involves degeneration of the neuronal elements themselves.

Meningovascular syphilis may involve either the leptomeninges or the pachymeninges; the former are affected more frequently. Leptomeningitis occurs most often at the base of the brain; the meninges become swollen and thickened, and occasionally small patches of gummatous necrosis may be seen. Cranial nerve involvement is not uncommon and the process may also obstruct the foramina of the fourth ventricle and thus cause hydrocephalus. Pachymeningitis may occur over the surface of the cerebral hemispheres and also in relation to parts of the spinal cord, where blood vessel involvement can cause patchy necrosis. These conditions are now seen very rarely.

Parenchymatous neurosyphilis occurs as two quite distinct sets of lesions and clinical syndromes. The first, termed **tabes dorsalis**, is characterized by degeneration of certain sensory fibres in the posterior nerve roots and posterior columns of the spinal cord. This leads to atrophy; the posterior columns are seen to be shrunken and greyish in colour (instead of white) at post mortem examination. The overlying leptomeninges are thickened and the posterior nerve roots are also atrophic.

On microscopic examination the posterior columns show fibre loss and demyelination. Similar changes may occur in more proximally situated parts of the nervous system (e.g. the optic discs and the third cranial nerve). The degeneration leads to severe loss of function, especially in relation to **deep pressure sensation, vibration sense, position sense** and **coordination**. Patients may develop a characteristic 'stamping' gait, as they cannot feel the ground beneath their feet. Deep tendon reflexes disappear and there may be episodes of very severe shooting pains in the limbs, known as 'lightning pains'. The lack of sensation may lead ultimately to disorganization of large joints such as the knee (Charcot's joints).

The pathogenesis of tabes dorsalis is still unknown. It is not likely to be related to proliferation of the organisms at a time when cell-mediated immunity is deficient, as organisms are very scanty in the lesions.

The second type of parenchymatous lesion seen in neurosyphilis is known as **general paresis of the insane (GPI)**. It was once one of the commonest causes of long-term admission to mental hospitals. GPI is a chronic treponemal inflammatory disorder in which, in contrast, to tabes dorsalis, it is reasonably easy to identify organisms. The brain is shrunken and the cerebral cortices are disorganized, the graphic term 'windswept cortex' being applied by some writers. The structural changes in the brain consist essentially of degeneration of nerve cells and their fibres, especially in the grey matter, with an associated proliferation of astrocytes and glial fibres. The small intracerebral blood vessels show the expected perivascular cuffing by lymphocytes and plasma cells, and swelling of the endothelial lining.

In the early stages the clinical picture is characterized by deterioration in personality and changes in mental function. This may express itself in the form of delusions, which may be at once bizarre and grandiose. If unchecked by treatment, the mental changes may proceed inexorably to complete dementia. Disturbances related to other functions may also be seen. These include tremors of the lips and tongue, general weakness, minor convulsive seizures and disturbances of finer movements.

Congenital syphilis

The presence of treponemas in the blood of a pregnant woman exposes the fetus to the hazard of transplacental infection. This usually occurs in about the fifth month of pregnancy. Depending on the number of spirochaetes in maternal blood, the fetus may be aborted or the child may die at birth, the lesions of congenital syphilis may appear early in the neonatal period, or the infection may remain latent for quite long periods.

If the infection is sufficiently severe to cause lesions in the perinatal period, the clinical picture tends to be dominated by skin and mucous membrane lesions in which severe loss of surface epithelium may occur. These lesions are intensely infective and contain many organisms. Typical inflammatory changes are seen at the growing ends of bones and in relation to the periosteum. Severe deformities of bone may result, including the formation of periosteal new bone over the anterior surface of the tibia which gives rise to a sabre-like appearance.

The **liver** may be diffusely affected by the syphilitic inflammatory reaction. This leads to an equally diffuse scarring where individual liver cells or small groups of such cells are surrounded by fine bands of fibrous tissue. Severe interstitial fibrosis may occur in the **lung**, leading to a marked narrowing of air spaces and, in the most severe cases, to a relatively airless lung.

The **cornea** is often the seat of an inflammatory reaction, and the **teeth** can show a characteristic deformity, the incisors being 'screwdriver' or 'peg' shaped (Hutchinson's teeth).

If the congenital infection manifests after a prolonged latent period, the features are usually similar to those seen in the tertiary stage of an acquired infection, although the presence of inflammation of the cornea together with tertiary features should suggest the possibility of transplacental infection.

SPECIFIC GRANULOMATOUS DISORDERS

- **Tuberculosis** is one of the most common and is potentially most lethal of the granulomatous diseases (2 million deaths annually). It is strongly associated with immune suppression, whether due to under-nutrition or HIV infection.
- The causal organism, *Mycobacterium tuberculosis*, has a lipid-rich coating which, when stained, resists decolorization by acid and alcohol.
- The characteristic extensive tissue damage is caused by immune reactions, which can both enhance elimination of the organisms and produce caseation necrosis (hypersensitivity). The T cell response determines which reaction is dominant. A mixed T helper cell response is associated with increased tissue damage.
- Primary infections (usually in childhood) produce small tissue lesions which are often associated with involvement of draining lymph nodes (Ghon complex). Spread with multi-organ involvement may occur.
- Adult (secondary) infections usually cause localized disease associated with significant caseation necrosis.
- Another important disorder is **leprosy** (caused by *M. leprae*). This is rare in the West but not uncommon in Asia and sub-Saharan Africa. The form of the disease mirrors the degree of cell-mediated immunity.

16 Amyloid and the amyloidoses

Amyloidosis is a disparate set of disorders showing a single common feature: extracellular deposition of proteins arranged in the form of β-pleated sheet fibrils, these being known as amyloid. Organs in which large amounts of amyloid are deposited are:

- **larger**
- **firmer**
- **paler**

than normal.

Amyloid shows the same reaction with iodine as does starch; the term amyloid (literally 'starch-like') was therefore coined, and the term has persisted despite the recognition that amyloid is proteinacious.

Identification of amyloid in tissue

Organs containing abundant amyloid are larger, paler and much firmer than normal. They appear somewhat waxy and the cut edges of solid viscera are much sharper than normal. It is sometimes possible to recognize the sites of amyloid deposition by staining portions of tissue with Lugol's iodine, the amyloid staining a rich brown colour.

Microscopic features
Amyloid is recognized by:

a) Its **eosinophilia and apparent lack of structure**, as seen in sections stained with haematoxylin and eosin.

b) Its ability to bind the dye **Congo Red**, which stains amyloid orange-red. In polarized light, this Congo Red-positive material has a characteristic green–yellow birefringence, termed **dichroism**. This is a fairly sensitive method and, apart from electron microscopy, is the most reliable everyday diagnostic method. *Treatment of sections with potassium permanganate helps to differentiate between two forms of amyloid: amyloid of immunoglobulin light chain origin and amyloid derived by cleavage of an acute-phase reactant, serum amyloid A (SAA).* In the case of the latter, Congo Red binding is abolished by permanganate treatment.

c) Its ability to exhibit **metachromasia** when sections are stained with **methyl violet**, amyloid staining red. This is not very satisfactory because the dye does not bind permanently to amyloid and tends to leach out into the mounting medium.

Electron microscopy. On electron microscopy amyloid is shown not to be structureless but to consist of bundles of fibrils varying in width from 7 to 14 nm and measuring up to 1600 nm in length. High-resolution electron microscopy shows pentagonal subunits along the filaments, consisting of **amyloid P component**, a glycoprotein coded for on chromosome 1.

P component belongs to a family of pentameric glycoproteins known as **pentraxins**, of which the acute-phase reactant C-reactive protein is a member. Amyloid P concentration in plasma increases under the same circumstances as other acute-phase proteins; its physiological role has not been determined, although in vitro it has some inhibitory effect on elastase. It binds in a calcium-dependent fashion to a number of ligands including fibronectin and amyloid fibrils, but the significance of this is not yet known.

The close association of the P component with amyloid fibrils in systemic amyloidosis can be made use of: serum amyloid P component linked with radioactive iodine, when injected intravenously, binds to amyloid deposits. Thus it may be possible to use scintigraphy to locate deposits and to monitor their extent.

The β-pleated fibril is the unifying feature of the amyloidoses

It is well known that diseases associated with amyloidosis are widely disparate. Equally, modern methods of protein analysis show the existence of several widely differing amyloid proteins, each one characteristic of a certain group of disorders. The common and unifying factor in this complex situation is the fact that **all amyloid proteins have a β-pleated sheet structure**.

Vertebrate proteins in general, normally exhibit an α-helical structure, and β-pleating is normally inconspicuous. The β-pleated configuration causes:

- the characteristic **reactions with Congo Red**
- the **fibrillar ultrastructure**
- the **relative resistance of amyloid fibrils to dissolve in normal physiological solvents and to proteolytic digestion**.

CLASSIFICATION

Classification of the amyloidoses is most rationally based on identification of the protein precursor involved. Older classifications of the amyloidoses, based on clinical and pathological criteria, show certain inconsistencies:

1) **Primary amyloidosis** was defined by the presence of a tendency for nodular deposition of amyloid with a special predilection for mesenchymal tissues and, most importantly, an absence of any recognizable preceding or concurrent disease. The only distinction between this and the entity known as 'amyloidosis associated with myelomatosis' was the presence in the latter of osteolytic lesions. In fact, both the distribution pattern of the amyloid and the protein involved are identical.

2) So-called **secondary amyloidosis** was characterized as such by the fact that it either followed or was associated with a wide range of **identifiable diseases**, many of which were chronic inflammatory disorders.

It seems more rational to propose instead a scheme of classification based on simple set theory (*Fig. 16.1*). Any individual case of amyloidosis can be regarded as representing the common set of three sets:

- the **nature of the amyloid protein**
- whether the amyloidosis is **acquired or inherited**
- the **distribution pattern of the amyloid deposits**.

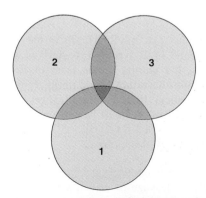

Fig. 16.1   A basis for classification of the amyloidoses.

1, The nature of the protein involved (e.g. immunoglobulin light chain); 2, anatomical distribution; 3, whether inherited or acquired.

SYSTEMIC AMYLOIDOSIS

AMYLOIDOSIS OF IMMUNE ORIGIN (AL TYPE)

This form shows the following characteristics:

- *The protein precursor is an immunoglobulin light chain and/or its homologous amino-terminal fragment.*
- *The disorder is acquired.*
- *The amyloid is systemically distributed.*

Amyloidosis of immune origin occurs in association (not surprisingly, in view of the nature of the amyloid protein) with **monoclonal proliferations of B lymphocytes or plasma cells** which may be overtly neoplastic. The most striking of these is **myelomatosis**, which accounts for about 20% of AL cases. Amyloidosis of immune origin occurs also in association with Waldenström's macroglobulinaemia, heavy chain disease and, occasionally with agammaglobulinaemia.

The amyloid protein

Analysis of amyloid proteins in this disorder shows them to consist of:

- an **intact immunoglobulin light chain**
- the **amino-terminal fragment of such a chain**
- on some occasions, a mixture of the two.

These amyloid proteins are called **AL proteins**. The majority of the light chains are of the **lambda (λ) type**. Anti-idiotypic antibodies raised against the amyloid protein of a given patient with AL amyloidosis react only with that patient's amyloid light chain, indicating patient specificity. In 90% of patients with this disease, the antibodies also react with soluble proteins in the plasma. This plasma reactant is an intact circulating light chain or **Bence Jones protein**.

Thus the cellular source of amyloid fibrils of the AL variety is almost certainly a **single clone of B lymphocyte-derived cells** whose protein product circulates in the plasma in the form of Bence Jones protein. Deposition of these light chains as amyloid fibrils requires their **conversion from a normal α-helical to a β-pleated sheet configuration**. Thus amyloidogenesis, in this context, must be a two-step process. Step 1 is the secretion of excess amounts of a single type of light chain (monoclonal) and step 2 is conversion to the β-pleated form.

How do soluble light chains undergo this change?

Progressive proteolytic cleavage of certain λ light chains can yield fibrils identical with amyloid fibrils. Not all λ light chains behave in this way. Inherent in the variable portion of some λ light chains is the capacity to assume a β-pleated sheet configuration when that part of the light chain is enzymatically cleaved.

The features separating so-called 'amyloidogenic' light chains from those that cannot be induced to form amyloid fibrils are not known. What is certain is that the characteristic features of amyloid depend on its configuration: β-pleated fibrils such as the natural product of the silk moth and synthetically created β-pleated fibrils derived from poly-L-lysine show the same tinctorial and ultrastructural features as amyloid.

Clinical features (*Fig. 16.2*)

Amyloidosis of immune origin is a disorder of middle life and old age; it affects males more often than females. Some 90% of patients show a plasma or urinary monoclonal immunoglobulin associated with a Bence Jones protein and, in some cases, only a Bence Jones protein is present. The bone marrow contains an excess number of plasma cells. While the clinical expressions are protean, certain symptom complexes strongly suggest amyloidosis.

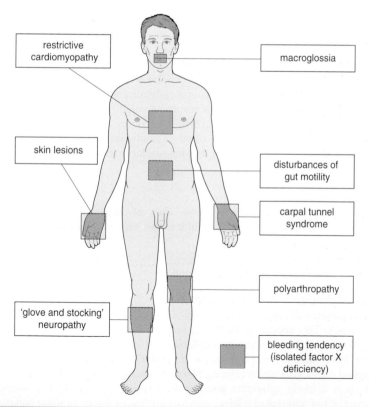

Fig. 16.2 Spectrum of clinical features in amyloidosis of immune origin.

Neuropathy

A peripheral and an autonomic neuropathy resembling that seen in diabetics may occur. Manifestations of autonomic neuropathy such as impotence, orthostatic hypotension, disturbances of gastrointestinal motility and abnormalities of sweating may be prominent. A peripheral neuropathy with a characteristic 'glove and stocking' distribution may also be seen, and can be associated with intermittent attacks of pain.

Restrictive cardiomyopathy

Restrictive cardiomyopathy is caused by extensive infiltration of the amyloid between the heart muscle fibres leading to an increase in the stiffness of the heart muscle and, thus, to a lessening of diastolic compliance. The clinical features of right-sided cardiac failure tend to dominate the picture and an incorrect diagnosis of constrictive pericarditis may be made. Patients with cardiac amyloidosis are extremely sensitive to digitalis, and fatal arrhythmias have been recorded following its administration. Even in the absence of digitalis treatment, there is an increased risk of arrhythmias, conduction disturbances and sudden death. Pulmonary deposition of amyloid has also been described in association with amyloidosis of the heart, and its presence strongly indicates an immune origin for the amyloidosis.

Skin manifestations

There are two main skin changes. The first, known as 'pinch purpura', is due to amyloid deposition in the basement membranes of small cutaneous blood vessels. Pinching of affected areas results in small haemorrhages. In addition, nodules of amyloid may occur within the dermis, giving an appearance somewhat resembling small drops of white candle wax on the skin. Areas of baldness and patchy thickening of the skin similar to that seen in scleroderma may also occur.

Polyarthropathy

Large joints tend particularly to be sites of amyloid deposition; the distribution of the arthropathy is similar to that seen in rheumatoid disease.

Enlargement of the tongue (macroglossia)

Macroglossia may be an early manifestation.

Isolated deficiency in clotting factor X

Some patients develop a coagulation disorder characterized by factor X deficiency. This appears to be due to very rapid clearance of factor X from the blood. For this to occur two criteria must be fulfilled: (1) the amyloid must have binding sites for factor X; and (2) there must be sufficient amyloid exposed to the circulating blood for such binding to take place. The spleen is a likely candidate site for the exposure of amyloid to blood. Certainly, the removal of a large, amyloid infiltrated spleen in some patients affected with factor X deficiency corrects the clotting defect.

Carpal tunnel syndrome

Carpal tunnel syndrome results from pressure on the median nerve and is expressed by tingling in the median nerve distribution, followed ultimately by atrophy of the muscles in the hand supplied by this nerve. The carpal tunnel is affected not only in immune-mediated amyloidosis of the AL type but in one of the hereditary neuropathic amyloidoses and also in some patients who have been on long-term haemodialysis for chronic renal failure.

HAEMODIALYSIS-ASSOCIATED AMYLOID

After 7 years on dialysis, 30% of patients develop carpal tunnel syndrome; this proportion increases to 50% after 10 years. The amyloid is derived from β_2-microglobulin. Amyloidosis of this type develops only in the presence of a persistently high plasma concentration of this protein, a situation particularly likely to develop if cuprophane membranes are used for dialysis. β_2-Microglobulin shows some degree of homology for the constant region of both light and heavy chains of immunoglobulin and the protein is shed continuously from cell membranes into the plasma before being catabolized in the kidney. In very high concentrations, isolated and purified β_2-microglobulin can be precipitated as a material with a fibrillar ultrastructure and a capacity to bind Congo Red; it can therefore be regarded as a naturally 'amyloidogenic' protein.

REACTIVE SYSTEMIC AMYLOIDOSIS ('SECONDARY' AMYLOIDOSIS)

The basic characteristics of this form of amyloidosis are as follows. The protein precursor of the amyloid (known as the **AA type of amyloid**) is a circulating acute-phase reactant (**serum amyloid A, SAA**). This is a 12.5 kD protein produced chiefly by the liver.

Under basal circumstances SAA is present in only very low concentrations. In tissue injury and/or inflammation the concentration of SAA rises very sharply (sometimes more than 1000-fold). The signals that upregulate its production are interleukin (IL) 1, tumour necrosis factor α and probably IL-6. While the biological role of SAA as an acute-phase protein is still unknown, it is worth noting that SAA is an apolipoprotein in the HDL_3 fraction of high density lipoprotein. The amyloid protein itself (AA) appears to be a cleavage product of SAA, 28 amino acid residues at the carboxy-terminal having been removed from the SAA.

The disorder is acquired in most cases, and is associated with a wide range of chronic inflammatory diseases and some neoplastic ones. However, AA protein deposition in the same distribution pattern as for reactive systemic amyloidosis occurs in association with the autosomal recessive disorder, familial Mediterranean fever (see pp. 287–288).

The distribution pattern is a systemic one: the **kidneys**, **liver**, **spleen** and **adrenals** are sites of predilection. The main cause of death in this variety of amyloidosis is **chronic renal failure**. Many other tissues may be involved; biopsy of the rectal mucosa or the gum can be a useful way of establishing a firm tissue diagnosis.

Disease associations of reactive systemic amyloidosis

- **Chronic inflammatory diseases in which infection is known to play a part**. The most common of these are tuberculosis, leprosy, syphilis, chronic osteomyelitis and bronchiectasis.
- **Chronic inflammatory diseases in which infection probably plays a part**, e.g. Reiter's syndrome, Whipple's disease.
- **Chronic inflammatory diseases of uncertain aetiology** such as rheumatoid arthritis and its variants, other connective tissue disorders, ulcerative colitis and Crohn's disease.
- **Long-standing paraplegia**, probably because of the high risk of recurrent urinary tract infections.
- **Neoplasms**, especially **renal adenocarcinoma**. Reactive systemic amyloidosis has also been reported with various other solid tumours and in association with Hodgkin's disease.

Chronic inflammatory diseases constitute the major causally related association of reactive systemic amyloidosis. With the advent of antibiotic treatment, the incidence of such disorders as chronic osteitis and bronchiectasis has declined and the introduction of successful chemotherapy for **tuberculosis** has led to a fall in the frequency of tuberculosis-associated amyloidosis. However, in parts of the world where tuberculosis still occurs on a large scale, it remains a far from negligible cause of amyloidosis.

Leprosy, because of the large number of sufferers world-wide, still ranks high as a cause of reactive systemic amyloidosis and is responsible for a significant proportion of the deaths caused by this disease.

In Western countries, the most common group of disorders associated with reactive amyloidosis is **rheumatoid disease**. In systemic-onset juvenile arthritis the frequency of amyloidosis is estimated to be 10%. Morbidity and mortality in these patients is high because of the baneful effect on the kidneys: the patients first develop a nephrotic syndrome and ultimately chronic renal failure.

The association between **long-standing paraplegia** and a high risk of reactive systemic amyloidosis has been known for many years; in one series of paraplegics coming to autopsy, the prevalence of amyloidosis was found to be 40%.

Pathogenesis of reactive systemic amyloidosis

The pathogenesis of reactive systemic amyloidosis is still unclear. *Overproduction of SAA is clearly necessary for amyloidosis to develop but it does not appear to be a sufficient cause, and other unknown factors must play a part*. At the genetic level, more than one gene can code for SAA and it is possible that one form may be more 'amyloidogenic' than another.

It has also been suggested that an **'amyloid enhancing factor'** may exist. This is a blanket term for a group of chemical species that can be extracted both from the tissues of animals in which amyloidosis has been induced and from human tissues in which amyloid fibrils are present. It appears in the tissues of experimental models before there is microscopic evidence of amyloid deposition.

Some specific patterns of organ involvement in reactive amyloidosis

The principal organs involved are the spleen, liver and kidney.

The spleen. The amyloid frequently deposits in the white pulp, giving the cut surface of the organ a speckled appearance classically termed 'sago spleen'.

The liver. The liver may be hugely enlarged and is firm and pale. Amyloid is usually deposited in the space of Disse (between the liver cells and the sinusoidal endothelium). Because amyloid fibrils resist digestion, the liver cell columns eventually become atrophic but, owing to the large functional hepatic reserve, the clinical effects are not usually great.

The kidney. Here the amyloid is deposited in the walls of the glomerular capillaries, and in relation to the basement membranes of the arterioles and renal tubules. In most cases the kidney is enlarged, firm and pale on naked-eye examination but in a few cases secondary ischaemic changes dominate the picture leading to irregular scarring and shrinkage of the kidney. Amyloidosis involving the glomeruli leads first to the appearance of the nephrotic syndrome (massive proteinuria, hypoproteinaemia and oedema) proceeding inexorably to chronic renal failure.

HEREDITARY SYSTEMIC AMYLOIDOSES

The hereditary systemic amyloidoses are rare, affecting fewer than 1/100 000 population in the USA annually. The syndromes associated with hereditary amyloidosis can be divided into three main groups:

- neuropathic
- cardiopathic
- nephropathic.

The **neuropathic group** is characterized by progressive systemic polyneuropathy. This occurs in three forms, the classification being based partly on the distribution of the neuropathy and partly in relation to the location of the affected families. Thus there is:

a) a group in which the lower limbs are first and predominantly affected; this has been found in Portugal, Japan and Sweden

b) a group in which the nerves of the upper limb are particularly affected; this has been found in Germany and Switzerland
c) a group in which the neuropathy affects the face; this has been reported only in Finland.

The **cardiopathic form** has been found in one Danish family and in a kindred in the Appalachian region of the USA of German–Irish–English origin.

Two forms of the **nephropathic group** have been reported:

a) familial Mediterranean fever
b) urticaria–deafness syndrome.

With the exception of familial Mediterranean fever, which is inherited in an autosomal recessive fashion, all these disorders are autosomal dominant.

Amyloid proteins in hereditary systemic amyloidosis

With one exception – Finnish familial amyloid polyneuropathy where the amyloid precursor protein has been described as being antigenically and structurally similar to **gelsolin**, an actin-depolymerizing protein – in both the neuropathic and cardiopathic forms the amyloid protein consists of an abnormal form of a plasma protein known until recently as **prealbumin**. This is a misnomer: the sole connection of prealbumin with albumin is that it migrates in front of albumin in electrophoretic strips. Prealbumin has now been renamed **transthyretin**, a name that has the virtue of telling us something about its function:

- *trans*port of about 25% of plasma *thy*roxine
- transport of *retin*ol (vitamin A).

The transthyretin molecule has 127 amino acid residues. All patients with the Portuguese form show a single amino acid substitution: methionine for valine at position 30. About 20 mutations have been discovered in the transthyretin molecule, indicating point mutations in the gene coding for this protein. Each of these is associated with a fairly distinctive clinical picture, although a certain degree of overlap is present.

The significance of mutations in the gene coding for transthyretin has been confirmed by a study in which mice were made transgenic by introduction of a mutant transthyretin gene cloned from a patient with the familial Portuguese type of polyneuropathy. Amyloid deposition started in these mice at 6 months of age and by 2 years was extensive.

The tertiary structure of transthyretin is unusual in that it is normally β-pleated. The molecule tends to form dimers and this is followed by fusion of a pair of dimers to form tetramers. The presence of a mixture, within a single tetramer, of normal and mutated forms of the protein appears to promote the joining up of several hundred tetramers to form an amyloid fibril.

Senile cardiovascular amyloidosis and transthyretin

A transthyretin amyloid precursor has also been identified in the non-familial and quite common disorder of senile cardiac amyloidosis. Cardiac amyloidosis of this kind occurs frequently in old individuals, about 25% of subjects over 80 years being affected. The patients present with signs and symptoms of congestive cardiac failure, often with a low-voltage electro-cardiogram, recurrent syncope and a high risk of arrhythmias. Although this disorder is most commonly termed senile cardiac amyloidosis, there is increasing evidence that extracardiac sites are frequently involved and that the condition should be regarded as a variant of systemic amyloidosis.

Other forms of amyloid in the elderly involving only the cardiovascular system are:

- Isolated atrial amyloidosis in which the amyloid protein precursor appears to be atrial natriuretic peptide.
- Aortic amyloidosis, which was found to be present in 100% of patients in a necropsy study of patients aged over 80 years. The amyloid is deposited mainly in the inner one-third of the tunica media. The nature of the protein precursor is still unknown but it does not react with antisera raised against transthyretin.

Nephropathic forms of familial systemic amyloidosis

Familial Mediterranean fever

This is by far the commonest form of hereditary systemic amyloidosis, with one clinic alone in Israel caring for more than 1500 sufferers. The disease is transmitted as an **autosomal recessive** trait and is seen in Jews of Sephardic ancestry, Anatolian Turks, Armenians and Middle Eastern Arabs. The gene frequency is very high, reaching 1 in 22 among North African Jews and 1 in 14 among Armenians living in Los Angeles. Recently a gene believed to be responsible was mapped to the short arm of chromosome 16.

Familial Mediterranean fever expresses itself in one or both of two forms:

1) Rather short-lived (24–48 hours), self-limiting febrile attacks associated with pain mimicking that of peritonitis, pleurisy or synovitis.
2) Amyloidosis which, in some of the groups mentioned above, may manifest itself very early in life. In the youngest fatal case reported, the patient died at the age of 5 years from renal failure, the amyloidosis having been obvious since the age of 2 years. Very few affected patients have survived beyond the age of 40 years, unless treated at an early stage or given a renal transplant.

The amyloid protein in familial Mediterranean fever is of the **AA type**; plasma concentrations of SAA are usually raised between attacks, although they also increase very steeply during febrile bouts. The amyloidosis obviously has a preclinical phase as it is only when glomerular function has been compromised significantly that proteinuria appears. *Early diagnosis is*

*important because the development of amyloidosis can be inhibited in 90%
of patients by administration of 1–2 mg colchicine daily.* Not only can amyloid deposition be inhibited *ab initio* but even in patients with established
proteinuria the process can be halted in most, and even reversed in a small
number.

Familial nephropathic amyloidosis with febrile urticaria and nerve deafness

In 1962 Muckle and Wells described an unusual, autosomally transmitted
syndrome in a single English family. Over four generations, nine of the 18
individuals at risk were affected.

The syndrome manifests during adolescence; its first expression is in the
form of febrile attacks associated with an itchy or painful urticarial skin rash
and with malaise, rigors and pains in the limbs. The second manifestation is
progressive nerve deafness. This is followed, in some patients, by the onset
of proteinuria leading to a nephrotic syndrome and eventually to death from
chronic renal failure. Autopsy shows widespread amyloidosis, the kidneys
being particularly affected. Interestingly, in view of the nerve deafness, no
amyloid was found in the inner ear or cochlear nerve.

Extraction of the amyloid protein from the fixed tissues of a single patient
and subsequent sequence analysis showed it to be homologous with AA
protein in respect of 28 of its amino acid residues.

LOCALIZED AMYLOIDOSIS

ENDOCRINE-RELATED AMYLOID

It has been known for a long time that certain endocrine glands, most notably
the pituitary and the pancreatic islets, can be infiltrated by amyloid under
certain circumstances. In the case of the pituitary, age seems to be the most
important associated factor, whereas pancreatic islets frequently show the
presence of amyloid deposition in patients with non-insulin-dependent
diabetes mellitus.

Certain neoplasms of endocrine glands are associated with the presence of
amyloid deposited solely within the stroma of the tumours and *not* appearing
systemically. One tumour most consistently associated with stromal amyloid
deposits is **medullary carcinoma of the thyroid**, derived from the
parafollicular or thyrocalcitonin-producing cells of the thyroid gland. *The
amyloid precursor protein in this case is the 9–19 amino acid portion of
the calcitonin molecule.*

The situation is equally intriguing in relation to the amyloid appearing in
the islets of patients with non-insulin-dependent diabetes and with insulin-
producing islet cell tumours. In acidic solutions, freezing and thawing of
insulin can produce fibrils and it was initially thought that islet of
Langerhans amyloid was related to the insulin molecule. More recent analy-

sis has shown that, both in islet cells tumours and in diabetes, the amyloid shows homology with the vasodilator **calcitonin gene-related peptide** (amylin).

INTRACEREBRAL AMYLOIDOSIS

Central nervous system amyloidosis is by far the commonest localized form of the disease occurring in Alzheimer's disease, the commonest form of dementia. The amyloid is derived from a protein known as A4, the function of which is unknown. It forms the centre of lesions known as senile or neuritic plaques. Amyloid also occurs in the spongiform encephalopathies, in the dementia occurring in some boxers and in some hereditary haemorrhagic syndromes.

Spongiform encephalopathies are a group of disorders occurring in many species and characterized by a common histological picture showing:

- neurone loss
- a spongy appearance in affected areas of brain due to the formation of small cysts
- reactive proliferation of astrocytes
- amyloid deposition in the afected areas and in neighbouring blood vessels.

Other characteristic features include transmissibility both within and across species and modification of a host protein into amyloid. The transmissible agent is an abormally folded protein encoded on chromosome 20. These have been called **prions** (proteinacious infective particle).

In humans prion-associated diseases, all of which cause dementia, include:

- Creutzfeldt–Jakob disease (can be sporadic, inherited or transmitted)
- Gerstmann–Straussler–Scheinker syndrome (inherited)
- kuru (due to ingestion of abnormal prion proteins in the course of ritual cannibalism)
- fatal familial insomnia
- new variant Creutzfeldt–Jakob disease (transmitted).

These human diseases have animal homologues in the form of scrapie (in sheep) and bovine spongiform encephalopathy (BSE). The latter is of particular importance since not only did it affect more than 170 000 of the British cattle herd but it seems almost inescapable that a variant form of Creutzfeldt–Jakob disease in young humans has been caused by eating beef containing abnormal prion proteins.

Cystatin C

This was the first cerebral amyloid protein to be characterized biochemically. It is found as the principal protein in the amyloid fibrils deposited in the cerebral blood vessels in an autosomal dominant disorder known as

hereditary cerebral haemorrhage with amyloidosis of Icelandic type (HCHWA-I). This disorder has been found in 128 individuals in eight families in a certain area of Iceland and is characterized by the presence of amyloid in small arteries and arterioles in the cerebral cortex and lepto-meninges. The patients usually die before they reach the age of 40 years from massive intracerebral haemorrhage.

AMYLOID AND THE AMYLOIDOSES

- Amyloidosis is a set of disorders characterized by extracellular deposition of protein arranged in the form of β-pleated sheet fibrils. If amyloid is present in large amounts the affected organs become enlarged, pale and firmer than normal.
- Amyloidosis may be acquired or inherited, systemic or local.
- Microscopically, amyloid appears structureless and eosinophilic. It binds the dye Congo Red, this stained material showing yellow-green birefringence in polarized light. Electron microscopy shows all amyloid to exist in the form of a meshwork of long, narrow fibrils. These structural features are the expression of the β-pleated configuration of the proteins.
- Systemic amyloidosis may represent over-production of immunoglobulin light chain by an expanded clone of B lymphocytes, as in myelomatosis (amyloidosis of immune origin), or a reaction to the presence of chronic inflammation or certain neoplasms (reactive systemic amyloidosis).
- The most common and important site for local amyloidosis is the brain, where it is associated with Alzheimer's disease and spongiform encephalopathies.

17 General pathology of viral infection

Viruses are obligate intracellular parasites, accounting for 60% of all infections. The spectrum of viral diseases ranges from the trivial to lethal or crippling situations. The range of tissue responses evoked is similarly wide.

GENERAL CHARACTERISTICS OF A VIRUS

SIZE

Viruses are the smallest infectious agents known. The largest are just visible with the light microscope; the majority can be seen only on electron microscopy, their diameters ranging from 20 to 300 nm (1 nm = 10^{-3} μm).

Genome

A virus contains only a **single** nucleic acid as its genome, either **DNA** or **RNA**; the type of nucleic acid forms one of the bases for viral classification. The nucleic acid is covered by a symmetrically arranged protein shell, known as the **capsid**. This consists of clusters of polypeptides forming ultra-structurally recognizable units called **capsomeres**. Capsid arrangement falls into two distinct structural patterns. It may confer either an **icosahedral** (20-sided) appearance to the virus or a **helical** one. All viruses in which the nucleic acid is **DNA** are icosahedral (apart from the **poxviruses**); **RNA** viruses may be either icosahedral or helical.

Infective particle

The mature infective virus particle is called a **virion**. In some viruses this may refer to the nucleic acid genome and the capsid only, but in others there is a glycoprotein **envelope**. Most DNA viruses have no envelope (with the exception of the **herpesviruses**); most RNA viruses are enveloped (with the exception of **picornaviruses** and **reoviruses**).

INTERACTION BETWEEN VIRUS AND HOST SPECIES

The production of a viral illness involves several steps. The virus must have an appropriate route of access to the host and there must be a mechanism or mechanisms for the virus to reach its ultimate target, for example the anterior horn cells in poliomyelitis. Routes of access to the host include the skin and subcutaneous tissues, the conjunctiva, the respiratory tract, and the genital and gastrointestinal tracts. These and the possible outcome of viral entry are shown in *Figs 17.1* and *17.2*.

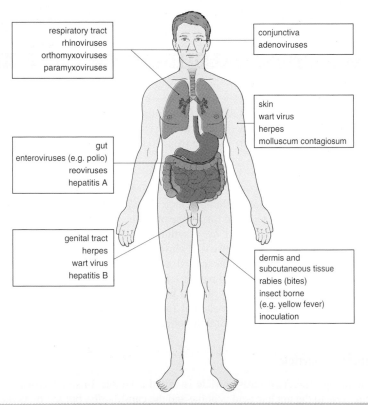

respiratory tract
rhinoviruses
orthomyxoviruses
paramyxoviruses

conjunctiva
adenoviruses

skin
wart virus
herpes
molluscum contagiosum

gut
enteroviruses (e.g. polio)
reoviruses
hepatitis A

genital tract
herpes
wart virus
hepatitis B

dermis and
subcutaneous tissue
rabies (bites)
insect borne
(e.g. yellow fever)
inoculation

Fig. 17.1   Portals of entry of some human viruses.

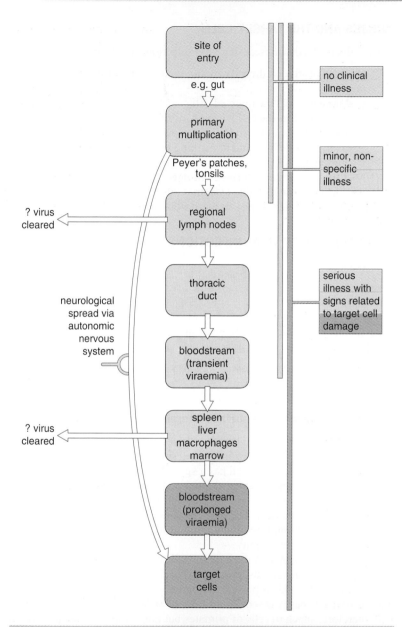

Fig. 17.2   Pathogenesis of a viral disease such as poliomyelitis.

VIRUSES AND THE TARGET CELL

The effects of a disease-causing viral infection stem from:

1) **changes produced directly by the virus in the host cell**; the virus may:
   - **damage** or **kill** the infected cell
   - **persist within the cell without injuring it** (persistent infection)
   - **transform** the cell, rendering it capable of an indefinite number of passages in culture, and of forming tumours in susceptible animals (tumorigenicity; see pp. 534–539)
2) **host tissue reactions to these changes**
3) **responses of the immune system**, both to the presence of the virus and to the cellular changes it has produced.

TRANSMISSION OF VIRAL INFECTIONS

This may be:

- vertical, i.e. the infection is transmitted from mother to child either in utero or perinatally
- horizontal, i.e. from person to person via **respiratory** (aerosol borne), **gastrointestinal** (faecal–oral), **genitourinary** (sexual) or **percutaneous** routes.

Entry into a host must be followed by **entry into susceptible host cells** and **viral replication** within them.

1. Virus attaches to cell surface membrane

Contact between viruses and target cells occurs more or less randomly. However, attachment of the virion to a cell surface will not take place unless the surface membrane of the cell has a **specific viral receptor site which is complementary to an attachment site on the viral surface**. The complementarity of ligands on the viral surface and receptors on the cells reflects configurational similarities. These similarities probably arose by chance in the course of evolution. It is of fundamental importance in determining cell tropism and viral pathogenicity.

This is well illustrated in the case of **poliovirus**. For poliovirus to attach to a target cell, the latter must possess a specific **lipoprotein receptor** on its plasma membrane. This is present in neurones and cells lining the intestinal tract in primates but is absent from those of rodents. The poliovirus virion will, therefore, attach to cells of primates but not to those of rodents, which cannot therefore be infected by poliovirus.

Similarly, the **influenza** virus attaches to cells via a specific glycoprotein cell surface receptor, **N-acetylneuraminic acid** (**NANA**). The receptor binds a **haemagglutinin** (so called because it causes red cells to clump) carried on the envelope of the influenza virus. This receptor can be destroyed by treating cells in culture with bacterial neuraminidase (sialidase); influenza virus will not attach to cells treated in this way.

Epstein–Barr virus is a herpesvirus which causes infectious mononucleosis and is also implicated in the causation of two neoplastic diseases, Burkitt's lymphoma and nasopharyngeal carcinoma; it binds to the receptor for the third component of complement (C3R) on B lymphocytes. **Rabies virus** recognizes acetylcholine receptors, and **human immunodeficiency virus** (**HIV**) binds to the CD4 receptor on T helper lymphocytes.

Not all viral attachment is specific. Both **orthomyxoviruses** and **paramyxoviruses** attach to sialic acid residues of host cell surface glycoproteins and glycolipids found on the membranes of most cells including those not susceptible to infection.

2. Virus penetrates the cell

Once attachment has occurred, the virion is engulfed within the cell by a process akin to receptor-mediated endocytosis. This is a temperature- and energy-dependent step and can be inhibited by treating the target cells with various metabolic poisons. In the case of some enveloped viruses, the viral envelope fuses with the plasma membranes of the cell and the nucleoplasmid is released directly into the host cytoplasm.

3. Viral nucleic acid is uncoated

The term 'uncoating' denotes physical separation of viral nucleic acid or, in some instances, the nucleocapsid from outer structural proteins, this being accompanied by loss of infectivity. Sometimes uncoating commences during the attachment stage. More commonly, however, it occurs within the host cell cytoplasm; lysosomal enzymes are thought to play a part in the process. In the case of a few viruses of the **reovirus** family, uncoating may never be completed.

From this point, viral replication differs depending on whether the nucleic acid genome is DNA or RNA.

4. Viral replication

DNA virus replication

Viral DNA is transcribed in two stages, giving rise to messenger RNA (mRNA) at two points in time, characterized as **early** and **late**.

Early transcription from the viral DNA takes place in the nucleus of target cells. The mRNA produced reaches the cytoplasm and is then translated by the host ribosomes into **early proteins**. These are required for the synthesis of **new viral DNA**, which again takes place in the host cell nucleus.

Late mRNA is then transcribed. This leaves the nucleus and is translated in the cytoplasm into **late proteins**, which constitute the material from which the capsomeres are made.

These proteins then enter the nucleus where virions are assembled before leaving the host cell. This last move is accomplished by a bursting open of the cell, with release of the new virions into the surrounding extracellular environment.

All DNA viruses replicate in this way, with the exception of the poxviruses which do so entirely within the host cell cytoplasm. The polymerases concerned in the transcription of viral DNA are derived from the host cell in most instances. The poxviruses, however, have their own DNA-dependent RNA polymerase.

RNA virus replication

With two exceptions, all classes of RNA viruses **replicate within the cytoplasm of the host cell**. **Orthomyxoviruses** (responsible for influenza) and **retroviruses** replicate within the host cell nucleus. Because normal cells do not copy RNA, the RNA viruses need to have their own **RNA-dependent polymerase** for replication. The details of RNA replication vary depending on the nature of the viral RNA, both new viral RNA and mRNA being produced from the original viral genome.

After uncoating, viral RNA may serve as its own mRNA. This is then translated, resulting in the formation of an RNA polymerase, which in turn is necessary for the formation of a replicative intermediate form of the viral RNA. This is double stranded, containing one strand from the parent RNA and one that is complementary to it.

At this time a series of **inhibitors** is formed; these effectively switch off the normal synthetic processes of the host cell.

From the double-stranded 'replicative' RNA, single-stranded viral RNA molecules are formed. These may then function in three ways:

1) They may serve as templates for further viral RNA synthesis.
2) They may serve as mRNA for capsid protein synthesis.
3) They may themselves become encapsidated forming mature virions.

Retroviral replication

In one group of RNA viruses, the **retroviruses**, which cause acquired immune deficiency syndrome and are also known to produce neoplasms in many animal species, the pattern of replication is different. Genetic information derived from the virus is inserted into the **host genome** and this inserted segment must, of course, be DNA. The existence of this DNA means that **viral RNA must be copied into DNA**. For viral replication, mRNA must be transcribed from this newly formed DNA in order for new viral proteins to be synthesized.

The formation of the DNA replica from the viral RNA is accomplished by a unique enzyme system known as **RNA-dependent DNA polymerase (reverse transcriptase)**. This DNA replica, the proviral DNA, is then integrated into the host cell DNA. Transcription from the provirus is mediated by host cell RNA polymerases. The transcribed RNA then serves both as mRNA for the synthesis of viral antigens and as genomic RNA which is packaged into new virions.

The properties of an archetypal retrovirus, HIV-1, are described on pp. 191–196.

During all the events that follow penetration of the virions into the host cells, virus particles cannot be detected within the infected cells. This is known as the **eclipse phase**. Its length varies from virus to virus, ranging from minutes in the case of certain bacterial viruses (**bacteriophages**) to hours in the case of some viruses infecting more complex life forms.

Once new viruses have been assembled they are **released** from the infected cell. This may occur by:

- bursting or lysis of the host cell
- budding from the host cell membrane.

In budding the host cell is not destroyed and the virus frequently becomes enveloped. The viral glycoproteins constituting the envelope are inserted into the plasma membrane of the host cell in the form of spikes. Beneath this there may be a matrix protein (M protein) which serves as an attachment point for the nucleocapsid. This altered segment of the host cell plasma membrane is wrapped round the nucleocapsid and the completed virion can then bud off from the cell in which replication has taken place (*Fig. 17.3*).

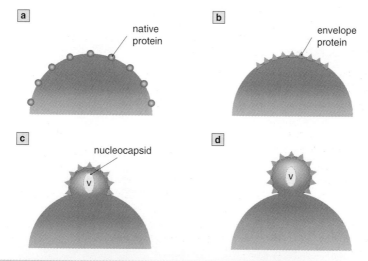

Fig. 17.3 **Release of an RNA virus by budding from the cell surface.**

a Surface membrane of the host cell with 'native' proteins. **b** A segment of the host cell membrane expresses the virally coded envelope proteins. **c** The nucleocapsid adheres to the altered segment of the host cell surface membrane. **d** The altered segment of the cell surface membrane becomes wrapped round the nucleocapsid.

MORPHOLOGICAL AND FUNCTIONAL EFFECTS OF VIRUSES ON HOST CELLS

The range of structural changes produced by viral infections is extensive (see *Fig. 17.4*).

No change

Cells in which the viral infection is of the **latent** variety show no structural abnormalities.

Cell death

Cell death is an extremely common outcome of viral infection. The type of cell affected may play a dominant role in determining the clinical pattern of the disease, as for example in poliomyelitis where death of neurones in the anterior horn of the spinal cord leads to flaccid paralysis. In cell culture systems, the morphology of the changes leading to cell death produced by different viruses may be so distinctive as to be useful in diagnosis.

The cause of cell death in viral infections is not always obvious. Sometimes it may be due to **cell lysis** caused by the release of large numbers of newly formed virions. More often, however, cell death is caused by **cessation of the normal synthetic activity** of the target cell due to

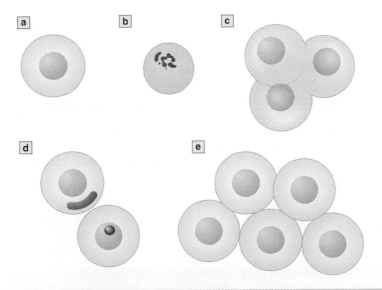

Fig. 17.4 **The effects of viruses on their target cells.**

a No change (latency); **b** cell death; **c** cell fusion; **d** formation of inclusion bodies; **e** cell proliferation.

suppression by virus-specified proteins, not all of which are components of the virion.

Cell death is not always caused directly by replicating virus. In some instances, the presence of virus may lead to the expression of virally coded proteins on the cell surface. These are recognized as foreign by the immune system and immune-mediated lysis of the infected cells follows (see pp. 177–178).

Alterations to cell surface membranes

Some viruses, especially certain members of the paramyxovirus group, cause **fusion** between infected and non-infected cells, with the formation of multinucleated giant cells. This is seen not uncommonly in the tissues of patients suffering from **measles**, the giant cells being found chiefly, but not exclusively, in lymphoid tissue. The highly characteristic mulberry-like giant cells are known as **Warthin–Finkeldey cells** and may be useful in the diagnosis of measles in tissue sections from patients dying from measles pneumonia.

Formation of inclusion bodies

An inclusion body is a localized change detected on light microscopy in the staining properties of either the nucleus or cytoplasm of cells that have been infected by certain viruses. *Inclusion bodies are rounded, sharply demarcated areas which usually show a marked affinity for acid dyes and are thus strongly eosinophilic in sections stained with haematoxylin and eosin.*

Intracytoplasmic inclusions are found in cells infected by **poxviruses**, paramyxoviruses and reoviruses. In one of the rhabdoviral infections (rabies), pathognomonic inclusions are present in neurones within the brain and spinal cord (**Negri bodies**).

Intranuclear inclusions may be present in cells infected by herpesviruses and adenoviruses.

Inclusion bodies can be helpful in the diagnosis of certain viral infections. For example, if difficulty were experienced in distinguishing between a severe case of chickenpox (varicella) and smallpox, examination of cells scraped from a lesion would reveal intranuclear inclusions in the former and intracytoplasmic ones in the latter. These criteria for diagnosis have been largely superseded by electron microscopy. Most inclusion bodies have been shown either by immunofluorescent or electron microscopic studies to be sites of viral synthesis within the cell. However, sometimes, as in herpesvirus infections, the inclusions do not consist of viral elements and may represent accumulations of byproducts of viral replication.

Cell proliferation

Independent of any tumour-producing effect, some viral infections can cause cells to proliferate. This is seen in a very common self-limiting disorder,

infectious mononucleosis, in which the patients, usually young adults, present with malaise, sore throat and enlarged lymph nodes. Infectious mononucleosis is caused by a herpesvirus, the **Epstein–Barr virus**, the target cell of which is the B lymphocyte. B lymphocytes proliferate and develop new antigens on their cell surface membranes. These virally coded antigens elicit a cytotoxic T-cell reaction which brings the virus-induced B-cell proliferation to an end.

Neoplastic transformation

Viruses are directly implicated in the causation of many neoplastic disorders in non-human species and in some human tumours. This question is discussed in the section dealing with oncogenesis (pp. 536–539).

NATURAL HISTORY OF VIRAL INFECTIONS

Viral infections may be divided into two main groups:

1) Infections that cause **lesions only at the portal of entry** (e.g. influenza and other viral infections of the respiratory tract).
2) Infections associated with **systemic spread**. In this case, viruses travel from the **portal of entry** to the **target organ**, producing the typical disease (e.g. poliomyelitis). In certain viral infections, both local and systemic lesions may occur.

Many of the effects of a viral infection (whether local or systemic) depend on the rate at which viral replication proceeds and whether the infected host cells are killed, either by lysis or by inhibition of their own synthetic processes by viral proteins.

KEY POINTS: CHARACTERISTICS OF VIRUSES

A true virus possesses several basic biological characteristics:

- It contains only **one type of nucleic acid**.
- Viral replication is controlled entirely by this nucleic acid.
- Unlike bacteria, viruses cannot undergo binary fission.
- Viruses lack the genetic information required to produce energy-generating systems.
- Viruses **replicate only intracellularly** and make use of the ribosomes of the host cell in the course of replication. This ability to replicate within host cells is an essential attribute of viral pathogenicity.
- Viral tropism depends on attachment to specific molecules on target cells.
- DNA viruses (with the exception of the poxviruses) replicate within the nucleus of the infected cell.
- RNA viruses (with the exception of orthomyxoviruses and retroviruses) replicate within the cytoplasm.

ACUTE PRODUCTIVE INFECTIONS

When a virus replicates actively within an infected cell and new viruses are released from such a cell, the infection is spoken of as being **productive**. This may lead to an acute illness, often febrile, whose clinical picture is modified by the nature of the cells that are killed. Within a few weeks either the virus is eliminated or the infected person dies.

Not all acute infections, however, produce a clinically apparent disease. In many instances viral infections are subclinical and the only objective evidence that they have occurred is the presence of appropriate antibodies in the plasma.

FAILURE OF VIRAL ELIMINATION

Failure to eliminate virus from an infected host may lead to a number of different situations. Such infections can be:

- **Latent**, in which the virus is not normally detected. The infection persists in an occult, quiescent form with episodes of reactivation in the form of acute, self-limiting illnesses.
- **Chronic**, in which virus may be detected continuously in the host; symptoms may be mild or absent. This is seen typically in infants infected in utero by hepatitis B virus (HBV).
- **Persistent** and **slow**, in which the infection persists and causes a prolonged disease which is slow to develop and often inexorable in its progress.
- **Oncogenic**, in which part of the viral genome is incorporated into the host genome, resulting in malignant transformation.

Latent infections

True latency implies the persistence of virus in such small amounts that ordinary methods fail to detect its presence. However, the virus will usually appear if the infected tissue is cultured, and may be identified by means of labelled viral probes.

Latent infections tend to occur particularly with viruses of the **herpes** group. Amongst the commonest clinical expressions of this are the 'cold sores' or 'fever blisters' that affect many people at frequent intervals throughout their lives (*Fig. 17.5*). These are due to infections with the **herpes simplex virus**, which produces clusters of little vesicles, usually at the mucocutaneous junctions of the lips. The vesicles rupture, leading to painful ulcers that heal without scarring. At various times, often in association with fever, sunburn, menstruation, etc., the vesicular lesions recur, always at the same site. Between these clinical episodes the virus can be recovered only with difficulty or often not at all.

The virus remains latent within the cells of the trigeminal ganglion between attacks and is released from the cells of the ganglion when they are

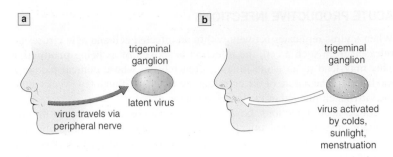

Fig. 17.5   Herpes simplex: an example of latency in viral infection.

a Primary infection leading to latency. **b** Recurrent infection following activation of latent virus ('cold sore').

cultured. The trigeminal ganglion is believed to harbour the herpesvirus in about 80% of adults.

Another virus of the herpes family, the **varicella zoster virus**, provides another common example of latency with occasional reactivation. The latter manifests as herpes zoster or shingles. This is characterized by a painful rash, usually limited to an area of skin or mucous membrane served by a single sensory ganglion. It occurs for the most part in individuals over 50 years of age **and is found only in those who have had chickenpox (varicella) in the past**.

Zoster and varicella are two distinct manifestations of infection by a single virus. Varicella represents the primary infection, and zoster the reactivation of the virus that has lain latent in sensory ganglia since the attack of the varicella, which may have occurred many years before.

Zoster is infectious to those who have not had varicella; infection in such an individual leads to an attack of chickenpox, not of shingles.

Zoster seems to increase in frequency in relation to X-irradiation, and a similar increase is seen in patients suffering from Hodgkin's disease. This suggests that the expression of infection and the appearance of clinical manifestations are controlled by the state of immunity of the host.

Persistent infections

These may be due to:

- well-characterized viral agents such as measles or hepatitis virus
- agents whose nature is unknown.

In the first, the virus is not eliminated from the host and goes on replicating inside infected cells, usually at a rate that does not cause any direct tissue damage. Often the infected individual will **carry** the virus in blood or other tissue fluids; such a patient may be a dangerous source of infection to others. Roughly one-third of patients who have an acute episode of hepatitis due to HBV will become carriers, and there are many more carriers with no history of a diagnosable episode of jaundice.

It is estimated that there may be as many as 300 000 000 carriers of HBV in the world. Obviously there is a considerable risk of the virus being passed on through the medium of blood transfusions, etc., screening of donors for this and, indeed, other carrier states is clearly important. Other types of viral infection in which this asymptomatic carrier state can develop include **cytomegalovirus** and **Epstein–Barr virus** infection.

In some instances chronic asymptomatic infections may lead eventually to the appearance of serious, clinically apparent, disease. An example of this is **lymphocytic choriomeningitis** in the common household mouse. The virus (one of the **arenavirus** family) is transmitted vertically from generation to generation, the infection being acquired in utero. This infection appears to be associated with low zone tolerance in which T lymphocytes are tolerant but B lymphocytes are not. Low levels of antibody to viral antigens are produced and eventually cause the appearance of glomerulonephritis in old mice. The tolerance that develops is associated with the fact that the lymphocytic chorio-meningitis infection occurs during the perinatal period. If mature, immuno-logically competent, mice are infected with this virus, they develop a severe inflammation in the brain (**encephalitis**).

A rather different type of chronic infection is seen in a small number of patients as a result of infection with **measles virus**. The disease, which can follow the very long-continued localization of measles virus in the brain, is known as **subacute sclerosing panencephalitis** (**SSPE**). The peak inci-dence of this, happily rare, condition is during adolescent life. Affected patients present with increasing reduction of intellectual function, motor abnormalities and fits. An inexorable downward path is followed by death within a year of the appearance of symptoms. The patients' brains show degenerative features with loss of myelin and a mild increase in the support-ing glial fibres. There is also evidence of an encephalitis in the form of a perivascular lymphocytic infiltrate. Cerebrospinal fluid contains high titres of measles antibody and viral antigen, and nucleocapsid material can be identified in cells within the brain as well as within lymph nodes. It has been suggested that the disorder is an expression of an aberrant T-cell response to the presence of virus in the brain, but this is still a matter of debate.

Slow progressive infections

The term 'slow virus infection' describes certain very slowly developing and chronic diseases in sheep, originally observed in Iceland, caused by members of the **lentivirus** group: **visna** and **maedi**.

In animals, slow virus infections occur in three disorders:

- maedi
- visna
- Aleutian mink disease.

Maedi produces a slowly progressive pneumonia in Icelandic sheep. **Visna** produces a progressive demyelinating disease, also of sheep. Both these diseases are caused by retroviruses and are transmissible, with incubation periods of several years.

Aleutian mink disease is a slowly developing syndrome caused by chronic infection by a member of the **parvovirus** group. There is a humoral immune response but this does not succeed in eliminating the virus.

Soluble immune complex formation is a prominent feature and most affected animals develop an immune complex-mediated glomerulonephritis. Other evidence of a disturbance in the regulation of the immune response is present in the form of hypergammaglobulinaemia and antibodies directed against red cell antigens.

Slow infections may be caused by conventional viruses

Subacute sclerosing panencephalitis, described above as a chronic infection, could just as well be regarded as a slow virus infection, because the onset of symptoms usually follows on a considerable period after the original measles infection.

Another slow viral infection in humans is **progressive multifocal leuco-encephalopathy**, a rare disease of the brain leading to focal demyelination in many areas of the white matter. It is caused by infections with members of the **papovavirus** group and occurs only in patients who are immuno-suppressed. Such immunosuppression may be seen in patients with neo-plastic disease involving the lymphoid system, such as Hodgkin's disease, and also in those who are receiving cytotoxic chemotherapy in the course of treatment for malignant disease. The papovaviruses isolated from the brains of affected individuals (the JC virus) are widespread, at least in Europe and the USA, and papovavirus infections in the general population are usually acquired fairly early in life.

Creutzfeldt–Jakob disease and other transmissible spongiform encephalopathies

There is a group of slow, relentlessly progressive, dementing disorders of the central nervous system which occur in both humans and animals. While they are clearly **transmissible**, they do not appear to be caused by agents with the characteristics of true viruses or indeed of any living agent. These disorders have been termed the **spongiform encephalopathies** because of the histo-logical changes seen in the central nervous system.

The 'infective' agents concerned are unique in that they have not been shown to contain any nucleic acid and consist of protein only. They have been given the name **prions** (proteinacious infective particles) and are closely related to normal intracerebral proteins encoded by a gene, PrP, on chromosome 20. Prions represent abnormal forms of the PrP proteins and appear to produce their effects by causing abnormal folding (β-pleating) of normal PrP protein.

Human prion-related diseases may be:

- inherited (Gerstmann–Sträussler–Scheinker syndrome, fatal familial insomnia, some cases of Creutzfeldt–Jakob disease)
- sporadic (Creutzfeldt-Jakob disease)
- related to ingestion of abnormal prions (kuru, bovine spongiform encephalopathy [BSE], new variant Creutzfeldt–Jakob disease which is believed to be acquired through eating beef from animals with BSE)
- related to transmission of abnormal prion-related proteins via hormone replacement (human growth hormone), insertion of allogeneic human tissue (dura mater and cornea).

Transforming infections

Viruses can produce **malignant neoplasms** in a variety of animal species and play a part in the induction of some human neoplasms. They can also induce transformation of cells (chiefly of connective tissue origin) in culture. Viral transformation of this type is discussed on pp. 489–491.

PROTECTIVE RESPONSES OF HOST CELLS AGAINST VIRAL INFECTIONS

INTERFERONS

The term **viral interference** is used to describe the situation in which a viral infection appears to protect against subsequent infections by another virus in the same animal.

In 1957, Isaacs and Lindemann showed that cells infected with inactivated influenza virus released soluble compounds into the culture medium which inhibited replication of influenza virus within other cells. The blanket term 'interferon' (IFN) has been applied to these inhibiting host-coded proteins, which constitute an important line of defence against viral infections.

Many interferons exist and are classified broadly into three groups known as:

1) IFN-α, which is released chiefly from leucocytes
2) IFN-β, released chiefly from fibroblasts
3) IFN-γ, released by activated T lymphocytes.

Despite this tendency to identify certain interferons predominantly with certain cell types, it is likely that all cells can produce α and β interferons when suitably stimulated.

The most important inducers of IFN-α and IFN-β release are viral infections, although production can be triggered by rickettsiae, protozoa, bacterial endotoxins and even certain synthetic polynucleotides.

Interferons produced by viral infection are **species specific** (i.e. chick interferon will not protect rat or monkey cells against infection), but are not virus specific. They appear between 12 and 48 hours after infection, and shortly after their appearance viral replication starts to decline. They are extremely powerful; it has been estimated that fewer than 50 molecules of interferon per infected cell suffice to inhibit viral replication.

The stimulus to interferon production in virus-infected cells appears to be foreign double-stranded RNA formed in the course of viral replication. How this induces the formation of the interferons is not known (*Fig. 17.6*).

Action of interferon

The protective effect of interferon is not limited to a single virus because, unlike antibody, it does not interact directly with the virus. The interferon secreted by an infected cell diffuses from that cell and binds to a membrane receptor on the surface of neighbouring non-infected cells. IFN-α and IFN-β bind to the same receptor, that for IFN-γ being quite distinct. IFN binding triggers tyrosine kinase activity, leading to the transcription of genes encoding enzymes that block viral replication.

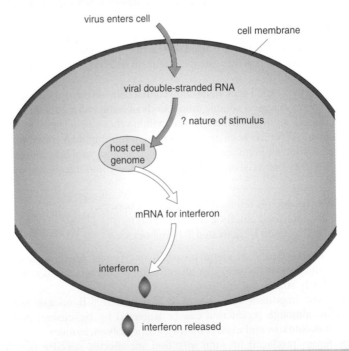

Fig. 17.6 Production of interferon in a cell infected by a virus.

There is no inhibition of viral attachment or penetration of the cell to which the interferon has bound. The protective effect is mediated by blocking the translation of viral mRNA in the host cell polyribosomes. There are two ways in which this can be done.

1) Cells to which interferon has bound contain increased amounts of an adenine trinucleotide, which activates a ribonuclease that can destroy certain mRNAs.
2) Bound interferon stimulates a protein kinase which phosphorylates and thus inactivates a protein initiation factor, thus inhibiting synthesis of viral protein.

In both these situations double-stranded RNA is required, so that the inhibition of translation occurs only in cells infected by a virus (*Fig. 17.7*).

Other effects of interferon

In addition to the protection of cells against viral infection outlined above, the interferons have other actions. At high dose levels some interferons, especially IFN-α, can inhibit cell proliferation and this has drawn attention

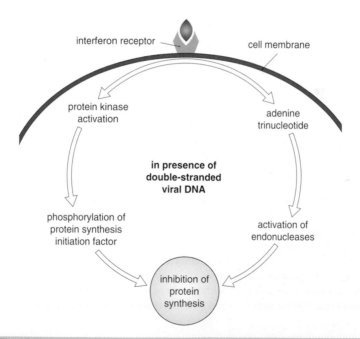

Fig. 17.7 Interferon binds to a non-infected cell and blocks translation of the viral messenger RNA.

to a possible role for them as **antitumour agents**. Unfortunately, high doses of interferons are associated with a number of unpleasant side-effects such as nausea, loss of hair, fever, and depression of platelet and leucocyte production by the bone marrow. The interferons also have an effect on some immune functions, being associated with increased T-cell and natural killer cell activity and decreased antibody formation.

PROTECTIVE RESPONSE OF THE IMMUNE SYSTEM

The ways in which the elements of the immune system respond to viral infections are discussed in Chapter 10.

A BRIEF CLASSIFICATION OF VIRUSES

Most known viruses can be separated into clearly defined groups on the basis of a number of criteria:

- the type and form of the nucleic acid genome
- the size and morphology of the virus
- the natural method of transmission from host to host
- susceptibility to a variety of chemical and physical agents
- viral preference for certain hosts, tissues and cells
- the diseases they cause (see *Table 17.1*).

DNA-CONTAINING VIRUSES

Poxviruses

The poxviruses are divided into two subfamilies depending on whether they affect vertebrates or not. In humans the variola virus caused **smallpox** (now eradicated), and others cause **vaccinia** (cowpox), **alastrim** and a curious disorder characterized by waxy nodules on the skin and trunk known as **molluscum contagiosum**.

Many poxviruses infect non-human species exclusively; some, however, such as the viruses causing **orf**, **cowpox** and **monkeypox**, may rarely cause disease both in animals and humans.

Some poxviruses, notably vaccinia, produce a growth factor that shows homology with both epidermal growth factor and transforming growth factor α; indeed the vaccinia growth factor has been shown to enhance wound healing. This growth factor production by poxviruses may be associated with the recognized ability of some of them to cause proliferative lesions in animals (e.g. Shope fibroma) and humans (molluscum contagiosum).

Table 17.1 Viruses and the diseases they cause

Disease	Virus
General diseases, in which blood spread of viruses occurs and many organs are affected	Vaccinia Measles Rubella Chickenpox Yellow fever Dengue Enteroviruses
Localized diseases	
Nervous system	Poliovirus Coxsackie Echoviruses Rabies Insect-borne encephalitides Herpes simplex Mumps Measles Vaccinia Papovaviruses (JC and BK)
Respiratory tract	Influenza Parainfluenza Respiratory syncytial virus Adenovirus Viruses causing the common cold
Skin and mucous membranes	HSV type 1 (mainly oral) HSV type 2 (mainly genital) Molluscum contagiosum HPV (warts) Herpes zoster
Eye	Adenovirus (conjunctivitis) Herpesvirus (keratoconjunctivitis) Enterovirus 70 (epidemic haemorrhagic conjunctivitis)
Liver	Hepatitis A Hepatitis type B Hepatitis type C Hepatitis type D Hepatitis type E Yellow fever In the newborn: Herpesvirus Enteroviruses Rubella virus
Salivary glands	Mumps Cytomegalovirus
Sexually transmitted diseases	HSV Hepatitis B HPV Molluscum contagiosum HIV-1 and HIV-2 Cytomegalovirus
Gastrointestinal tract	Rotavirus Norwalk virus Enteric adenoviruses

HSV, herpes simplex virus; HPV, human papillomavirus.

KEY POINTS: POXVIRUSES

- The viruses of the pox group are the largest and most complicated known.
- They are brick-shaped or elliptical and contain double-stranded DNA.
- The nucleocapsid is enveloped by a double membrane.
- Poxviruses are unique in that they replicate solely within the cytoplasm of the host cell, where the site of the viral replication may appear as an inclusion body.

Herpesviruses

Herpesviruses are classified on the basis of their biological activities. Thus we have:

- α-herpesviruses – fast growing, cytolytic and tending to establish latent infections in neurones
- β-herpesviruses – slow growing and causing enlargement of the cells they infect (cytomegaly)
- γ-herpesviruses which infect lymphoid cells and cause them to proliferate (e.g. Epstein–Barr virus).

Herpesviruses are responsible for **cold sores** and **genital blistering** (herpes simplex virus), chickenpox (varicella) and **shingles** (zoster), **infectious mononucleosis** (Epstein–Barr virus) and cytomegalovirus-associated disorders, some of which occur in the context of intrauterine infections of the fetus with severe consequences. Herpesvirus type I can also produce a severe **encephalitis**, **keratoconjunctivitis** characterized by keratitis and/or corneal ulceration, and **Kaposi's varicelliform eruption** (a severe and extensive blistering disorder of the skin that tends to occur in those with chronic eczema). The Epstein–Barr virus (a γ-herpesvirus) probably also plays a role in the induction of Burkitt's lymphoma and nasopharyngeal carcinoma. Evidence has also appeared recently that a novel type of herpesvirus (herpesvirus VIII) is implicated in Kaposi's sarcoma.

KEY POINTS: HERPESVIRUSES

- Viruses of this group are large (the nucleocapsids measuring 90–110 nm and the enveloped forms 120–200 nm in diameter).
- The viral genome consists of double-stranded DNA.
- The capsid possesses icosahedral symmetry and is surrounded by a lipid-containing envelope.
- There is little DNA homology among the different herpesvirus types and even different strains of the same type show considerable DNA differences. This has made possible the epidemiological tracing of different strains.
- The virus forms intranuclear inclusion bodies (known as Cowdry type A bodies), which are rich in DNA and virtually fill the nucleus.

Adenoviruses

Adenoviruses can be divided into seven main groups on the basis, inter alia, of the animal species whose red cells they agglutinate. They can be further subdivided into 33 subtypes on the basis of antigenic differences in hexon and fibre proteins. Of the subtypes that cause infection in humans, many exhibit **latency** and may survive in lymphoid tissue such as the tonsil for many years.

The disorders caused in humans by adenoviruses are summarized in *Table 17.2.*

Table 17.2 Adenoviral diseases

System affected	Disease
Respiratory tract	**Acute febrile pharyngitis:** affects infants and children most commonly; usually caused by group C viruses. Patients complain of stuffy nose, cough, sore throat and fever.
	Pharyngoconjunctival fever: symptoms as above but conjunctivitis is also present. This disorder tends to occur in outbreaks in closed communities such as children's summer camps. Usually caused by group B viruses.
	Acute respiratory disease: characterized by fever, pharyngitis, cough and malaise. Tends to occur in young military recruits and is associated with overcrowding and fatigue. Caused by group B viruses.
	Pneumonia: this is a complication of acute respiratory disease. It may affect children as well as young adults and the mortality rate among the former is high (8–10%). Severe adenoviral pneumonia also occurs in immunocompromised individuals such as post-transplant patients.
Eye	**Mild self-limiting conjunctivitis** associated with respiratory and pharyngeal syndromes.
	Follicular conjunctivitis resembling that caused by Chlamydia; self-limiting.
	Epidemic keratoconjunctivitis: acute conjunctivitis associated with enlargement of the preauricular nodes. This is followed by corneal inflammation with the formation of subepithelial corneal opacities, which last for up to 2 years.
Gut	**Infantile gastroenteritis:** this can occur in the presence of infection by two adenovirus serotypes (40 and 41).
Other	**Acute haemorrhagic cystitis:** this occurs in boys and is particularly associated with infections by types 11 and 21.

KEY POINTS: ADENOVIRUSES

- Like the herpesviruses, the adenoviruses are also medium sized (70–90 nm).
- They contain double-stranded DNA and are icosahedral.
- Most of the 252 capsomeres are hexons but 12 are pentons in which the cytotoxic potential of these viruses resides. From the pentons that form the corners of the virion, fine fibres project, each terminating in a knob-like structure. These terminal knobs are responsible for the agglutination of red blood cells and for adhesion to host cells.
- The nucleocapsid is not enveloped and the virus resists treatment with ether.
- Viral replication occurs within the host cell nucleus.

Papovaviruses

This family derives its name from its three members:

- *pa*pillomavirus
- *po*lyomavirus
- *va*cuolating virus in monkeys.

Gene products of these viruses may bind with proto-oncogenes and activate them. For example, the middle T antigen of simian virus 40 (SV40) complexes with the c-*src* gene product and activates its tyrosine kinase function. Similarly, gene products of both polyoma and papilloma viruses can bind with the gene products of tumour suppressor genes and inactivate them (see pp. 504, 506).

KEY POINTS: PAPOVAVIRUSES

- These viruses are small (43–53 nm) and contain double-stranded DNA arranged in a circular pattern.
- In animals, papillomaviruses cause a variety of neoplasms; in humans they cause the common wart and almost certainly have a role in the pathogenesis of cervical neoplasia and other squamous neoplasms of the genital region.
- Polyomavirus infections (JC virus) are also associated with **progressive multifocal encephalopathy**, a rare degenerative condition of the cerebral white matter seen in immunosuppressed patients, usually with malignant lymphomas.

Parvoviruses

Human parvovirus B19 is the cause of a number of diseases.

KEY POINTS: PARVOVIRUSES

- As their name implies (*parvus*, small), these are very small viruses with a diameter of about 20 nm.
- They contain single-stranded DNA and their replication takes place in the nucleus of the infected cell.
- Parvovirus infection in humans causes:
  a) temporary erythroid aplasia in patients with chronic haemolytic anaemia (e.g. sickle cell disease)
  b) a common rash illness of childhood (erythema infectiosum or 'fifth disease')
  c) one variety of gastroenteritis occurring particularly in cold weather ('winter vomiting disease').

Hepadnaviruses

There is only one virus in this group causing disease in humans: the hepatitis B virus. There are many types, however, that cause hepatitis in animals such as woodchucks, squirrels and ducks. The small number of susceptible species reflects a lack in most species of cell surface receptors for the lipoprotein envelope of the virus.

The viral DNA is arranged in a peculiar pattern with one long circular strand containing the whole genome and an incomplete complementary strand comprising 50–70% of the genome. There are four open reading frames, three of which encode the surface and core antigens and DNA polymerase; the product of the fourth ORF is not yet known. In addition to DNA polymerase, the viral core contains two antigens: the core antigen (HbcAg) and the e antigen (HbeAg). The presence of e antigen in serum indicates:

- active viral replication
- infectivity of the serum
- on-going liver cell damage.

The viral core is enclosed in a surface coat composed of lipid, protein and carbohydrate expressing a surface antigen (HbsAg). This surface coat may be synthesized in excess and appear in serum, under the electron microscope, as either small spherical particles or tubules. The complete virion may also appear in plasma as a 43 nm diameter double shelled particle with an electron-dense core (the Dane particle).

Viral transmission occurs via two principal routes:

- *vertical*, i.e from mother to infant at or shortly after birth
- *horizontal*, i.e between adults following exposure to infected blood, blood products or body fluids such as semen and saliva.

Horizontal transmission occurs under the following circumstances:

- use of infected needles by drug abusers
- in the course of tattooing
- as a result of sexual intercourse.

The range of effects of infection by the hepatitis B virus is shown in *Fig. 17.8*. Chronicity is an important sequel: 300–400 million people are believed to have a chronic HBV infection.

Several other hepatotrophic viruses exist; these are discussed in larger texts.

RNA-CONTAINING VIRUSES

Picornaviruses

This group is divided into the enteroviruses and the rhinoviruses.
Enteroviruses include:

- three types of **poliovirus**.
- 29 types of **coxsackievirus**.
- 32 types of **echovirus** (enteric cytopathic human orphan virus); the term 'orphan' refers to the fact that for some time they were regarded as 'viruses in search of a disease'.

The enteroviruses cause a wide range of diseases in humans, including **poliomyelitis**, **aseptic meningitis**, **myocarditis** (chiefly in the newborn), **myositis**, **herpangina** and **upper respiratory tract infections**.

Infection occurs via both the **alimentary** and **respiratory** tracts, the former being much more important in the case of poliovirus infection. There is no natural animal host. This has interesting implications in respect of poliovirus, of which there are only three types. Vaccines have been prepared against all of these and it is quite possible that, following widespread immunization, the disease may be eliminated in a similar way to smallpox.

Most poliovirus infections are symptomless but the virus, which is cytocidal, may spread to involve the anterior horn cells with resulting paralysis. (The pathogenesis of full-blown poliovirus infections of this kind is shown in *Fig. 17.2*.)

Rhinoviruses cause the common cold.

KEY POINTS: PICORNAVIRUSES

- Picornaviruses (*pico*, small) are very small (2–30 nm), non-enveloped, icosahedral viruses.
- They contain single-stranded RNA and are resistant to treatment with ether.
- This family includes important human pathogens, including the viruses responsible for poliomyelitis and the common cold.
- The picornaviruses are divided into two genera: the **enteroviruses** and the **rhinoviruses**.

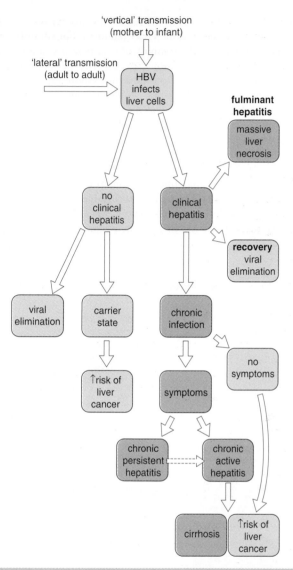

Fig. 17.8   Consequences of HBV infection.

Orthomyxoviruses

The acute respiratory disease caused by the **influenza virus** in humans can be fatal. Influenza may occur in very large-scale local epidemics, usually every 2–4 years, or even on a world-wide basis (pandemics) every 10–20 years. A single influenza virus infection does *not* confer lifelong immunity to the disease. An important part of the reason for this curious epidemiological behaviour lies in the fact that the **viral genome is continually changing**.

Minor changes in the haemagglutinins of a particular strain may occur as a result of a series of point mutations; over a long period, this process is called **antigenic drift**. From time to time a much more fundamental change occurs in which multiple alterations suddenly appear in the antigenic make-up of the viral strain, probably as a result of recombination of genome segments. This is known as **antigenic shift**. The appearances of new subtypes of influenza virus as a result of antigenic shift are likely to be associated with the occurrence of pandemic outbreaks. Of the three types of influenza virus – A, B and C – A is the most likely to undergo antigenic shift and is responsible for most epidemics of influenza. Type B and C viruses do not undergo antigenic shift, C being the most stable.

The pathogenesis of influenza is shown in *Fig. 17.9*. Sporadic cases are usually fairly mild and self-limiting. Sometimes, especially in the elderly,

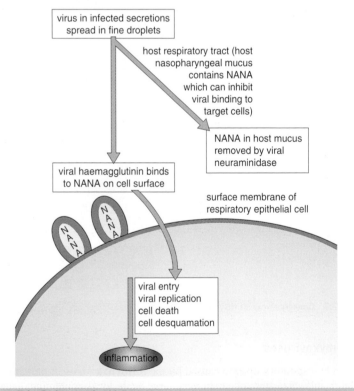

Fig. 17.9   Pathogenesis of influenza.

NANA, *N*-acetylneuraminic acid.

severe pneumonia supervenes. This is most commonly due to a secondary bacterial infection, although in rare instances it is a primary viral pneumonia in which intrapulmonary haemorrhage is a conspicuous feature.

KEY POINTS: ORTHOMYXOVIRUSES

- As defined currently, the orthomyxoviruses contain only viruses that cause human influenza.
- They are medium sized with a helically arranged capsid, contain single-stranded DNA and are enveloped. The lipid envelope is somewhat unusual in that it is studded with spike-like projections called peplomers. These are of two varieties, the first being a viral haemagglutinin which binds to the NANA on the surface membrane of most cells, and the second being a neuraminidase.
- In morphological terms they are pleomorphic, some viruses being spherical in shape whereas others are filamentous.
- The arrangement of the RNA is distinctly unusual. Instead of being a continuous thread, it exists in the form of eight segments, each of which represents a single gene. These eight gene segments code for 10 or 11 viral proteins, this being explained by the pattern of splicing of two of the mRNAs.

Paramyxoviruses

Viruses of this group cause:

- sore throats and croup (parainfluenza virus)
- measles
- mumps
- infections of the lower respiratory tract (respiratory syncytial virus).

In animals, paramyxoviruses cause Newcastle disease in birds, distemper in dogs, and rinderpest in cattle.

One of the interesting characteristics of viruses of this family is that they promote cell fusion with the formation of multinucleate cells (see p. 299). This feature has been used extensively in the production of hybrid cells, the virus employed for this purpose being Sendai virus (which causes parainfluenza in mice). The ability to promote cell fusion is conferred on the virus by its possession of a spike on the envelope glycoprotein. This glycoprotein is also necessary for penetration of the target cell; strains that lack the F glycoprotein are not infective.

KEY POINTS: PARAMYXOVIRUSES

- These viruses were originally grouped with the orthomyxoviruses because of the morphological features that they share.
- They are roughly cuboid in shape.
- They are somewhat larger than orthomyxoviruses, but share with them a number of characteristics such as the presence of haemagglutinins and neuraminidase (which, in contrast to what is seen in the influenza virus, coexist on the same 'spike' on the envelope).

Rhabdoviruses

Rabies

Many warm-blooded animals such as dogs, foxes, bats, skunks and jackals are reservoirs for rabies virus. Victims of the disease are infected by the bite of a rabid animal, the virus being present in the saliva. The rabies virus appears to have a special affinity for nervous tissue and travels slowly up the peripheral nerves to reach the central nervous system where it causes the encephalitis characteristic of the disease.

In experimental rabies infections, where it is possible to examine specimens of peripheral nerves, viral particles have been seen in the axons on electron microscopy.

KEY POINTS: RHABDOVIRUSES

- Viruses of this group have a curious shape, being flattened at one end and rounded at the other.
- The genome consists of single-stranded RNA.
- The nucleocapsid is enclosed in an envelope which bears spikes of about 10 nm in length.
- This group includes the rabies virus, which causes one of the most serious of all viral infections.

Arenaviruses

Arenaviruses derived their name from the Latin word *harenaceus* meaning 'sandy'. This term was coined because of the electron-dense granules that can be seen within the virions on electron microscopy.

The natural hosts of arenaviruses appear to be rodents, which are often persistently infected. Humans are infected more or less by accident on exposure to rodent excretions. The resulting infections include some of the most lethal viral disorders known: Lassa fever and Argentinian and Bolivian haemorrhagic fevers. The natural host of the Lassa fever virus is a West African rodent, the multimammate rat, which is persistently but apparently harmlessly infected.

Another example of arenavirus infection in animals discussed earlier in this chapter is the virus that causes **lymphocytic choriomeningitis** in mice (see p. 303).

Coronaviruses

Viruses of this family include several which cause the common cold. They are medium sized, rather pleomorphic, viruses with widely spaced club-shaped peplomers in their lipoprotein envelope; it is the arrangement of these 'clubs' that gives this virus its distinctive appearance and its name.

Togaviruses

Togaviruses are spherical, closely enveloped, RNA viruses containing single-stranded RNA. They multiply within the cytoplasm of target cells and mature by budding from cytoplasmic membranes. All togaviruses, with the exception of rubella, belong to a larger grouping known as the **arboviruses** (*ar*thropod-*bo*rne viruses). Arthropods are not only the vectors for these viral infections, but are the primary natural **hosts** in which viral multiplication occurs before transmission to a secondary vertebrate host by insect bite. These vertebrates act as a **reservoir** for the viruses and are unaffected by the presence of the arboviruses. However, when humans (an unnatural host) are infected, serious and often lethal disorders arise, such as **yellow fever**, various encephalitides and some of the haemorrhagic fevers. In the course of biting, the virus in the saliva of the insect is injected into human capillaries. Viral multiplication occurs in the first instance in the vascular endothelium and in the fixed phagocytic cells of the reticuloendothelial system. There is a short-lived viraemia, which may be followed by a variety of clinical developments, depending on the precise nature of the virus and its localization. In the haemorrhagic fevers, bleeding occurs from many sites and death may result from hypovolaemic shock. In yellow fever, the liver and kidneys are affected, leading to jaundice and impaired renal function. There is massive necrosis in the mid-zones of the liver lobules and, as a consequence, a decrease in the synthesis of clotting factors formed in the liver.

Rubella

Rubella virus is a member of the togavirus family but is not transmitted via an insect vector and is classified as being in the genus **Rubivirus**. Infection by the rubella virus has no serious consequences unless it occurs in utero, especially in the first three months of pregnancy. When this happens there is a high risk that the infant will be born with a wide range of congenital defects, most notably in the heart, ears (nerve deafness) and eyes (cataract). Many other organs may be affected, and hepatitis and pneumonia in the neonatal period are quite common. The risks are so serious that rubella occurring in the first three months of a pregnancy constitutes good grounds for termination of that pregnancy. To prevent intrauterine infection with the rubella virus, girls may be immunized with an attenuated viral vaccine in their early teens. Alternatively, the vaccine may be given to all children in an attempt to eliminate the infection altogether.

Reoviruses

The acronym reo is derived from respiratory, enteric and orphan. This is because the initial sites of isolation were the respiratory and gastrointestinal tracts, and because no diseases were known to be associated with this group of viruses (hence 'orphan'). Three genera are known, of which only two, **rotavirus** and **orbivirus**, cause disease in humans.

- **Orbivirus** is an arbovirus and causes Colorado tick fever.
- **Rotavirus** has a curious double-layered capsid, the outer layer appearing smooth on electron microscopy and the inner layer symmetrically 'roughened'. This gives the virion a wheel-like appearance, hence the name (L. *rota*, wheel).

Rotaviruses are an important cause of gastroenteritis, mainly in young children. They also cause a similar syndrome in a variety of young animals. Diagnosis of gastroenteritis caused by these viruses can be made by examining stool samples, either by electron microscopy, as the highly characteristic virions are present in large numbers in the faeces, or by immunological methods.

The severe diarrhoea is caused by a viral protein (NSP4) which acts like a viral 'exotoxin' causing severe fluid and electrolyte loss. Rotavirus is said to cause 125 million episodes of diarrhoea annually in children in developing countries, and almost 1 million of these children die.

Retroviruses

Retroviruses occur in many vertebrate species and are implicated in many diseases. All have a diploid RNA genome which encodes **reverse transcriptase** (RNA-dependent DNA polymerase). The retroviral genome consists of at least three genes: *gag*, *pol* and *env*. *Gag* encodes a precursor protein that is cleaved, yielding internal structural proteins; the reverse transcriptase is encoded by *pol* and the two disulphide-linked envelope proteins by *env*.

The retrovirus family is divided into three subfamilies:

1) oncovirinae, which includes tumour-producing viruses
2) lentivirinae, which includes HIV and the non-primate viruses causing maedi and visna
3) spumavirinae or foamy viruses.

Human retroviruses

Four major classes of human retroviruses are recognized:

- human T-cell lymphotropic oncoviruses: HTLV-1 and HTLV-2
- human T-cell lymphotropic lentiviruses: HIV
- foamy viruses; these may be implicated in causing a granulomatous thyroiditis (de Quervain's thyroiditis) but this is not proven
- endogenous retroviruses.

Only HIV and HTLV are clearly linked with human disease (see pp. 190–196).

Oncornaviruses

These are oncogenic RNA viruses belonging to the family Retroviridae. They are responsible for the production of a wide variety of neoplasms of connective, lymphoid and haemopoietic tissue in a number of different animal species. They are also capable of inducing malignant transformation in cultured cells. This involves insertion of part of the viral genome into the genome of the target cell. As the viral genome consists only of RNA, clearly some mechanism must exist for transcribing DNA from the viral RNA; this is accomplished via the action of a virally coded enzyme system known as **reverse transcriptase**. The activity of these viruses is discussed on pp. 489–493).

GENERAL PATHOLOGY OF VIRAL INFECTION

- Viruses are very small, obligate, intracellular parasites.
- They are responsible for over 60% of infectious illnesses.
- A virus possesses only one type of nucleic acid, either DNA or RNA; unlike bacteria it cannot undergo binary fission and so it uses the ribosomes of infected cells to synthesize and assemble viral proteins
- Viruses may kill, persist within, or transform infected cells so that they proliferate to an abnormal degree.
- Some of the cell injury that occurs in certain viral diseases returns from the reaction of the immune system to viral proteins expressed on the surfaces of infected cells (e.g. hepatitis B).
- Many viruses infect only certain cell types (**viral tropism**). This is due to binding between viral surface molecules and target cell receptors (e.g. HIV binds to glycoprotein receptors on T helper cells and by destroying these cells causes immune deficiency).
- In addition to the actions of the cells of the immune system, cells protect themselves in many viral infections by releasing glycoproteins known as **interferons**.

18 The pathological bases of ischaemia I: atherosclerosis

Ischaemia defines a state in which the arterial perfusion of an organ or tissue falls short of its metabolic needs.

Any pathological change that either narrows or blocks an artery is likely to produce ischaemia in the tissue it supplies distal to the point of narrowing or occlusion. In arteries, such narrowing is usually brought about by a widely prevalent disease of the wall of large elastic and muscular arteries known as **atherosclerosis**.

Occlusion of arteries is caused by **platelets**, first adhering to an abnormal vascular surface and later aggregating to form a plug capable of blocking the artery. Such a plug, which can form very rapidly is a **thrombus** – a solid mass formed within the heart, arteries, veins and capillaries from the components of streaming blood. The process of thrombus formation is known as **thrombosis** and is a frequent complication of atherosclerosis.

In the Western World the complications of atherosclerosis kill more people than any other single disease, including all the forms of cancer. More than 150 000 patients die each year in Britain alone from the effects of coronary artery narrowing and occlusion (about 25% of all deaths).

WHAT IS ATHEROSCLEROSIS?

The term atherosclerosis is derived from two Greek words – '*sclerosis*' (hardness) and '*athere*' (gruel or porridge). A commonly used synonym is **atheroma**. It owes its adoption to the fact that many atherosclerotic lesions, which consist essentially of localized thickenings in the arterial intima, contain soft material in their deeper portions. This lipid-rich material can ooze out into the arterial lumen and be carried away in the bloodstream if the more superficial parts of the atherosclerotic lesions rupture.

These processes together lead to the formation of the raised, fully developed, advanced **fibrolipid plaque**. Such lesions are common and do not necessarily cause symptoms. Fibrolipid plaques are the archetype of atherosclerosis. The more extensive they are in a given population, the greater is the frequency of acute occlusive arterial events. However, it should be remembered that there will always be a few unfortunate individuals who have few fibrolipid plaques but who develop acute ischaemic heart disease because of thrombosis occurring in relation to a single strategically placed lesion.

Injury to the plaque cap results in acute thrombus formation. This may be clinically silent and lead either to further plaque growth and hence more severe stenosis of the affected arterial segment or to one of the acute syndromes of coronary heart disease.

THE LESIONS OF ATHEROSCLEROSIS

LOW DENSITY LIPOPROTEIN AND THE FATTY STREAK

The earliest morphologically identifiable atherosclerotic lesion is the **fatty streak**. These start as small, lipid-rich, minimally elevated, yellowish dots 1–2 mm in diameter. In the descending aorta, these small lesions lie roughly parallel to the direction of the blood flow and eventually coalesce to form long streaks.

Fatty streak formation starts quite early in life, being present in 45% of infants dying in the first year of life. There is good evidence, from both human and animal studies, that fatty streaks may progress to form advanced plaques. This progression is not inevitable, however, as shown by the fact that the marked geographical differences existing in the extent and severity of arterial involvement by mature fibrolipid plaques are *not* seen in relation to fatty streaks.

Microscopically, fatty streaks show mild intimal thickening associated with an increase in the intimal cell population. The cholesterol-rich lipid is chiefly intracellular at this stage; most of the fat-laden cells are macrophages, though some lipid-containing smooth muscle cells are often present as well. On scanning electron microscopy, the early stages of fatty streak formation in hyperlipidaemic animals are characterized by the appearance of large subendothelial 'humps' covered by an intact layer of endothelial cells. Transmission electron microscopy shows this surface deformation to be due to a mass of lipid-filled cells within the intima. A minority of these are smooth muscle cells but most of the lipid-laden cells are macrophages in which residual bodies containing partly oxidized lipid can be seen. In some instances macrophages lie between separated endothelial cells, half within the intima and half within the arterial lumen. This supports the view that a two-way traffic of monocyte–macrophages exists between the blood and the arterial wall.

The initiation phase of fatty streak formation is best studied in hyper-lipidaemic animals (the Watanabe or St Thomas's rabbit, or fat-fed pri-mates), though identical appearances are seen in humans. Lesion formation is preceded by adhesion of monocytes and T lymphocytes to an intact endo-thelial surface at sites of predilection for lesion development (*Fig. 18.2*). This adhesion is associated with the expression by endothelial cells of adhe-sion molecules of the immunoglobulin gene super-family and selectin type. The adherent cells then migrate into the subendothelial space, differentiate into macrophages and ingest large amounts of lipid, thus becoming 'foam cells'.

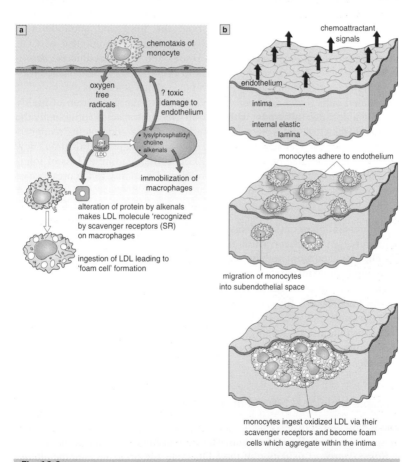

Fig. 18.2

a LDL modification within the arterial intima and its functional effects. **b** Interaction between vessel wall and monocytes in fatty streak formation.

Unlike many other cell types, macrophages cannot bind low density lipo-protein via the LDL receptor. Indeed, both humans and animals with inherited absence or defects of LDL receptors (familial hypercholesterol-aemia in humans) develop very severe and premature atherosclerosis in the lesions of which numerous foam cells are present. Instead, macrophages recognize and bind intra-intimal LDL via a family of novel receptors (**scavenger receptors**) which bind only chemically modified LDL.

Acetylation of LDL leads to its uptake by macrophages. It is now known that incubation of LDL with either endothelial or smooth muscle cells renders the LDL similarly recognizable to macrophages. This is due to the ability of the cultured cells to initiate lipid peroxidation of the LDL.

In vivo the chemical change believed to occur in LDL is **oxidation**; this is probably mediated through the release of reactive oxygen species from endothelium. The oxidation affects both the lipid and apolipoprotein moieties of the LDL molecule. Initially, the lecithin component of LDL phospholipid undergoes conversion to lysolecithin. Lysolecithin is chemo-tactic for monocytes, causes monocytes to become immobilized once they are within the arterial intima and, in ex vivo systems at least, is cytotoxic for endothelial cells. Fatty acid peroxidation leads to the generation of highly reactive aldehydes (**alkenals**) which modify the amino acids (principally the lysine residues) of apoprotein B100 and render the apoprotein 'recogniz-able' to the scavenger receptors. In the course of this modification, new epitopes are generated on the apo B100 molecule, leading to loss of toler-ance for the molecule and antibody formation in response to the presence of modified LDL in the arterial intima.

Evidence supporting the significance of oxidation includes the following:

- Administration of anti-oxidants to congenitally hyperlipidaemic rabbits inhibits fatty streak formation to a considerable extent.
- LDL extracted from both human and rabbit lesions shows the features of having been oxidized.
- Many humans show the presence of antibodies within their plasma which are specific for epitopes of oxidized LDL.
- Some epidemiological evidence exists that there is an inverse correlation between the risk of developing ischaemic heart disease and the dietary consumption of anti-oxidants such as vitamin C, vitamin E and β-carotene.

Possible biological effects of oxidized LDL

The interaction between reactive oxygen species and LDL may be followed by several potentially atherogenic effects other than foam cell formation.

Some degree of oxidation of the LDL molecule occurs before the altered molecule is recognized by the scavenger receptors on the macrophage. At this stage, the LDL is spoken of as being *minimally oxidized*. This minimally oxidized LDL is capable of stimulating the release of a number of potent chemical signals from aortic endothelial cells in culture. These include the stimulators of leucopoiesis – M-CSF, GM-CSF and G-CSF – which may account for the increase in monocyte release from bone marrow occurring in hyperlipidaemic animals. Minimally oxidized LDL can also stimulate secretion of monocyte chemotactic protein 1 (MCP-1) when added to endothelial and smooth muscle cells; in vivo, when it is injected into mice it increases the mRNA expression of the mouse homologue of MCP-1.

Oxidized LDL may also influence arterial functions not directly related to atherogenesis such as the regulation of vascular tone and the platelet and coagulation systems. It impairs the nitric oxide-mediated vasodilatation that occurs in response to such agents as acetylcholine, bradykinin and thrombin, though the precise mechanism of this action is still not understood. In addition oxidized LDL appears to increase the release of tissue factor from macrophages and also increases the release of plasminogen activator inhibitor 1 (PAI-1).

THE FIBROLIPID PLAQUE OR 'RAISED' LESION

Fatty streak progression is associated with the accumulation of a core of extracellular lipid and the migration of smooth muscle cells into the intima where they proliferate and secrete connective tissue proteins thus forming a 'cap' on the luminal side of the lipid core. These processes may result in the formation of large fibrolipid plaques, rich in both connective tissue and lipid. Much of the core lipid is believed to be derived from the release of the intracytoplasmic contents of dead macrophages.

The raised fibrolipid plaque is clearly the substrate on which acute thrombotic complications develop. In a sense, all fibrolipid plaques are the same since all are comprised of the two basic elements: a superficial collagen-rich cap and an underlying, lipid-rich, 'atheromatous' pool or lipid 'core'. In an equally valid sense, all fibrolipid plaques are different since the proportions of 'cap' and 'core' differ from plaque to plaque. The relative proportions of these components are vitally important in the natural history of any fibrolipid plaque. A large 'pool' and a relatively thin 'cap' are associated with a higher risk of plaque injury and consequent thrombosis than is the case where there is a thick cap and comparatively inconspicuous pool.

Important also in this context is the degree to which the **circumference** of any affected arterial segment is involved. If the entire circumference is involved the plaque is termed **concentric**; if only part of the circumference is affected, the plaque is termed **eccentric** (*Fig. 18.3*). In concentric plaques, the splinting effect of the plaque and the atrophic changes in the underlying media lead to a failure to vary the lumen diameter in response to vasomotor signals. Luminal variation is achievable, however, in eccentric lesions. The eccentric variety is heavily over-represented in plaques which have sustained injury with consequent acute thrombosis.

The connective tissue formation characteristic of fibrolipid plaques is mediated by arterial smooth muscle cells. The greater the volume of the

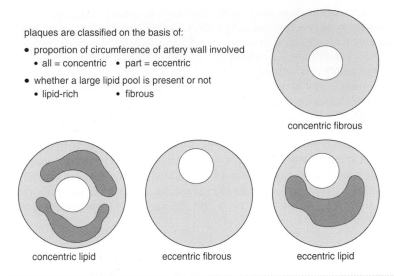

plaques are classified on the basis of:

- proportion of circumference of artery wall involved
  - all = concentric • part = eccentric

- whether a large lipid pool is present or not
  - lipid-rich   • fibrous

concentric fibrous

concentric lipid   eccentric fibrous   eccentric lipid

Fig. 18.3   Types of atherosclerotic plaque.

connective tissue plaque 'cap', the greater the number of smooth muscle cells is likely to be. Smooth muscle cells are often seen in the normal intima of young animals and in humans, in areas of either diffuse or focal non-atherosclerotic intimal thickening. This intimal population of smooth muscle cells is thought to derive from medial cells migrating through gaps in the internal elastic lamina marking the boundary between intima and media.

The role of the smooth muscle cell in atherogenesis and indeed in the response to virtually any form of arterial injury stems from the fact that it can exist in at least two contrasting phenotypes: **contractile** and **synthetic** (*Fig. 18.4*). The functional repertoire of contractile cells appears to be limited to contraction and relaxation; they respond to vasoconstrictor or vasodilator signals such as nitric oxide, prostaglandins, angiotensin II, various neuro-peptides and leukotrienes. The turnover of cells in the contractile phenotype is extremely slow. When medial smooth muscle cells, which represent the archetype of the contractile phenotype, are cultured only about 3% of the cells incorporate tritiated thymidine at any one time and mitoses are not seen in smooth muscle cells of normal arteries.

In contrast, expression of the synthetic phenotype is associated with very rapid proliferation of the smooth muscle cell population in the affected area. In the synthetic state, the smooth muscle cells express genes for a number of growth-regulating factors and cytokines and their response to such growth factors is altered by the expression of appropriate receptors. The very considerable increase in intimal thickness which can occur in non-athero-sclerotic areas as a result of injury or in relation to atherosclerotic plaques over which mural thrombi have formed, is due less to the increase in number

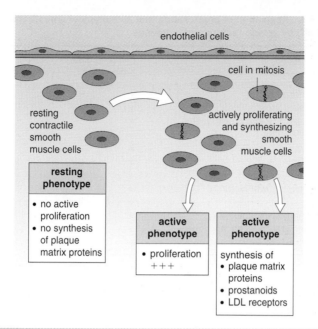

Fig. 18.4   Contrasting functional phenotypes of arterial smooth muscle cells.

of smooth muscle cells than to synthesis and secretion of the extracellular matrix proteins which are found in plaque connective tissue.

This phenotypic modulation of arterial smooth muscle cells is of importance not only in relation to lesion progression but also in relation to the intimal responses leading to re-stenosis following coronary artery angioplasty. Thus, the factors which influence this process are of very great interest.

Migration, proliferation and the stimulation of extracellular matrix synthesis in relation to arterial smooth muscle cells is controlled by a complex web of growth factors, cytokines, vasoactive agents, prostaglandins, leukotrienes, extracellular matrix components and the wide range of receptors for these chemical signals. Both growth factors and cytokines are proteins but it is conventional to distinguish between them, using the term 'cytokine' for those species which, among other functions, regulate immune responses, and the term 'growth factor' for those molecules whose function relates primarily to the control of cell proliferation. It is important to understand that these molecules have many functions and thus a single molecule can produce a wide range of cellular changes at many different levels

To date, no fewer than 30 chemical species which regulate smooth muscle cell growth, migration and phenotype have been identified (see *Table 18.1*).

Table 18.1 Regulation of proliferation and phenotype of smooth muscle cells (SMC) by growth factors and cytokines

Chemical species	Effect on SMC proliferation	Effect on SMC migration
Epidermal growth factor	+	
Basic fibroblast growth factor	++	0
Heparin-binding EGF-like growth factor	++	+
Insulin growth factor-1	+	+
Interferon γ	±	
Interleukin-1	+	
Interleukin-6	+	
Platelet-derived growth factor	+	+
Thrombin	+	
Transforming growth factor α	+	
Transforming growth factor β	±	+
Tumour necrosis factor α	+	

Platelet-derived growth factor as a paradigm for the control of smooth muscle cell proliferation

Much of current knowledge of the impact of growth regulatory factors on smooth muscle cell proliferation and phenotype stems from the studies of Russell Ross and his colleagues in Seattle, who showed that the mitogenic effect of serum derived from clotted whole blood on arterial smooth muscle cells in culture was due to a factor released from platelets (platelet-derived growth factor – PDGF). This term is a misnomer since PDGF is produced by endothelial cells, macrophages and smooth muscle cells themselves, the latter situation representing an autocrine loop (*Fig. 18.5*).

PDGF is a cationic, dimeric protein with a molecular weight of 28–32 kD. The dimer is composed of two homologous polypeptide chains A and B encoded by genes on different chromosomes. The B chain shows a marked degree of homology with the gene product of the proto-oncogene *c-sis*. PDGF binds to high affinity receptors on arterial smooth muscle cells, fibroblasts and other mesenchymal cells, though to date, no receptors have been identified on endothelium. Like other growth factors and cytokines, the expression of PDGF may be modulated by autocrine induction so that PDGF itself induces locally the expression of the genes which code both for the growth factor and its receptor. Cytokines such as IL-1, TNF-α and TGF-β, which are macrophage products, also induce PDGF expression; this suggests that there is a dual mechanism by which macrophages within an atherosclerotic plaque may contribute to the growth of that lesion.

Binding of PDGF to its receptor on smooth muscle cells leads rapidly to a series of intracellular events, only some of which are related to cell migration and proliferation, since smooth muscle cells stimulated by PDGF show an increase in endocytosis, cholesterol synthesis and expression of

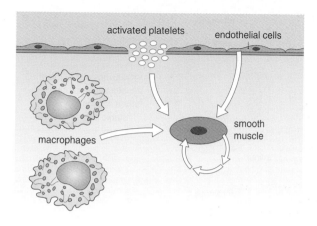

Fig. 18.5   Sources of platelet-derived growth factor in atherogenesis.

LDL receptors. So far as cell proliferation in smooth muscle cell cultures is concerned, exposure to PDGF leads to an increase in DNA synthesis which is maximal between 18 and 24 hours; the cell population doubles within 30 hours. Occupation of the binding site on the smooth muscle cell by the growth factor causes the receptor to act as a tyrosine kinase. As a result cytoplasmic and membrane-associated proteins are phosphorylated and this is followed by expression of the proto-oncogenes *c-myc* and *c-fos*, *c-fos* transcription increasing 50-fold in a very short time. The gene products of both these genes are DNA-binding proteins and are known to be implicated in cell proliferation.

THE GENERATION OF SYMPTOMS IN ATHEROSCLEROSIS

Advanced plaques cause symptoms in three ways (*Fig. 18.6*):

- Plaque growth may cause lesion volume to become so great as to **interfere with blood flow** through the affected segment. Such a process is usually slow and leads to chronic symptoms such as stable angina.
- The plaque may be complicated by **thrombosis**. Major episodes lead to acute and major clinical disturbances. Minor episodes are subclinical but contribute to plaque growth by stimulating smooth muscle cell proliferation.
- Atherosclerosis can be associated with widepread **alteration in endothelial function**, such that **vasoconstrictor responses** occur in situations, such as exercise, where normal arteries would dilate.

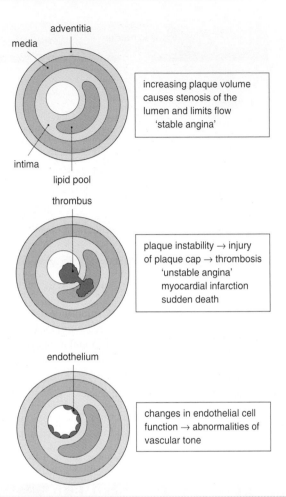

Fig. 18.6   The effects of atherosclerosis.

PLAQUE INJURY AND THROMBOSIS

In most cases, the morphological correlate of potentially life-threatening events such as unstable angina or myocardial infarction is **thrombosis** arising in relation to plaques which have been termed '**unstable**'. The antecedent to such thrombosis is plaque injury, which may be of two types: '**superficial**' or '**deep**' (*Fig. 18.7*).

Superficial plaque injury

Superficial injury can be defined as denudation of the surface endothelium and the most superficial strands of collagen of a fibrolipid plaque. It

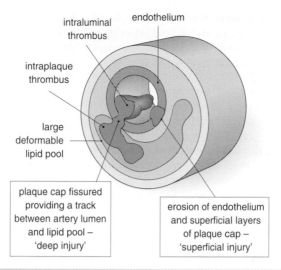

intraluminal thrombus

endothelium

intraplaque thrombus

large deformable lipid pool

plaque cap fissured providing a track between artery lumen and lipid pool – 'deep injury'

erosion of endothelium and superficial layers of plaque cap – 'superficial injury'

Fig. 18.7   Deep and superficial plaque injury and thrombosis.

represents progression of the process of focal endothelial denudation that is very commonly seen on the surface of coronary artery plaques. When large areas of denudation develop, mural or even occlusive thrombi may form. This type of plaque injury precedes about 25% of the thrombi that occur in relation to damaged fibrolipid plaques. Plaques in which such superficial injury occurs tend to be those in which the superficial collagen fibres of the plaque cap are separated by large numbers of foamy, lipid-filled macrophages.

Deep intimal injury (plaque disruption)

The defining criterion of deep intimal injury is the development of a split or tear extending from the plaque surface deep down through the connective tissue cap into the soft underlying atheromatous pool. Blood from the artery lumen enters the plaque and comes into contact with various thromboplastic components, leading to activation of platelets and the clotting cascade. Thus the initial formation of thrombus takes place **within the substance of the plaque itself** and, in some instances, may never extend through the plaque fissure into the lumen of the artery. In other instances the thrombus grows up rapidly through the fissure into the lumen where it may propagate against and/or with the direction of blood flow. Both mural and occlusive thrombosis may occur in this way. It is not without interest that the intra-plaque portion of such a thrombus is usually platelet-rich while the intraluminal part is often relatively poor in platelets and rich in fibrin, a fact which may have considerable implications for the success of thrombolytic therapy.

The **unstable plaque** in which such fissuring is likely to occur is one in which there is a large lipid-rich pool (more than 40% of the plaque volume) especially where this pool is lacking in collagen 'struts' passing from the undersurface of the plaque cap to the deep margins of the pool. Such a large, relatively unsupported pool constitutes a highly deformable region within the plaque (*Fig. 18.8*). Deformation leads to a marked degree of stressing of the plaque connective tissue, especially in the region where the cap connective tissue fuses with lesion-free parts of the arterial intima. In addition these lesions show a significant reduction in the ratio of smooth muscle cells to lipid-filled macrophages. This change in the proportions of these two cell types reflects an absolute increase in the volume of the plaque occupied by macrophages and a corresponding decrease in that occupied by smooth muscle cells. Plaque instability therefore appears to be a function of:

- large amounts of extracellular lipid
- a decrease in the number of smooth muscle cells, and thus a decrease in the amount of extracellular matrix protein which might otherwise serve to stabilize the plaque
- large numbers of lipid-filled macrophages.

An interesting question is whether these lipid-filled macrophages merely constitute a **marker** of unstable plaques or whether they actually cause instability. This area of the natural history of atherosclerosis deserves much fuller investigation than it has received to date. A reduction in plaque instability may have an effect on mortality and morbidity much greater than may be achieved by what is usually understood as plaque regression, i.e. a reduction of luminal stenosis seen on angiography.

Epidemiological studies of the effects of substantial lowering of plasma lipid concentrations show a much greater effect in terms of a decrease in clinical events and a decrease in mortality than in terms of angiographic improvements. This constitutes support for the hypothesis proposed above.

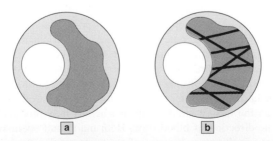

Fig. 18.8   High- and low-risk eccentric coronary artery plaques.

a is devoid of collagen crossing the lipid pool. It is therefore more deformable and its cap is more likely to rupture than that of **b**.

RISK FACTORS IN RELATION TO ATHEROSCLEROSIS

Any variable associated with a significant increase in the chance of developing either a specific disease or a specific lesion can be regarded as a risk factor. The risk factor concept is an important one for prevention of disease rather than cure. If such primary prevention is to be brought about, the identification of potentially reversible risk factors must be of great importance. However, it must be borne in mind that not all the factors that have been found to be associated with the prevalence of a given disorder have a direct causal relationship. Thus the removal or reversal of such a factor may not materially affect the frequency and severity of the disease.

Many risk factors have been canvassed in the development of occlusive arterial disease and hence, by implication, in the development of atherosclerosis. Apart from such inescapable variables as **age**, **sex** and **race**, which are discussed briefly below, the most important of these appear to be:

- hyperlipidaemia
- hypertension
- cigarette smoking
- diabetes mellitus.

Age

Age has the strongest and most constant association with atherosclerosis. Different arterial areas are affected at different rates. Lesions appear in the aorta in the first decade of life, in the coronary arteries in the second, and in the cerebral vessels in the third. It would be useful to know whether the fact that the lesions are closely age-related is due to some intrinsic ageing process or whether it is simply a reflection of the time during which other factors can exert their effect. It seems likely that the second of these possibilities is true since population groups exist whose lifespan is not significantly different from the human species in general and in whom ageing is not accompanied by clinical manifestations of atherosclerosis.

Sex

Clinical events related to atherosclerosis are far commoner in males than in females during the middle decades of life. With increasing age this difference diminishes but never disappears. These clinical differences are, to a considerable extent, mirrored by differences in the prevalence and severity of arterial lesions as seen at necropsy. It is obviously tempting to describe these differences in terms of a role for sex hormones. In human males the use of oestrogens in a large scale secondary prevention study has not proved encouraging. Some sex differences appear to exist in lipid metabolism and merit further exploration. In females taking oral contraceptives, the effect on plasma lipids depends on the type of compound: high doses of oestrogen increase the plasma concentrations of high density lipoproteins, while the reverse is true of progesterone and its analogues. However, in post-menopausal females, hormone replacement treatment appears to delay the appearance of atherosclerosis-related clinical disease.

Race

The prevalence of atherosclerosis-related clinical disease is strikingly influenced by geography. These differences correspond roughly to the distribution of various racial groups and are also mirrored in the prevalence and severity of atherosclerotic lesions. Within individual racial groups, quite steep gradients exist in the extent and severity of coronary artery atherosclerosis; these large intra-group variations suggest that membership of one or other racial group does not *per se* confer relative immunity from or increased susceptibility to atherosclerosis. This view gains strength when the experience of immigrant groups is considered. They appear to acquire a risk for the development of atherosclerosis-related disease much closer to that of their host population than to that of the community from which they came.

Lipid metabolism and atherosclerosis

A vast amount of literature exists relating to the association between lipid metabolism, atherosclerosis and occlusive arterial disease. Despite the complexity of this subject, this association can be expressed in a number of simple propositions:

1. Atherosclerotic lesions contain far more lipid than adjacent non-involved areas of the intima. Most of this lipid, in mature plaques, is derived from the plasma.
2. Increasing the plasma concentrations of certain lipid classes in a variety of animal species by dietary and/or pharmacological means leads to the appearance of focal intimal lesions resembling those of human atherosclerosis.
3. In populations in which the prevalence of atherosclerosis-related diseases and/or raised fibrolipid plaques is high, plasma concentrations of certain lipids (notably cholesterol in the form of low density lipoproteins) are also high. Where the prevalence of such lesions is low, the reverse is true.

Plasma concentrations of two complex proteins – **low density lipoprotein** and **high density lipoprotein** – are related to the risk of coronary heart disease and hence, by implication, to atherogenesis. *There is a strong positive association between the risk of coronary heart disease and high levels of low density lipoprotein (LDL).* In contrast, there is a strong **inverse** relationship between high plasma concentrations of high density lipoprotein (HDL) and coronary heart disease risk.

LDL concentrations are affected by both genetic and environmental factors

It is believed that some 30% of the variance in plasma cholesterol concentrations (which correlate closely with LDL concentrations) in a given population may be due to genetic determinants. This excludes a number of diseases in which **single mutant genes** with powerful effects can cause elevated levels of LDL, or absence of LDL. In **familial hyperlipidaemia type IIa**, the increased LDL plasma concentration is due to absence or a reduction in the function of cell surface receptors for low density lipoprotein. These receptors are responsible for much of the catabolism of LDL. This variety of hyperlipidaemia is transmitted in an autosomal dominant manner. Homozygotes are relatively rare and most of them die from coronary heart disease by the time they reach their early 20s. The incidence of the heterozygous form of familial type IIa hyperlipidaemia is about 2 per 1000 in most communities.

Much more common is **familial combined hyperlipidaemia**, in which a familial clustering of different forms of hyperlipoproteinaemia is found. The primary defect here may be excess secretion of one of the carrier proteins (apoprotein B) leading to an overproduction of LDL and very low density lipoprotein (VLDL). Coronary heart disease is strongly associated with this disorder.

Environmental factors

The most important environmental factor regulating LDL concentrations is diet. The intake of fat and the type of fat consumed are the most powerful dietary factors though dietary cholesterol, fibre, protein and carbohydrate all affect plasma lipids. There is a strong correlation between plasma cholesterol concentrations and the intake of saturated fatty acids.

High density lipoproteins (HDL)

High plasma concentrations of HDL are inversely related to the risk of subsequently developing coronary heart disease. Similarly, low concentrations constitute an efficient predictor for coronary heart disease. The question arising from this is whether HDL has some protective role and can partially inhibit the development of atherosclerosis, or whether it functions merely as a predictor. It has been suggested that HDL may take up free cholesterol from extrahepatic tissues. The free cholesterol is then esterified, transferred to LDL and returned to the liver, where the cholesterol esters are hydrolysed. The free cholesterol so formed in the liver enters a pool of free cholesterol which is available for removal of bile, conversion into bile acids which can also be removed, or re-incorporated into lipoprotein.

Plasma concentrations of HDL are increased by agents inducing microsomal enzymes, including phenobarbitone, phenytoin and certain insecticides. Alcohol also produces a rise in HDL levels and this may well be due to the same mechanism. Any factor increasing adipose tissue lipoprotein lipase activity, such as insulin or physical exercise, tends to increase HDL concentrations. HDL levels tend to be low in obese people and increase following weight reduction.

Genetic factors also play a part in regulating the plasma levels of this lipid fraction and are believed to be of more importance here than in determining LDL concentrations. Interestingly enough, in this respect, a familial syndrome has been recognized in which HDL levels are very high and this is associated with longevity.

Hypertension

It is quite clear from a number of studies that high blood pressure is associated with an increased risk of death from coronary and cerebral artery disease. While this does not necessarily indicate that hypertension also increases the degree of atherosclerosis, careful necropsy studies show that this is the case. There are significant differences in raised lesions between hypertensive and non-hypertensive cases at all ages, in both sexes and in both the aorta and coronary arteries.

High blood pressure may affect the development of atherosclerosis in a number of ways, however, no convincing evidence exists to persuade us that factors other than the raised pressure itself are responsible. In patients with coarctation (congenital segmental narrowing) of the aorta, atherosclerosis develops in the high pressure area proximal to the stenosis but not distal to it where the pressure is normal. A fascinating experiment of nature which reinforces this view is a rare congenital anomaly in which the left coronary artery originates from the pulmonary artery and is thus perfused at low pressure. In patients with this abnormality who survived to middle age, atherosclerosis was present in the right coronary artery but not in the left.

Cigarette smoking

Cigarette smoking correlates strongly with a high risk of occlusive arterial disease affecting both coronary arteries and arteries of the lower limb. British data show that the risk of dying from coronary heart disease in men aged between 45 and 54 is **trebled** if they smoke more than 15 cigarettes per day. The risk seems to be related to the number of cigarettes rather than to the duration of the habit. The increase in risk diminishes fairly rapidly in those who give up smoking. This suggests that smoking may have an effect over and above an increase in atherosclerosis, though postmortem studies have shown that the extent and severity of atherosclerosis is greater in smokers than in non-smokers.

Many possibilities have been canvassed in the search for mechanisms to account for any effects of cigarette smoking on the arterial wall. These include a possible direct effect of nicotine, high carbon monoxide levels in the blood, the action of free radicals, and possible hypersensitivity to glycoprotein antigens in tobacco. At this time it is impossible to say whether any, all or none of these plays a role.

Diabetes mellitus

In over-privileged Western communities there is no doubt that diabetes is a powerful additional risk factor for atherosclerosis-related clinical disease. A certain pre-existing background level of atherosclerosis appears to be necessary since, in those parts of the world where atherosclerosis is not a serious problem, diabetes does not produce any significant increase in frequency of the major clinical syndromes associated with atherosclerosis. The question of whether diabetes increases the severity of artery wall disease is not easy to answer. Ideally one would need to compare two groups coming to necropsy who were alike in every way other than in respect of the presence or absence of diabetes. Such data as do exist suggest that there is a real difference between diabetics and non-diabetics in respect of raised atherosclerotic lesions in both the aorta and coronary arteries.

ATHEROSCLEROSIS

- Atherosclerosis is a disease affecting large elastic and muscular arteries; its complications – **coronary heart disease**, **stroke** and **peripheral vascular disease** – kill over 10 million people annually.
- The lesions of atherosclerosis (**plaques**) are focal thickenings of the inner lining of arteries (intima). They consist of a newly formed connective tissue 'cap' covering, accumulations of fat-filled macrophages and areas of tissue necrosis.
- The most dangerous complication is thrombosis. This happens because of either splitting or erosion of the connective tissue of the plaque cap, which is most likely to occur in lesions with large accumulations of lipid-filled macrophages and extracellular lipid.
- Risk factors include hyperlipidaemia (inherited or acquired), high blood pressure, cigarette smoking and diabetes mellitus.
- Macrophages entering the intima from the blood probably play a role at all stages of the natural history, in that they are responsible for lipid accumulation, triggering the growth of new connective tissue and in producing unstable plaques that are likely to rupture and be complicated by thrombosis.

19 The pathological bases of ischaemia II: thrombosis

A thrombus is a solid mass or plug formed within the heart, arteries, veins or capillaries from the components of the streaming blood.

Thrombosis and clotting are not synonymous. It is important that the fundamental differences between the two processes should be appreciated (*Fig. 19.1*). In **clotting** the activation of a protein cascade system within the blood leads to the generation of thrombin and thus to the conversion of soluble fibrinogen to insoluble fibrin. The process of **thrombosis** involves both platelet activation and clotting, the mechanisms being identical to those occurring in haemostasis.

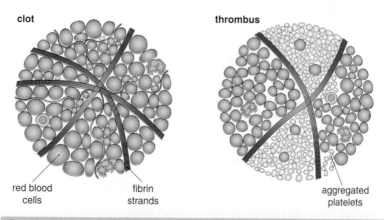

Fig. 19.1 The essential differences between clot and thrombus.

In the former the only process involved is conversion of soluble fibrinogen to insoluble polymerized fibrin. In the latter the various phases of platelet activation constitute an essential element.

PLATELETS AND HAEMOSTASIS (*Fig. 19.2*)

The contribution of platelets to haemostasis is mediated via:

- **adhesion of platelets to the underlying vessel wall**
- **release of pharmacologically active compounds**

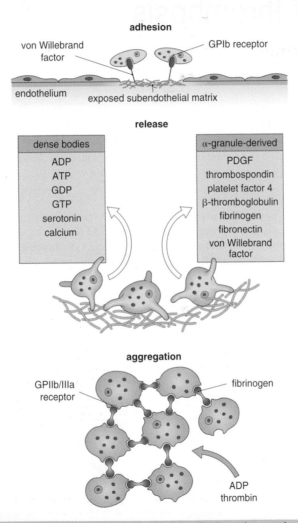

Fig. 19.2   The three phases of platelet activation: adhesion, release and aggregation.

GP, glycoprotein; ADP, adenosine 5′-diphosphate; ATP, adenosine 5′-triphosphate; GDP, guanosine 5′-diphosphate; GTP, guanisone 5′-triphosphate; PDGF, platelet-derived growth factor.

- **aggregation (platelet to platelet) to form a plug**
- **provision of co-factors for clotting.**

Adhesion

Platelets adhere to damaged endothelial cells or exposed subendothelial tissues when vessel wall-derived ligands bind to glycoprotein receptors on the platelets. Collagen, which is exposed when a vessel is damaged, binds to a glycoprotein receptor (GPIa); von Willebrand factor (vWf), a large multimeric glycoprotein synthesized by the endothelial cells, binds to GPIb. *Deficient production of von Willebrand factor (as is seen in von Willebrand disease) or an absent Ib receptor (Bernard–Soulier syndrome) must lead to defective adhesion of platelets and will be reflected in an abnormally prolonged bleeding time.*

Von Willebrand's disease, characterized by a prolonged bleeding time, is inherited for the most part as an autosomal dominant trait which has variable penetrance. The platelets themselves are normal, as are all their post-adhesion functions.

Laboratory findings in von Willebrand's disease

- A prolonged bleeding time.
- Low plasma concentrations of vWf.
- Low plasma concentrations of factor VIII.
- Defective ristocetin-induced platelet aggregation. Ristocetin is an antibiotic, now withdrawn since it causes thrombocytopenia, which causes aggregation of normal platelets in vitro.

Release

Adherent platelets change shape and release several pre-formed and newly formed molecules which may affect both haemostasis and the metabolism of the underlying vessel wall. Platelets contain two types of storage granules – **α-granules** and **dense bodies** – the latter having a dark, electron-dense centre and a less dense peripheral zone. A wide range of active chemical species is released from these (see *Table 19.1*). The release reaction is usually triggered by exposure to either collagen or thrombin (*Fig. 19.3*).

Table 19.1 Compounds released from platelet granules following activation

Granule type	Contents
α-Granule	PDGF, thrombospondin, platelet factor 4, β-thromboglobulin, fibrinogen, fibronectin, vWf, etc.
Dense body	ATP, ADP, GDP, GTP, serotonin, calcium

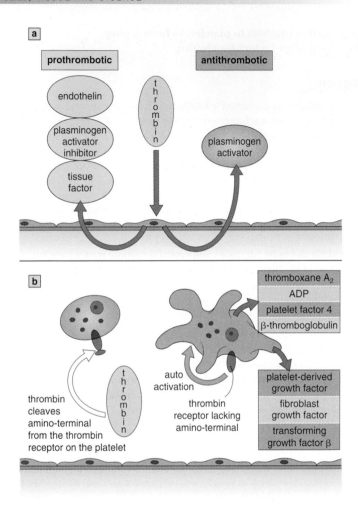

Fig. 19.3

a Some effects of thrombin on endothelium. Thrombin upregulates the synthesis and release by endothelium of certain prothrombotic molecules such as endothelin, plasminogen activator inhibitor I (PAI-I) and tissue factor. It also upregulates production by endothelial cells of the antithrombotic plasminogen activator. **b** Platelet activation by thrombin. Thrombin activates platelets by binding to a specific receptor on the platelet surface. It cleaves the amino-terminal from the receptor. The truncated receptor now acts as an auto-activator for the platelet, causing release of stored compounds from within the granules.

In addition to the release of stored compounds, probably mediated through the activation of protein kinase C, collagen and thrombin also initiate the release of **arachidonate** from the platelet membrane. This is the first step in the synthesis of **prostaglandins**, including the powerfully anti-aggregatory **prostacyclin**, and the equally powerful pro-aggregatory **thromboxane A$_2$** (*Fig. 19.4a*).

Aggregation

In aggregation, platelets form a mass through the agency of fibrinogen 'bridges' between adjacent platelets. Fibrinogen binds to receptors formed

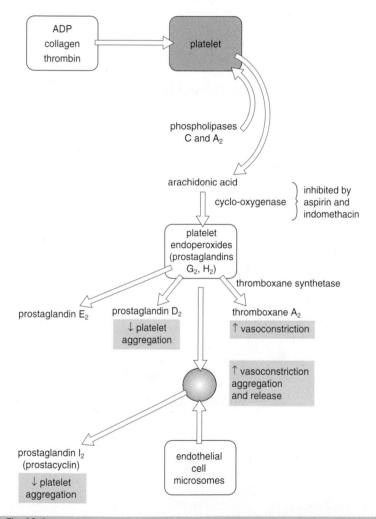

Fig. 19.4a

Platelet activation causes arachidonic acid to be cleaved from membrane phospholipids and stimulates arachidonic acid metabolism with release of prostaglandins and thromboxanes.

by a rearrangement of two platelet surface glycoproteins, IIb and IIIa, which are members of the integrin family. This receptor also binds to vWf and may thus make a contribution to platelet adhesion as well. *The stimuli for aggregation are ADP and thromboxane A_2.*

Provision of co-factors for clotting

Platelets also interact with clotting cascade proteins such as factors V, VIII, IX and X. Following activation, phospholipids that are normally present on the internal layer of their plasma membranes are 'flipped' to the external aspect of the cell, playing an important part in prothrombin activation by factor Xa, and in factor X activation by the factor IXa–VIIa complex.

THE MICRO-ANATOMY OF THE PLATELET

Understanding platelet physiology and pathology is made easier by some knowledge of platelet structure. The platelet is so small that only ultra-structural studies are capable of providing this essential information (*Fig. 19.4b*).

The platelet circulates in the blood as a flat disc. If such a disc is cut in the equatorial plane, **four major zones** can be seen on examination with the electron microscope. These are:

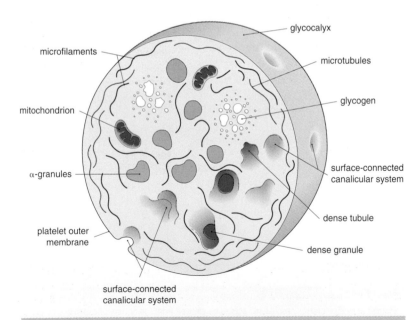

Fig. 19.4b   **Microanatomy of a platelet.**

1) the **peripheral** zone
2) the **sol-gel** zone
3) the **organelle** zone
4) the **membrane** zone.

The peripheral zone

This consists of the surface membranes and structures closely associated with the surface. There is an **exterior coat** or **glycocalyx** rich in glyco-proteins. This houses receptors for signals triggering platelet activation, and substrates for adhesion and aggregation reactions. Several different glyco-protein receptors have been identified and some clearly serve important roles in relation to platelet–platelet and platelet–vessel reactions.

Platelets from patients with **thrombasthenia** lack glycoproteins IIb and IIIa and thus cannot bind fibrinogen and aggregate normally. In **Bernard–Soulier syndrome**, platelets aggregate normally but fail to adhere to damaged blood vessels in vivo, or to bovine fibrinogen or the antibiotic ristocetin in vitro. This indicates that the glycoprotein Ib, which is absent from these platelets, is the receptor for the von Willebrand factor.

Another peripheral zone component lies just deep to the unit membrane. It contains a system of filaments similar to microfilaments. They are believed to contribute to maintenance of the normal discoid shape of the unstimulated platelet and also interact with other elements of the platelet's contractile system.

An important element is the open canalicular system. These invaginations of the cell surface ramify deeply within the platelet and thus markedly increase its surface area, rather like a sponge. The functions of the open canalicular system are closely interrelated with those of the membrane system, but structurally it shares the same features as other portions of the cell surface membrane.

The sol-gel zone

This zone contains fibres of various types; changes in the state of polymer-ization and movement of these fibres are intimately related to maintenance of the discoid form and to internal contraction. At least three systems of fibres are present:

1) the submembrane fibres mentioned above
2) microtubules
3) microfilaments.

The **microtubules** are arranged as a circumferential band near the peripheral zone, which suggests that their role is to contribute to the support of the discoid shape of the unstimulated platelet. Agents (e.g. colchicine) that interfere with assembly of microtubules (see pp. 83–84), dissolve platelet microtubules and cause loss of the discoid shape.

The **microfilaments** exist in a dynamic balance of sol-gel transformation and, like microfilaments in other cells, appear to consist of actin and myosin.

The organelle zone

Like many other cells, platelets contain **mitochondria**, **lysosomes** and **peroxisomes**. There are, in addition, two other types of organelle peculiar to platelets.

The α-granule

The contents of this organelle are listed above in Table 19.1. A rare defect (**the grey platelet syndrome**) is characterized by absence of α-granules. These platelets lack all the proteins listed above. None is essential for platelet aggregation so long as the plasma concentration of fibrinogen is adequate. The only abnormalities noted are a somewhat prolonged bleeding time and easy bruising.

The dense body

This, as its name suggests, is much more electron-dense than the α-granule. Its contents are also listed in Table 19.1. Dense bodies may be absent from platelets in a number of rare inherited syndromes, including the Hermansky–Pudlak syndrome (associated with albinism and accumulation of partly oxidized lipid in macrophages) and the Wiskott–Aldrich syndrome (see p. 186). The lack of releasable adenosine diphosphate (ADP) has its main effect on **aggregation**, but bleeding problems are generally not severe since aggregation can be induced via other pathways.

The membrane zone

Two elements make up this part of the platelet structure. The first of these is the so-called **surface-connected open canalicular system** which tunnels through the cytoplasm of the platelet in a serpentine manner. These channels remain open whether the platelet is inactive and discoid in shape, or activated, contracted and changed in shape. This suggests that the canaliculi serve not only as a means for increasing the surface area of the platelet susceptible to chemical signals, but also as a series of conduits for secretions produced by platelets in the course of the **release** phase.

There is an additional membrane-related system of tubules known as the **dense tubular system**. These tubules consist of smooth endoplasmic reticulum derived from the parent megakaryocyte. In some areas within the cell the membranes of the dense tubular system and those of the open canalicular system are closely apposed in a manner similar to the relationship between sarcotubules and transverse tubules in muscle cells.

The role of these membrane systems can be appreciated most easily if one regards the platelet as being in some respects rather like a muscle cell, in that it contracts on stimulation. The contraction of platelet actin and myosin, as in other situations, is modulated by calcium flux. In the platelet calcium is sequestered in the dense tubular system when the cell has not been activated. Signals reach the platelet interior via the open canalicular system and the connections between this and the dense tubular system lead to the extrusion of calcium from the dense tubular system into the cytoplasm. This is followed by contraction of actomyosin and a change in the shape of the platelet. When the platelet is not activated by a chemical signal, the cytoplasmic calcium is maintained at low levels by the operation of a calcium pump which transports cytoplasmic calcium into the dense tubular system, and which appears to be essential for maintaining the platelet in its resting, discoid form. If there is a rise in intracellular cAMP, the activity of the calcium pump is enhanced. It is not without interest that chemical agents which appear to inhibit platelet activity, such as the anti-aggregatory prostaglandins E_1, D_2 and I_2, act by stimulating the platelet adenylate cyclase to produce a rise in intracellular cAMP. In addition to its role in modulating contractile functions, the dense tubular system also appears to be the site of prostaglandin synthesis within the platelet.

MECHANISMS OF PLATELET ACTIVATION

Adhesion

During both haemostatis and arterial thrombosis, platelets react with exposed subendothelial tissue components. They then lose their normal discoid shape, becoming more rounded, and put out pseudopodia. Alternatively, if fibrin is present, they may adhere to fibrin strands and undergo a similar shape change; this is probably brought about by local accumulations of thrombin, which converts fibrinogen to fibrin. How collagen influences platelet behaviour is not clear. There does not appear to be a specific collagen receptor on the platelet surface, and it is possible that several sites on the platelet membrane are cross-linked by the collagen fibril.

The release phase

Shape change is associated with the release of the contents of the intracellular granules. Some of the compounds released at this point are believed to be deeply involved in **aggregation**, when platelets stick to one another to form a clump. Many substances promote platelet aggregation (at least in vitro) and most of these also induce the discharge of granule contents. These compounds include **ADP**, which can be released from activated platelets, damaged red cells or injured cells of the vessel wall, or formed from ATP, which is also released from platelets. Another powerful aggregator of platelets is **thrombin**, which can exert its effect via a number of different pathways. In addition, an important group of both pro- and anti-aggregatory compounds can be released from activated platelets as a result of metabolic pathways which have **arachidonic acid** as their starting point.

Products of arachidonic acid metabolism in the platelet

Activation of platelets leads to two phospholipases, C and A_2 acting on membrane phospholipids. Phospholipase C cleaves phospholipids, releasing diacyl-glycerol and phosphatidyl-inositol tri-phosphate; phospholipase A_2 frees the arachidonate from phosphatidyl inositol (aided by mono- and diglyceride lipases).

The arachidonate is converted via the cyclo-oxygenase pathway to the prostaglandin endoperoxides, prostaglandins G_2 and H_2. These are then converted to thromboxane A_2 by thromboxane synthetase. Other products formed in platelets from prostaglandin endoperoxides include prostaglandins D_2 and E_2. Prostaglandin D_2 is a powerful inhibitor of platelet aggregation because of its ability to stimulate adenylate cyclase. Thromboxane A_2 and its endoperoxide precursors are all platelet-aggregating agents and also cause contraction of vascular smooth muscle.

Just as certain prostaglandins are powerful promoting agents for platelet aggregation, so the most potent inhibitors of aggregation are those prostaglandins that stimulate the adenylate cyclase system and thus produce an increase in the platelet cAMP content. One of these, prostaglandin I_2, is produced by stimulated endothelial cells. Its effects are directly opposite to those of thromboxane A_2 and it is the most powerful inhibitor of platelet aggregation known. Prostaglandin I_2 formed locally may affect the extent of platelet accumulation at that site, though it seems unlikely that it can act as a circulating hormone.

Platelet factor 3 and surface glycoprotein receptors

When platelets undergo the release reaction, a phospholipoprotein, platelet factor 3, becomes available on their surfaces. This accelerates the thrombin generation by taking part in two steps of the intrinsic clotting pathway: the interaction of factors VIIIa and IXa to form factor Xa from factor X, and the interaction of factors Xa and Va to form thrombin from prothrombin.

FACTORS PROMOTING THROMBOSIS

Thrombosis may be likened to haemostasis occurring in the wrong place and at the wrong time. It is harmful rather than beneficial.

The complexity of the interrelating processes involved in platelet adhesion, release and aggregation suggests that several different circumstances may influence platelet/vessel wall behaviour. In the 1860s, when thrombosis was recognized (but not the existence of the platelet), Rudolf Virchow suggested that the factors likely to promote thrombus formation fell naturally into **three** major groups:

1) changes in the intimal surface of the vessel
2) changes in the pattern of blood flow
3) changes in the constituents of the blood.

These are known as **Virchow's triad**.

CHANGES IN THE VESSEL WALL SURFACE

Changes in the surface of the vessel wall are of major importance in the pathogenesis of arterial thrombi. The most important of these changes is undoubtedly unstable **atherosclerosi**s, as described in Chapter 18; however, injury (in the broadest sense), inflammation or neoplasms may also be associated with thrombosis-inducing damage to the vessel wall. Of all the vessel wall components the one most likely to be implicated in thrombosis is the **endothelial cell**. In any situation where there is actual loss of endothelial cells with exposure of the subendothelial collagen, platelet adhesion is the inevitable sequel. This certainly happens in complicated atherosclerotic plaques when either splitting ('deep injury') or fraying ('superficial injury') of the connective tissue plaque 'cap' occurs. Endothelial cell desquamation can also take place in the rare inherited metabolic disorder **homocystinuria**, and it has been claimed that endothelial cells can be identified in significant numbers in the blood following smoking.

Injury

Trauma to the endothelium sufficient to cause thrombosis can occur under a number of circumstances. At a rather extreme level, thrombosis can occur after burning or freezing (e.g. capillary thrombosis in 'frostbite'). Mechanical trauma to endothelium occurs in association with the presence of indwelling cannulae. Another type of much less easily provable endothelial trauma has been suggested as being one of the factors involved in the production of postoperative venous thrombi in the lower limb. During anaesthesia there is loss of the normal muscle tone, and the dead weight of the limb and the hard surface of the operating table might be sufficient to cause trauma to the venous endothelium. There is no direct evidence for such trauma at the moment, though surgery certainly appears to be a very potent thrombogenic stimulus as far as the veins are concerned.

Chemical injury to vessel walls certainly occurs, as seen in cases where thrombosis may follow infusion of certain compounds into veins. This fact is made use of in treating both varicose veins and haemorrhoids, where sclerosing chemicals are injected into the affected veins with the deliberate intention of causing thrombosis.

Inflammation

Thrombi occur frequently in situations where vessels or the heart are involved in an inflammatory process. This occurs in the heart valves in patients with either rheumatic or infective endocarditis. Arteries involved in an immune complex mediated inflammatory reaction such as occurs in **polyarteritis nodosa** or **temporal arteritis** are often thrombosed; veins and capillaries passing through an inflamed area may also be affected in the same way.

Neoplastic involvement

The invasion of small venules by malignant cells is often accompanied by thrombosis. There is evidence to suggest that fibrin formed in relation to the tumour cells in the course of this process may enhance their chances of survival and, hence, of multiplying.

CHANGES IN THE PATTERN OF BLOOD FLOW

The important changes in blood flow pattern which are believed to increase the risk of thrombus formation are:

- changes in the **speed** of normal laminar flow
- **loss of the normal laminar pattern** of flow and its replacement by a **turbulent pattern**.

Slowing of the speed of blood flow without loss of the normal laminar pattern appears to be of particular significance in relation to **venous** thrombosis, while turbulence plays a more important haemodynamic role in the **heart** and **arteries**.

A **reduction in the speed of blood flow** may be either a general or a local phenomenon. The first of these may occur in patients with severe congestive cardiac failure, in whom the circulation time can be reduced significantly. Local slowing tends to occur particularly in the veins of the leg under a number of different circumstances, of which the most important are:

- prolonged dependence of the limb
- reduced muscle pumping activity
- proximal occlusion of the venous drainage.

These circumstances are most likely to occur in a patient immobilized in bed, especially after surgery. So far as venous thrombosis is concerned, hospitalization is a very high risk factor. Dissection of the deep veins of the calf shows thrombi at necropsy in more than 30% of medical patients and in about 60% of surgical patients. Clinical diagnosis of such thrombi is difficult; only a small minority are correctly diagnosed during life by the presence of some swelling and tenderness in the affected calf and by pain in the calf being elicited on dorsiflexion of the foot (Homan's sign). Rational prevention aimed at minimizing changes in the pattern of blood flow is likely to be much more useful than treatment of an established thrombus. It should include routine physiotherapy with exercises emphasizing calf and thigh muscle contraction, early postoperative ambulation, and avoidance of prolonged dependency of lower limbs.

Stasis of blood can also occur in the heart and large vessels such as the aorta if either the cardiac chambers or a segment of a major artery are abnormally dilated. This is found in aortic and other arterial **aneurysms**, in the dilated chambers of the heart in a disorder of heart muscle known as **congestive cardiomyopathy**, and in the dilated atria of patients with mitral valve disease, especially if there is associated atrial fibrillation. A situation rather similar to this occurs in patients in whom **myocardial infarction** has occurred. The dead heart muscle is replaced by non-contractile scar tissue; this can lead to local disturbances of flow during ventricular systole and the formation of thrombi over the area of lost cardiac muscle.

Turbulent flow is of particular importance in relation to areas where arteries branch and to segmental narrowing of arteries, chiefly due to atherosclerosis. The haemodynamics at points of branching are such that platelets tend to collect on the outer walls of branches.

CHANGES IN THE CONSTITUENTS OF THE BLOOD

Platelets

It seems obvious that the function of platelets should be considered in relation to the three main components of their behaviour: adhesion, release and aggregation. In addition, their **concentration** within the blood should be determined; we know that a low platelet count is associated with abnormal bleeding and a high one with an increased risk of thrombosis.

In the laboratory the **aggregatability** of platelets to a given stimulus can be measured. ADP, collagen and thrombin are added to a suspension of platelets in a cuvette and the turbidimetric changes resulting from aggregation are measured. Platelet **adhesiveness** can also be measured: the suspension of platelets (of known concentration) is passed at a constant rate across glass beads and the drop in platelet numbers occurring as a result of this passage is determined. The **release reaction** can be monitored by measuring changes in concentration of two products derived from the α-granules – platelet factor 4 (an anti-heparin factor) and β-thromboglobulin. If sufficient care is taken in the sampling of the blood, a rise in the concentration of these compounds is *prima facie* evidence that thrombosis has taken place. However, the half-lives of both platelet factor 4 and β-thromboglobulin in plasma are very short and thus the timing of sampling is critical.

A hypercoagulable state is one in which the normal haemostatic equilibrium is tilted in such a way that thrombosis is favoured. In terms of the processes involved, an increased risk of thrombosis may therefore be due to:

- **up-regulation of platelet–vessel wall interactions**
- **an increase**, which may be general but is much more frequently local, **in procoagulant factors**, most notably fibrinogen and factor VII
- **a decrease in natural anticoagulant factors** such as antithrombin III or the protein C–S–thrombomodulin system
- **increased viscosity of the blood**
- **the presence of anticardiolipin antibodies** (lupus anticoagulants)
- **the presence of stasis** in the venous circulation, especially if this is associated with surgical trauma
- **the release into the blood of procoagulant compounds released from malignant tumours**, especially adenocarcinomas

- **an increase in the platelet count** (thrombocytosis)
- **an increase in platelet adhesiveness and aggregatability**.

Up-regulation of platelet–vessel wall interactions. The most important cause of this is atherosclerosis associated with either superficial or deep injury to the plaque cap. The presence of prosthetic heart valves or synthetic grafts also increases platelet reactions with the underlying vascular surface. Thrombosis may also be the consequence of endothelial damage in the rare inherited disorder of metabolism, homocystinaemia.

Increased viscosity of the blood. This may occur in individuals with elevated levels of fibrinogen in the blood or as a result of grossly elevated plasma concentrations of immunoglobulins such as may be seen in plasma cell dyscrasias like multiple myeloma. Similar increases in viscosity are seen in patients with polycythaemia.

INHERITED DISORDERS WHICH INCREASE THE RISK OF THROMBOSIS

Abnormalities of antithrombin III

This disorder is an autosomal dominant one. Most affected individuals are heterozygotes whose plasma, therefore, contains 50% of the normal concentration of functional AT III. In patients with a deficiency of normal AT III, there is an increase in the concentration of prothrombin fragments. This suggests that the coagulation system is in a constant state of very low grade activation, normally regulated and restrained by AT III.

AT III deficiency causes recurrent episodes of mainly venous thrombosis. As is usual with venous thrombi, leg veins are most frequently affected and complicating pulmonary emboli are common. In women thrombi often occur for the first time during pregnancy or in association with the taking of oral contraceptives. In men, there is often a history of antecedent injury or surgery. With increasing age, the frequency of the episodes of thrombosis increases.

PROTEIN C DEFICIENCY

Protein C deficiency is an autosomal dominant disorder. It is associated with a life-long increased risk of thrombosis. It occurs in two forms. In the first, **the amount of the protein in the plasma is decreased**; the functional deficit is proportional to the reduction of the protein concentration. In the second, the amount of protein C in the plasma is normal but there is a **gross functional defect**. Levels below 65% of normal are usually associated with an increased incidence of thrombosis. Clinically affected heterozygotes suffer from thrombosis in the deep leg veins and also have episodes of superficial thrombophlebitis.

Rarely the disorder may occur in a homozygous form. In this case the affected children have a 'devastating thrombo-embolic diathesis starting in infancy' which involves the renal and mesenteric veins and dural sinuses. The clinical picture may be complicated by **purpura fulminans** in which there are widely distributed skin haemorrhages associated with fibrin plugs occluding small skin vessels.

Protein S deficiency

This disorder presents with much the same clinical picture as C deficiency. It too is inherited as an autosomal dominant trait.

Deficiencies in proteins C and S can occur in association with acquired diseases. Both these molecules are dependent on vitamin K for their activation and may thus be functionally impaired in patients with vitamin K deficiency from any cause.

Protein C resistance

A syndrome characterized by recurrent, familial, venous thrombosis has been recognized, in which all the anticoagulant factors are present in normal concentration but in which there is **abnormal resistance to the normal biological effect of activated protein C** (*Fig. 19.5*). This phenomenon has been found by one group of workers in about one-third of patients referred for evaluation of venous thrombo-embolism. The abnormality is inherited in an autosomal dominant fashion and confers a seven-fold increase in the risk of developing venous thrombosis. The existence of this disorder implies that there must be a dysfunctional co-factor for activated protein C. This co-factor has been identified as factor V, which now seems to have an anticoagulant as well as a procoagulant role.

Recently a mutation has been identified in the gene encoding factor V which correlates with the presence of resistance to activated protein C. It is a single point mutation at nucleotide position 1691 at which there is a G → A substitution. In Holland where this mutation (factor V Leiden) was identified, its frequency in the population appears to be about 2%, which is at least ten-fold higher than that of all other genetic risk factors for thrombosis together. The combination of this mutation with other risk factors for thrombosis may be very powerful; e.g. women with mutated factor V who take oral contraceptives have a 30-fold increase in the risk of thrombosis.

Inherited disorders affecting the fibrinolytic pathways

Inherited disorders of fibrinolytic pathways are rare and include:

- dysfibrinogenaemia
- dysplasminogenaemia
- defective release of plasminogen activator from the vessel wall.

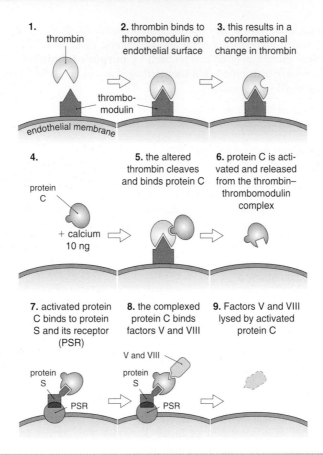

1. thrombin

2. thrombin binds to thrombomodulin on endothelial surface

3. this results in a conformational change in thrombin

thrombo-modulin

endothelial membrane

4. protein C

5. the altered thrombin cleaves and binds protein C

6. protein C is activated and released from the thrombin–thrombomodulin complex

+ calcium 10 ng

7. activated protein C binds to protein S and its receptor (PSR)

8. the complexed protein C binds factors V and VIII

9. Factors V and VIII lysed by activated protein C

protein S

PSR

V and VIII

protein S

PSR

Fig. 19.5   Normal working of the protein C–protein S system shown in nine steps.

Elevated plasma fibrinogen and factor VII$_c$ concentrations

The Northwick Park Heart Study, a prospective study relating certain factors to coronary heart disease risk, shows a strong positive association between plasma concentrations of fibrinogen and factor VII$_c$ and the risk of a first episode of coronary heart disease.

Fibrinogen levels increase with:

- increasing age
- obesity
- the use of oral contraceptives
- the onset of the menopause
- the presence of diabetes
- cigarette smoking.

With the exception of smoking, the same factors are associated with increased plasma levels of factor VII_c. In addition, there is a positive association between a diet high in fat, leading to high plasma cholesterol concentrations, and elevated plasma levels of factor VII_c. Whether high plasma concentrations of fibrinogen are entirely 'acquired' or whether there is a genetic component is still not known.

ACQUIRED DISORDERS AND ENVIRONMENTAL FACTORS WHICH INCREASE THE RISK OF THROMBOSIS

Oral contraceptives

The introduction of oral contraceptives was followed by the recognition that both arterial and venous thrombosis might complicate their use. Users of 'the pill' had a 3–5-fold increase in the risk of developing a myocardial infarct or a stroke, and oral contraceptives appeared to act synergistically with other known risk factors such as cigarette smoking or diabetes mellitus.

This increased risk of thrombo-embolic disease correlates with the amount of oestrogen in the compound. A decrease in the oestrogen content has been associated with a decrease but not with abolition of the increased risk of thrombosis. Contraceptives raise the plasma concentrations of fibrinogen and vitamin K-dependent clotting factors by about 10–20% and there is also a decrease in plasma AT III levels. Factor XII and prekallikrein increase causing an increased potential for contact factor-mediated fibrinolysis.

Malignancy

Patients with certain types of malignancy are at increased risk of thrombo-embolic disease as well as disseminated intravascular coagulation.

It appears that mucin-secreting adenocarcinomas, especially carcinoma of the pancreas, are a risk factor for recurrent venous thrombosis. Malignant cells may release tissue thromboplastin. There is also evidence that mucins released from certain adenocarcinomas, and proteases released from other tumours, can directly activate factor X without the extrinsic clotting pathway being involved.

The nephrotic syndrome

Venous thrombosis commonly complicates the nephrotic syndrome (average incidence 35%) and particularly involves the renal vein. Arterial thrombosis has also been recorded as an association but is much rarer.

The cause is not yet clear though quantitative changes in some clotting and anti-clotting factors have been noted. One of the most striking of these is a decline in the plasma concentrations of antithrombin III, the levels of which fall proportionally with the decline in serum albumin.

Correlations between risk factors for clinically evident thrombotic events and platelet function

Prostaglandins

Epidemiological studies among the Eskimos of North-West Greenland suggest that alterations in the plasma concentrations of certain lipids may influence the balance between thromboxane A_2 and prostaglandin I_2. The incidence of ischaemic heart disease in this Eskimo community is very low. They have low levels of cholesterol and low density lipoprotein in the blood and correspondingly high levels of high density lipoprotein. This plasma lipid pattern is not genetic in origin but appears to be brought about by the diet. In addition, platelet aggregatability is lower than in age- and sex-matched Danes, and the bleeding time is prolonged. One of the outstanding features of the Eskimo diet is a high intake of eicosapentaenoic acid (EPA) (which is present in fish), and Eskimos have high plasma concentrations of this fatty acid and low concentrations of arachidonic acid. Eicosapentaenoic acid is a starting point for the synthesis of prostaglandin I_3, which is anti-aggregatory, but the thromboxane derived from EPA is said not to be pro-aggregatory. Diets rich in cod-liver oil, which contains large amounts of EPA, have been shown to reduce the tendency to thrombosis in extra-corporeal shunts inserted into rat aortas.

Platelet aggregation and plasma lipid patterns

Other evidence that the pattern and concentrations of plasma lipids may influence platelet behaviour is derived from patients with type IIa hyper-lipidaemia. Their platelets are many times more sensitive to doses of aggregating agents such as collagen, ADP or thrombin than are those of normal subjects, though the lipid composition of the platelets themselves differs little, if at all. However, platelets from patients with hyperlipidaemia convert more arachidonic acid to thromboxane A_2 than do those from normal subjects.

Cigarette smoking and platelet function

There is a strong positive correlation between heavy smoking of cigarettes and the risk of one of the major clinical manifestations of occlusive arterial disease. Cigarette smoking could operate as a risk factor in a number of ways including vessel wall damage resulting from an increase in circulating free radicals.

THE EVOLUTION OF VENOUS THROMBI

The process of thrombus formation in a non-inflamed vein is usually termed **phlebothrombosis**. Thrombosis occurring in an inflamed vein is spoken of as **thrombophlebitis**. This is most commonly seen in superficial veins.

The site of initiation of phlebothrombosis is usually the valve pocket. If these areas are examined in sections of thrombosed veins, small clumps of platelets can be seen adhering to the luminal surface. It is a moot point whether this is preceded by damage to the endothelium in this area. No positive evidence has been presented that such damage occurs, but the technical problems of carrying out such a study are daunting and it is, perhaps, too early to write off endothelial injury as an important starting point for the process of venous thrombosis. Some workers have noticed the presence of leucocytes rather than platelets in these valve pockets and it is possible that these cells could bring about changes in the endothelium. Once platelets are aggregated, clotting factors are activated locally and fibrin strands stabilize the platelet aggregate and help to anchor it to the underlying vein wall. A second phase then begins in which a further batch of platelets are laid down over the initial aggregate. At this stage of the development of the thrombus, the platelets can be seen to have aggregated in the form of laminae projecting from the surface of the initial aggregate and lying across the stream of blood. As a result of the forces exerted by the streaming blood, these platelet laminae are bent in the direction of flow and form a somewhat coralline structure (*Fig. 19.6*). Between the platelet laminae are large numbers of red cells, some fibrin strands and a moderate number of leucocytes. The laminar

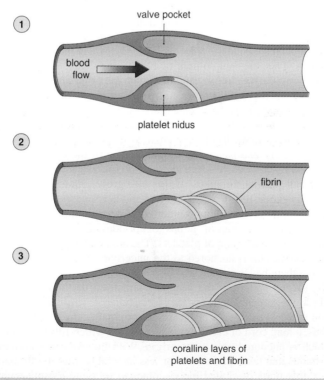

Fig. 19.6 Evolution of a venous thrombus.

arrangement of the platelets coupled with shortening of the fibrin strands between the laminae gives rise to a curious 'rippled' appearance when the thrombi are viewed from above. The appearances are reminiscent of what one sees when a wind has blown across a beach and produced rippling of the sand. In both instances the 'ripples' lie concave to the direction of the force; in the case of the platelet laminae this force is the bloodstream. These elevated ridges on the surface of the thrombi are known as **lines of Zahn** in commemoration of the pathologist who first described them. They are clearly visible with the naked eye, but may be seen best with the aid of a hand lens. The more rapid the streaming of the blood in the segment of vessel where thrombosis has occurred, the more prominent are the lines of Zahn. They are most easily seen, therefore, in large arteries such as the aorta.

At this stage the process may come to an end. The thrombus will then become covered by new endothelial cells and be incorporated into the structure of the underlying vessel wall. However, if the deposition of platelets and fibrin continues, a third phase ensues. As the coralline mass of platelets admixed with clotted blood continues to grow, the stream of blood through the affected segment slows still further and occlusion may ultimately occur. This phase is predominantly mediated by activation of the coagulation pathways rather than by platelet adhesion and aggregation.

Once a segment of vein is occluded in this way, the flow of blood cephalad to the occlusion stops. Thus a stagnant column of blood exists between the point of occlusion and the point cephalad to it where the next venous tributary enters. This stagnant column of blood coagulates and forms what is termed a '**consecutive clot**' in continuity with the original thrombus. This is the first step in a process known as **propagation** of the thrombus. This process may occur in two basic patterns.

In the first pattern, consecutive clot forms between the original occlusion and the tributary immediately cephalad to it. At this point blood enters from the tributary and passes across the surface of the clot. Platelets then adhere to the fibrin meshwork and aggregation follows with the formation of another small platelet thrombus. If this also grows enough to occlude the lumen, propagation may occur again and another segment of vein may fill with fresh clot. In effect, a long segment of venous drainage of the limb can become occluded in a series of 'jumps' or episodes of clotting, each of which is triggered by the adhesion of platelets. The mixed mass of platelet thrombi and consecutive clot is anchored to the underlying vein wall only at those sites where there has been adhesion of platelets.

In the second pattern, if the venous return from the limb as a whole is slowed down, propagation by the formation of consecutive clot may occur on a massive scale. Cephalad to the original occlusive platelet–fibrin thrombus, a long cord of clotted blood may form which fills the vein lumen and which is anchored only at its origin. With the eventual shortening of fibrin strands that takes place more or less inevitably after the formation of any clot, this mass of clotted blood comes to lie quite loosely within the lumen except at the point where the original thrombus is attached. If the thrombus becomes dislodged from its attachment point, then the whole mass is carried away in the systemic venous circulation until impaction takes place within the pulmonary arteries (pulmonary embolism).

THE NATURAL HISTORY OF THROMBI

Lysis

Some thrombi may undergo lysis through the action of plasmin and 'like some insubstantial pageant faded, leave not a wrack behind'. This is clearly the most desirable outcome, especially in relation to occlusive thrombosis within the arterial tree. If spontaneous lysis is unlikely, the process can be triggered by lytic agents such as streptokinase, or genetically engineered plasminogen activator.

Embolization

Thrombi may become detached from the underlying vascular wall, be it vein, artery or heart. When this occurs, the detached portion of thrombus travels at high speed in the systemic venous circulation (if its origin is a vein) or within the systemic arterial circulation (if the site of origin was an artery or the heart). At some point a vessel will be reached whose calibre is less than the diameter of the thrombotic material and impaction occurs. This embolization can have serious structural and functional consequences which will be discussed in Chapter 20.

If the thrombus persists, the processes of organization (see pp. 364–365) are triggered. Much will depend on whether the thrombus is occlusive or whether it lies in a plaque-like fashion on the surface of the vessel wall without seriously impeding the flow of blood. This latter case is known as a **mural thrombus**.

The organization of occlusive thrombi

If a segment of a vessel remains plugged by thrombus, new capillary vessels of granulation tissue type grow out from the vasa vasorum in the adventitia, across the media, into and across the intima and, ultimately, into the thrombus itself. At the same time, the removal of thrombotic material is proceeding, largely through the action of macrophages. Eventually, at the worst, the occlusive thrombus may be replaced by a solid plug of collagenous tissue and all chance of re-establishing flow is lost.

Recanalization

Fortunately, however, the picture is not by any means always so gloomy. Quite early on after the formation of an occlusive thrombus, clefts may appear within the thrombotic material. These clefts often lie in the long axis of the occluded segment and hence, by implication, in the same axis as the

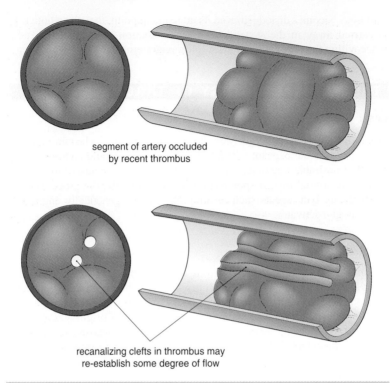

segment of artery occluded
by recent thrombus

recanalizing clefts in thrombus may
re-establish some degree of flow

Fig. 19.7   Recanalization of an occlusive thrombus.

blood flow. Not infrequently they link up with one another to form new channels which pass through the occluding plug of thrombus/granulation tissue from one patent segment of the vessel to another (*Fig. 19.7*). Within a few days the clefts become lined by flattened cells of mesenchymal origin which ultimately differentiate into endothelial cells. Occasionally some of the mesenchymal stem cells close to the new vascular channels differentiate into smooth muscle and arrange themselves round the clefts in a concentric fashion. The whole process by which a greater or lesser degree of blood flow is re-established through the occluded segment of vessel is known as **recanalization**.

The organization of mural thrombi

In this situation the pattern of organization is different because the patho-physiological circumstances are so different from those in an occluded segment of a vessel. Flowing blood passes over the surface of the mural thrombus and so the superficial portion of the thrombus is infiltrated by oxygenated plasma. Granulation tissue type capillaries derived from the vasa grow only very slowly, if at all, into the thrombus. The lack of this feature may be mediated, in part at least, by the normal intramural tension within the affected part of the vessel.

Many of the platelets disaggregate and are either washed away by the passing stream of blood or are phagocytosed. In arteries this means that, within a short time, the major part of the remaining thrombus consists of a spongy mass of polymerized fibrin which tends to become packed down onto the surface of the underlying vessel wall. Within a few days the surface of the thrombus becomes partly covered by a layer of flattened cells. Originally it was thought that these were new endothelial cells but there is some evidence to suggest that the cells making up the early new intima are smooth muscle cells.

As in other situations where organization is taking place, the mass of fibrin and platelets becomes vascularized. An unusual feature, however, is the fact that the new vascular channels, which can be seen within a few days of the thrombus being formed, are derived from the main lumen of the

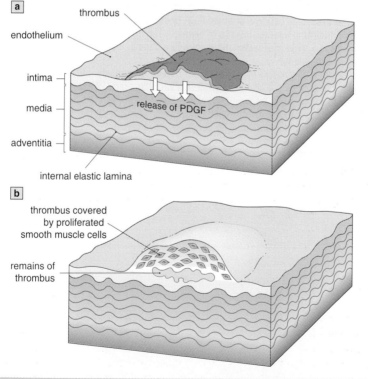

Fig. 19.8   Organization of a mural thrombus.

PDGF, platelet-derived growth factor.

vessel and grow down into the thrombus rather than upwards across the media from the vasa vasorum.

The picture is further complicated by the interaction of platelet-derived growth factor with smooth muscle cells in the underlying vessel wall. The major part of the proliferation of smooth muscle cells which ensues after the formation of a mural thrombus appears to take place on the luminal aspect of the thrombus, so that the thrombus eventually lies deep within the thick new intima (*Fig. 19.8*). The possibility that this process may play a part in the growth of atherosclerotic plaques is discussed in Chapter 18.

THROMBOSIS

- A thrombus is a mass formed in blood vessels from the components of streaming blood. It is the resultant of the interaction of two biological processes – aggregation of platelets and blood clotting – that are normally involved in haemostasis.
- Platelet activation involves their adhesion to a vascular surface, release from them of many biologically active compounds, and aggregation to form a plug.
- Factors promoting thrombosis include abnormalities in the blood vessel wall, abnormalities in patterns of blood flow, and abnormalities (qualitative or quantitative) in the constituents of blood.
- Stasis is a major risk factor for venous thrombosis, especially in the middle-aged and elderly.
- In arteries, atherosclerosis is the most potent abnormality, but platelet/vessel wall interactions are also up-regulated in vascular grafts, in relation to prosthetic valves in the heart and where blood homocystine concentrations are raised, thus causing endothelial damage.
- Hypercoagulable states may be acquired (as in myelomatosis) or inherited, as in protein C/S resistance.

20 The pathological bases of ischaemia III: embolism

An embolus is an abnormal mass of material, either solid or gaseous, which is transported in the bloodstream from one part of the circulation to another until it finally impacts in the lumen of a vessel of too small a calibre to allow the embolus to pass.

Emboli may consist of:

- thrombus
- mixed thrombus and blood clot
- air
- nitrogen
- fat
- small pieces of bone marrow
- debris from the base of atherosclerotic plaques
- groups of tumour cells (embolization constitutes an important means of tumour spread).

Most major emboli are derived from thrombus.

THROMBUS-DERIVED EMBOLI

Roughly 99% of emboli are derived from thrombus or from thrombus mixed with blood clot such as is found in the veins of the lower limb.

Pulmonary emboli

When the origin of the embolus is a venous thrombus, the end result must be impaction in the pulmonary arterial tree. This is one of the commonest and most dangerous forms of embolization. Some 600 000 cases of pulmonary embolization occur annually in the USA; 20 000 to 50 000 of these are fatal. In unselected necropsies, pulmonary emboli are present in about 10% of cases. If the necropsy sample is more selective (e.g. patients who have had

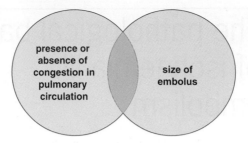

Fig. 20.1   Factors determining the outcome in pulmonary embolization.

orthopaedic operations on the lower limb, patients with severe burns or with fractures), the frequency of emboli rises steeply.

The effects of pulmonary embolization depend on the interaction between two principal factors (*Fig. 20.1*):

1) the **size** of the embolus and hence the degree of mechanical obstruction which it causes;
2) the presence or absence of **congestion** in the pulmonary circulation at the time of impaction.

Insofar as size is concerned, pulmonary emboli are classed as massive, small or medium sized.

Massive pulmonary emboli

Massive pulmonary emboli are derived from **thrombus occluding a long segment of the venous drainage of the lower limb**. In effect this means that the thrombotic process has involved the iliofemoral part of the venous system, but even then it must be remembered that the calibre of the main pulmonary arteries exceeds that of the iliac or femoral veins. In order for blocking of one of the major pulmonary vessels to occur, the length of the mixed thrombus and clot must be loosely bundled together to form a mass of the appropriate dimensions.

Clinically, massive pulmonary embolism usually presents suddenly. Often the symptoms appear when the patient is straining, for example at stool. Affected patients may die suddenly or complain of chest pain and experience shortness of breath. The signs of circulatory collapse are usually present. It is humiliating to have to confess that the mechanisms involved in the production of this dramatic clinical picture are still not well understood. It has been suggested that the sudden blockage to the flow of blood through one of the main pulmonary arteries with resulting excess acute strain on the right side of the heart is responsible. However, there are reasons to suggest that mechanical obstruction may not be entirely responsible for the acute right heart failure. Other possibilities canvassed include:

- a vagal reflex inducing spasm of the coronary and pulmonary arteries
- a reflex producing marked peripheral vasodilatation

- a reflex producing cardiac arrest
- a massive release of prostaglandins which can provoke vasospasm.

Small pulmonary emboli

Small emboli are usually clinically 'silent' and are often multiple and recurrent. Retraction of the emboli from the wall of the occluded vessel often occurs. The combination of such retraction with the organization described previously may leave small fibrous tissue cords, criss-crossing the lumen of the affected vessel in a web or band-like fashion, as the only marker of the embolic episode. In other cases the emboli retract so much that the thrombotic mass becomes packed down onto the vessel wall in the same way as occurs with a mural thrombus. These emboli then become covered by new endothelium and are incorporated into the vessel wall. This process of incorporation is accompanied by the proliferation of smooth muscle cells and the formation of a thicker than normal intimal layer. *If this sequence of events is repeated many times, the increased thickness of the intima in the pulmonary arterial bed leads to a decrease in the compliance of the vessels and ultimately to a rise in pulmonary artery pressure (pulmonary hypertension).*

Medium-sized pulmonary emboli

Under certain circumstances, pulmonary emboli of moderate size (i.e. large enough to block secondary or tertiary branches of the pulmonary arteries) may reduce the perfusion of a segment of lung tissue sufficiently to produce a localized area of necrosis. Such areas of necrosis secondary to ischaemia are known as **infarcts**; these are discussed in Chapter 21.

Systemic emboli

Most thrombotic systemic emboli are derived from the left side of the heart, especially the atrial appendages (this being particularly likely to occur in patients with atrial fibrillation). Intraventricular thrombi may occur as a consequence of transmural myocardial infarction or in congestive cardiomyopathy, a muscle disorder in which the myocardium is flabby and the ventricles are dilated. There is a marked decrease in the amount of blood expelled from the left ventricle with each contraction and thus a volume overload on the ventricular muscle. In life, the presence of these thrombi can be detected by echocardiography.

Thrombi affecting the heart valves of a size sufficient to give rise to significant emboli are usually due to **infective endocarditis**, a disorder produced by the combination of haemodynamically induced endocardial injury and bacteraemia. The infected thrombi, or **vegetations** as they are often called, may be bulky and liable to break up easily. Portions of the vegetations can break off readily and travel in the systemic arterial circulation until they impact. This may, of course, occur in a very large number of places, but the brain, lower limbs, spleen and kidneys are favoured sites.

When an infected thrombus impacts, it may set up a localized inflammatory reaction leading to partial destruction of the wall of the vessel in which impaction has taken place. This leads to a dilatation of the affected arterial segment, and rupture followed by haemorrhage may occur. Such a lesion is termed a **mycotic aneurysm**, a misleading term since fungi have nothing to do with the pathogenesis ('*mycos*', mushroom).

Small **platelet thrombi** occur quite commonly in relation to athero-sclerotic plaques at the point in the neck where the common carotid artery divides. Emboli derived from these platelet masses lodge in the cerebral circulation, often in small vessels, where they may give rise to permanent or transient neurological deficiencies.

GASEOUS EMBOLI

Air

Air may be introduced into the systemic circulation under a number of circumstances. These include:

- operations on the head and neck where a large vein is opened inadvertently
- mismanagement of blood transfusions where positive pressure is being used to speed up the flow of blood
- during haemodialysis for renal failure
- following the introduction of air into the fallopian tubes in the course of investigation of sterility
- interference with the placental site during criminal abortion.

The air enters the right side of the heart where, in the right ventricle, it is whipped up into a frothy mass. This mass can block the flow of blood through the pulmonary arteries. The clinical picture that develops closely mimics that of massive pulmonary embolization by thrombus derived from the leg veins. In some cases the froth may gain access to the systemic arterial circulation and impact there. The most frequent site for this is the brain, but cases have also been reported of embolization of vessels supplying the spinal cord, and patients being investigated for sterility have become quadriplegic following the introduction of gas into the fallopian tubes to check patency. As little as 40 ml of air can have serious clinical results and 100 ml can be fatal, though there have been rare cases in which 200 ml have been tolerated. If air embolism is suspected as the cause of death, it is necessary to place the heart and pulmonary arteries under water when they are opened, in order to detect the escape of the air bubbles from the blocked vessels.

Nitrogen

Nitrogen embolization occurs in **decompression sickness**, which is also known as '**caisson disease**'. It affects persons whose occupation causes them to work at very high atmospheric pressures and who may then be returned too quickly to normal atmospheric pressure (deep sea divers, tunnellers, etc.).

At high pressures, inert gases, particularly nitrogen, are dissolved in the plasma and in interstitial tissue, especially adipose tissue. If the person at risk returns too quickly to normal atmospheric pressure, the gas comes out of solution and small bubbles are formed within the interstitial tissues and blood; platelets are often associated with gas bubbles in the blood. These bubbles coalesce to form quite large masses. The clinical features are produced either by emboli in the circulating blood or by the presence of bubbles in the interstitial tissues, especially in tendons, joints and ligaments. Patients complain of excruciating pain (the syndrome being known as '**the bends**'). The central nervous system may be affected and the sudden onset of respiratory distress has also been described. The symptoms may be relieved by placing the patient in a compression chamber and forcing the gases back into solution. Once this has been done, slow and careful decompression should avoid a recurrence.

Occasionally the presence of nitrogen emboli in the systemic circulation is followed by ischaemic damage to the ends of long bones (aseptic necrosis); this is associated with secondary damage to the articular cartilages and joints.

FAT EMBOLI

Fat embolism is a common event occurring in 90% of patients who have sustained significant trauma. Significant clinical consequences are, happily, quite rare. It has been associated with:

- fractures of the long bones
- severe burns
- severe and extensive soft tissue trauma
- hyperlipidaemias
- ischaemic bone marrow necrosis in patients with sickle cell disease
- joint reconstruction
- cardio-pulmonary bypass
- acute pancreatitis
- intramedullary nailing in the course of certain orthopaedic procedures.

The fact that the syndrome can occur in the absence of trauma suggests a multifactorial pathogenesis, as discussed below. The two major theories of the pathogenesis of the fat embolism syndrome may be summed up as:

- the mechanical theory
- the biochemical theory.

The **mechanical theory** suggests that bone marrow-derived fat globules enter the venous system and lodge in the pulmonary vasculature as fat emboli. Droplets smaller than about 7–10 μm may pass through the pulmonary capillaries and eventually lodge in the systemic circulation. Indeed, urinary fat droplets are so common after injury that their presence is of little or no value in the diagnosis of the fat embolism syndrome.

The **biochemical theory** suggests that circulating free fatty acids directly affect cells lining the air spaces and thus produce abnormalities in gas exchange.

As is so often the case, it is likely that both these mechanisms act synergistically. The operation of the biochemical pathway would explain the occurrence of fat embolism syndrome **in the absence of trauma**. A rise in circulating catecholamines, which is seen in a number of pathophysiological situations including trauma and sepsis, promotes the release of free fatty acids from adipose tissue stores. In addition, an increase in the acute phase protein C-reactive protein causes chylomicrons to coalesce and form large fat globules.

Clinical fat embolism syndrome always manifests with pulmonary dysfunction in the form of low oxygen levels in blood and rapid breathing. This is the first manifestation of the syndrome. There is certainly convincing evidence that after, for example, reaming and intramedullary nailing of the femoral bone marrow compartment for the repair of fractures, material which can be detected by means of echocardiography passes into the right side of the heart and can cause the fat embolism syndrome.

Some patients present with predominant central nervous system involvement. They may become agitated at first and then lapse into coma; a high proportion of such patients die. At autopsy, if they have survived the onset of unconsciousness for a day or two, the brain shows oedema and **very many tiny haemorrhages**. These occur in both the grey and the white matter but are more easily seen in the latter site. Frozen sections of brain stained with fat soluble dyes show fat globules within the lumina of cerebral capillaries. There may be two explanations for the cases in which the nervous system is affected predominantly. The cerebral embolization may be due to the passage of emboli through a patent foramen ovale between the cardiac atria, an abnormality which is present in between 20–34% of individuals, or the emboli may be derived from the small droplets which can pass through the pulmonary capillaries.

Fat emboli occur more frequently than the fat embolization syndrome. Autopsies carried out on Korean war battle casualties dying within four weeks of having been injured showed evidence of fat embolization in 90% of cases. However, in only 1% could any part of the clinical picture in these patients be attributed to fat emboli.

BONE MARROW EMBOLI

Bone marrow emboli are not infrequently found on microscopic examination in post mortem samples of lung tissue from patients who have had episodes of cardiac arrest due to ventricular fibrillation and in whom the attempts at resuscitation have included external cardiac massage. In middle-aged and elderly people, in whom the costal cartilages have long since become ossified, repeated pressure on the rib cage usually results in the fracture of several ribs, and it is from these sites that the bone marrow is squeezed into the veins. It is not known what are the clinical effects, if any, of such emboli.

EMBOLI DERIVED FROM ATHEROMATOUS DEBRIS

Atheromatous emboli obviously occur only in the systemic arterial tree. They are derived from plaques which ulcerate and in which there is a massive basally situated pool of lipid and tissue debris, as described in Chapter 18. The emboli are usually found incidentally on histological examination of tissue and can be easily recognized since they consist of a mixture of thrombotic material and lipid-rich debris in which highly characteristic cigar- or torpedo-shaped cholesterol crystals are present.

EMBOLISM

- **Embolism** describes the transport of abnormal intravascular masses until they impact in a blood vessel smaller in diameter than they are.
- Emboli are of many types – solid and gaseous; by far the most common are those derived from **thrombus**.
- Emboli derived from venous thrombi impact in the pulmonary circulation; their effect depends largely on their size and, hence, the degree of obstruction to pulmonary blood flow that they cause.
- Large **pulmonary emboli** are frequently lethal; small, multiple emboli have chronic effects and may lead to pulmonary hypertension. Medium sized pulmonary emboli may cause areas of necrosis known as **infarcts**.
- **Systemic emboli** are most often derived from the left side of the heart. They may impact in any systemic vascular bed and cause ischaemia in any organ.
- **Fat emboli** occur most often after significant trauma. They may impact in any vascular bed but have the most serious consequences in the brain, where impaction is associated with multiple small haemorrhages.

Ischaemia and infarction

Ischaemia is the state that exists when an organ or tissue has its arterial perfusion lowered relative to its metabolic needs (Fig. 21.1). An **infarct** is a **morphological entity**: a large, localized area of tissue necrosis which is brought about by **ischaemia**.

Ischaemia is most often caused by some **local** interference with perfusion. On some occasions, however, the ischaemic state may be generalized. This is rare and is associated with a fall in cardiac output. Acute reductions in cardiac output are by no means uncommon, but they do not often cause ischaemic changes in individual tissues. Rarely, gangrene of the extremities may be seen following either extensive myocardial infarction or the sudden onset of a ventricular arrhythmia, both of which may be associated with a severe drop in cardiac output. Disorders of cardiac rhythm, including pathological changes in the conducting system, are not uncommon causes of cerebral ischaemia. An obvious and important example of this is **complete heart block**, in which sudden periods of unconsciousness (Stokes–Adams attacks) occur. If adequate perfusion of the brain is not restored within three to four minutes, irreparable damage to the neurones occurs.

LOCAL CAUSES OF ISCHAEMIA

The most important of the pathological bases of ischaemia – atherosclerosis, thrombosis and embolism – have been described in Chapters 18 to 20. In addition, arterial perfusion may be interfered with by arterial smooth muscle spasm or by pressure on the vessel from without. However, it is worth remembering that interruption of arterial blood flow is not the only way in which ischaemia may be produced; it can also be due to pathological changes affecting veins and capillaries.

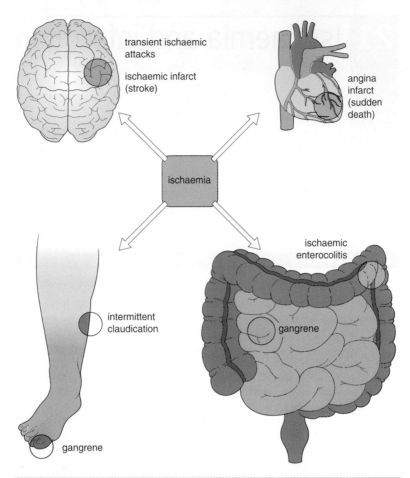

Fig. 21.1 Principal anatomic targets for ischaemia.

Ischaemia due to venous occlusion

The pathogenesis of ischaemia due to venous occlusion is outlined in *Fig. 21.2*. Ischaemia of this kind occurs only in anatomical situations where blood cannot bypass the obstruction via collateral drainage channels. Because of the interruption to venous return, affected tissues are likely to be **intensely congested** and possibly even **haemorrhagic**. Thus **venous infarction** is seen in:

- **extensive mesenteric venous thrombosis**, leading to small gut infarction
- so-called **strangulation of hernias**, where entrapment of bowel occurs leading to oedema and pressure on the draining veins

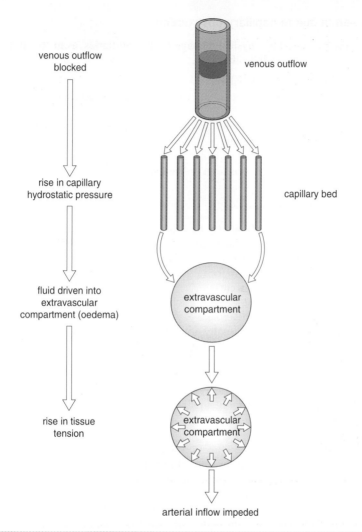

Fig. 21.2 Pathogenesis of ischaemia due to venous occlusion.

- **cavernous sinus thrombosis**, leading to thrombosis of the retinal vein and, ultimately, to blindness
- **thrombosis of the superior longitudinal sinus within the dura**; this can occur in severely dehydrated children and lead to patchy haemorrhagic necrosis in the cerebral cortex
- a very rare variant of **thrombosis in the iliofemoral system**, which may be followed by gangrene in the lower limb.

Ischaemia due to capillary obstruction

This may be caused by physical damage to the capillaries, as in 'frostbite'. Capillaries may be occluded by:

- parasites, as in cerebral malaria
- abnormal red cells, as in sickle cell disease or certain autoimmune haemolytic anaemias
- fibrin, where disseminated intravascular coagulation has occurred
- antigen–antibody complexes
- fat or gas emboli
- external pressure, such as is seen in '**bed sores**'.

Arterial obstruction

Obstruction of arterial inflow may be followed by a spectrum of functional and/or structural changes which ranges from no effect to extensive tissue necrosis. If neither functional nor structural changes occur, we can infer that the collateral arterial supply to the target area is good and that no significant reduction in perfusion has occurred.

Functional evidence of ischaemia

Functional disturbances are usually noted when the collateral supply is good enough to maintain adequate perfusion only so long as the metabolic demands of the tissue are at a basal level. If these demands are increased, as for example in the heart or the muscle of the lower limb during exercise, then ischaemia occurs and the patient will experience either substernal pain (**angina pectoris**) or a cramp-like pain in the calf (**intermittent claudication**). Cessation of activity leads, in most instances, to disappearance of the pain.

The eventual changes in the function of an ischaemic organ or tissue may result either from **loss of cells** or from **abnormal or deficient behaviour on the part of surviving cells**. In ischaemic myocardium, for example, there is a marked tendency for electrical disturbances to occur and these frequently give rise to fatal arrhythmias such as ventricular fibrillation. Indeed, at least half the patients who die in the course of their first 'heart attack', die in this way. Similarly ischaemia in sensory nerve bundles may lead to qualitative abnormalities in the sensory patterns interpreted within the central nervous system. It has been suggested that this mechanism may underlie the phenomenon of **persistent pain in patients with limb ischaemia**.

Structural changes caused by ischaemia

If the degree of ischaemia is greater than has been described above, then structural damage to cells and tissues will occur. This may take the form of patchy loss of parenchymal cells, such as is seen in the myocardium of patients with a long history of angina pectoris, or of massive necrosis. In either event, if the patient survives the ischaemic episode the lost tissue is replaced (except in the case of the brain) by fibrous tissue in a manner identical with that occurring in repair (see Chapter 8).

The degree of post-ischaemic necrosis is proportional to the degree of ischaemia; this, in turn, depends on the balance between the needs of an individual tissue and the decrease in arterial perfusion. When the ischaemia is slow in onset and chronic in nature, cell death characteristically affects either individual cells or small groups of cells.

Initially, affected cells show the changes of intracellular oedema or fatty change, eventually they die and are replaced by small foci of fibrous tissue. When such chronic ischaemia occurs in the heart it gives the muscle a curious flecked appearance because of the 'drop out' of small numbers of cells and their replacement by collagen fibres. In chronic lower limb ischaemia, the dermal papillae of the skin become flattened and both epidermis and dermis are thinned. Skin appendages such as hair follicles, sweat glands and sebaceous glands may also disappear. As a result of these changes, the skin appears shiny, hairless and dry.

THE DEGREE OF ISCHAEMIA

The degree of ischaemia is determined by a number of interacting variables (*Fig. 21.3*). These include:

- the metabolic needs of the underperfused tissue
- the speed of onset of arterial occlusion
- the completeness or otherwise of the arterial blocking
- the anatomy of the local blood supply
- the state of patency of the collateral blood supply.

Metabolic needs of underperfused tissue

Tissues vary in their capacity to withstand decreased arterial perfusion. The brain is the most sensitive in this respect; oxygen deprivation for

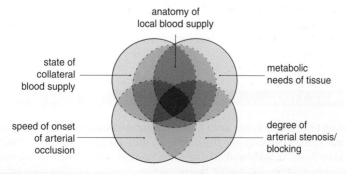

Fig. 21.3   Factors influencing the degree of ischaemia.

more than three to four minutes causes irreversible nerve cell damage. The myocardium is also very susceptible to ischaemic damage. It is doubly unfortunate that both brain and heart have rather poor collateral blood supplies and that neither heart muscle cells nor neurones are able to regenerate.

Speed of onset of arterial occlusion

If arterial occlusion takes place very rapidly as, for example, when an atherosclerotic coronary artery plaque ruptures, the effects of this are more severe than with slow narrowing of the same segment of artery, since there is little or no time for collateral vessels to open.

Completeness of the arterial blocking

Other things being equal, complete occlusion of an arterial lumen causes more extensive damage to the affected area than does severe stenosis. Equally, the more proximally the occlusion is situated in a given artery, the greater will be the area of tissue affected.

Anatomy of the local blood supply

Some organs or tissues have no collateral blood supply; arteries which perfuse such parts are known as 'end-arteries'. The retina is an example. It is supplied by a single vessel, the central retinal artery, which branches only once it has reached the retina. Unrelieved occlusion of the central retinal artery causes irreparable ischaemic damage within the retina. Smaller arteries within the cerebral cortex also function as end-arteries. In contrast, some tissues, such as the lung, have a double arterial supply. Occlusion of one part of this blood supply need not lead to ischaemic necrosis since the supply from the other source may be sufficient to maintain tissue viability.

Patency of the collateral blood supply

A good collateral supply can compensate for blockage in the main arterial tree only if the collateral vessels themselves are neither stenosed by athero-sclerotic plaques nor in spasm.

INFARCTION

An **infarct** is a **fairly large area of ischaemic necrosis** (usually coagulative in type). Blood may seep into the ischaemic area for some time, as a result of back flow from venules and oozing from vessels in the local microcircula-tion damaged in the course of the ischaemic process. Thus many infarcts contain a good deal of blood in the early stages of their natural history.

In spongy tissue, such as the lung, the escape of red blood cells and fibrin is a conspicuous feature and the ischaemic lung tissue becomes firmer than normal. At necropsy, infarcts of this type can be appreciated as wedge-shaped lumps on the pleural aspect of the lung. When the lung is cut into, the infarcted area tends to bulge from the surrounding normal lung. This outpouring or 'stuffing' of blood into the devitalized areas is merely an epiphenomenon and is not the core event in infarction. Failure of pathologists to appreciate this led to the introduction of the archaic and essentially unhelpful term '**infarct**', which is derived from the Latin verb '*infarcire*' meaning 'to stuff'.

With time the dying cells often swell. This tends to squeeze blood out of the interstitial tissue in the infarcted area and the infarct becomes much paler. In the heart, for example, it takes 24–36 hours for this process to become complete. The pallor is a useful marker for the macroscopic diagnosis of infarction at necropsy. However, because pallor takes a considerable time to develop, it may be difficult to make such a necropsy diagnosis in the early stages of the natural history of a myocardial infarct.

The division of infarcts into **pale** and **red** varieties other than in the brain is pointless. Many infarcts start off red and become pale as the blood is squeezed out of the infarcted area by swelling of the dying cells. Cerebral infarcts are usually pale from the outset (unless they are embolic in origin); infarcts in the spongy lung tissue remain red and undergo repair while still at that stage.

Dead parenchymal cells in the infarcted area undergo auto-digestion and the red blood cells that have escaped from damaged capillaries break and release their haemoglobin. The dead tissue elicits a brisk inflammatory reaction: first neutrophils and then macrophages infiltrate the necrotic tissue. Breakdown products of haemoglobin – haematoidin (bile pigment) and haemosiderin (aggregated molecules of ferritin) – may be deposited and are ingested by macrophages. At this stage, usually about one week after arterial occlusion, an infarct in a solid organ is generally firm in consistency and a dull yellow in colour, with a red zone of hyperaemia at the margins.

The large number of macrophages corresponds with the **demolition** phase of an inflammatory reaction, and is equally important in the context of infarction. In some tissues, for example the heart, dead parenchymal cells are removed rapidly; they are then rapidly replaced, first by granulation tissue and then by scar tissue. In other situations, such as the kidney, the infarct persists, sometimes for months, before being replaced by scar tissue. Histological examination of such an area shows the 'ghost outlines' of the architectural elements of the tissue, the tubules and glomeruli, although the constituent parenchymal cells are clearly dead. A slow but progressive ingrowth of connective tissue occurs even in these cases, and eventually the infarct becomes converted to a fibrous scar in which calcium salts may be deposited (dystrophic calcification).

The sequence of events described above may be interrupted, at any time, by the death of the patient.

INFARCTION IN SPECIFIC SITES

The central nervous system

The general description above of the natural history of infarcts does not apply to the brain. Here the processes involved after cerebral ischaemia are somewhat different. The necrosis is typically **liquefactive** rather than coagulative and this may, in the long term, lead to cavity formation.

Microscopic features

The early stages of the development of a cerebral infarct are characterized by a transient neutrophil response which is followed by a period of intense phagocytic activity by the **microglial cells**. These cells, which in their resting phase, are normally small, cluster in the infarcted area and phagocytose lipid liberated from degenerate myelin. The cytoplasm of the microglia therefore, increases markedly and appears foamy or granular in appearance. (Classically these swollen microglia are referred to as **compound granular corpuscles**.) Reactive astrocytes now gather at the margins of the infarct and synthesize new glial fibres, which eventually replace part or all of the infarcted tissue.

The heart

Cardiac ischaemia is the single most important cause of death in Western communities. Approximately 150 000 adults in the United Kingdom die every year from ischaemic heart disease (about 25% of all deaths). Myocardial ischaemia may express itself in a number of ways, and it is important to realize that different clinical pictures may be brought about by different pathogenetic mechanisms. The patients may:

- complain of angina on effort (**'stable' angina**) caused by an increase in myocardial oxygen and nutrient demand
- develop angina at rest (**'unstable' angina**) caused by a drop in perfusion rather than increased myocardial oxygen demand
- die suddenly as a result of a lethal **ventricular arrhythmia**
- develop **acute myocardial necrosis (infarction)** of different patterns and with different underlying pathogenetic processes
- develop **failure of muscle pumping activity** due to extensive muscle loss.

Stable angina pectoris

At autopsy on patients dying **with** rather than **from** angina pectoris, the myocardium may show no macroscopic abnormalities. In some instances there will have been ischaemic necrosis of small groups of heart muscle cells, shown by small flecks of fibrous tissue in the muscle wall of the left ventricle. The coronary arteries invariably show the presence of severe stenosis by atherosclerotic lesions.

Sudden death

Sudden death may be defined as death occurring from myocardial ischaemia within one hour of the onset of acute symptoms. In practice many of these deaths occur within a few minutes. Sudden death is a major part of the overall problem of ischaemic heart disease, since at least 50% of the deaths due to a first attack of ischaemia occur in this way and without the patient having the benefit of medical attention. Death is due to the onset of severe ventricular arrhythmias, most notably ventricular fibrillation with loss of cardiac output.

Of the patients who collapse with such severe arrhythmias and who are resuscitated, only 16% develop a Q wave on electrocardiography (suggestive of myocardial necrosis involving most of the left ventricular wall thickness); 45% show elevations in the plasma concentrations of enzymes derived from heart muscle. Thus a majority of these patients show no clinical or biochemical evidence of acute myocardial necrosis. Post mortem examination of the majority of patients dying suddenly in this way reveals evidence of acute, though not necessarily occlusive, thrombosis. The prevalence of **occlusive thrombi** is lower than in patients dying with myocardial infarction. Narrowing of the lumina of the coronary arteries by 80% or more is very frequent in these patients. *Thrombi are almost always present in those individuals who die in the course of their first attack.* In those who have survived a previous major ischaemic episode and who have scars in the myocardium, the onset of ventricular fibrillation is not necessarily associated with acute thrombosis: scar tissue alone seems sufficient to trigger the arrhythmia.

Acute myocardial necrosis

Acute myocardial necrosis occurs in two distinct patterns, although a combination of these may sometimes be seen. It is useful to distinguish between these patterns since the pathogenesis of each differs considerably.

Distinction between the patterns of acute myocardial necrosis requires the ability to identify irreversibly damaged heart muscle. If the heart is examined some 18 to 36 hours after the onset of severe underperfusion there is no problem. The ischaemic heart muscle shows all the features of coagulative necrosis; macroscopically the necrotic area is a dull, yellowish, 'wash-leather'-like colour with a hyperaemic zone at the periphery. However, if the patient dies earlier, recognition of ischaemic damage is much more difficult.

If the patient has survived 6–9 hours after the onset of the acute ischaemia, the difficulty can be overcome by using a simple histochemical technique. This depends on the fact (see p. 31) that an irreversibly damaged cell loses its intracellular water-soluble enzymes. Respiratory enzymes, such as succinic dehydrogenase, in normal heart muscle can be shown by immersing a slice of unfixed heart muscle in a solution of the dye nitroblue tetrazolium. This is a yellow dye which acts as a hydrogen acceptor. In the presence of a normal intracellular content of dehydrogenase, the yellow dye turns a bluish-purple colour and is deposited on the tissue at the site where the reaction has taken place. *Where a cell has been irreversibly damaged and has lost its intracellular dehydrogenases, no such colour reaction takes place.* Thus, viable and non-viable muscle can be distinguished from each other with relative ease.

Regional myocardial infarction.   The commonest pattern of acute ischaemic myocardial necrosis is regional infarction (*Fig. 21.4*). This is a large single area of coagulative necrosis, measuring at least 3 cm along one of its axes and **usually involving more than 50% of the thickness of the ventricular wall**. In more than 90% of cases this pattern is associated with occlusive thrombosis in the coronary artery segment supplying the affected area of muscle. The majority of these thrombi occur in relation to breaks in the connective tissue caps of underlying atherosclerotic plaques.

Subendocardial necrosis.   Subendocardial necrosis in its pure form is much less common than regional infarction at necropsy. Here the necrosis is confined to the **inner half** of the left ventricular myocardium, a very thin

regional transmural infarction   regional non-transmural infarction

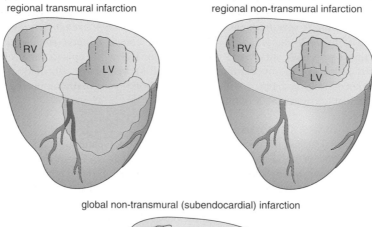

global non-transmural (subendocardial) infarction

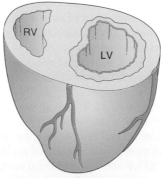

Fig. 21.4   Patterns of acute ischaemic necrosis.

layer of viable muscle immediately beneath the endocardium always being present (*Fig. 21.4*). The necrosis may be segmental or can extend to involve the whole circumference of the left ventricle. Occlusive thrombi in the coronary arteries are found in only about 15% of cases, though severe stenosing atherosclerosis is widespread within the coronary artery tree.

Subendocardial ischaemic necrosis is the morphological expression of a **generalized lowering of myocardial perfusion**. It can occur in the absence of coronary artery disease in such situations as severe aortic valve stenosis and incompetence. Its pathogenesis can be understood most easily if one recalls two facts. These are that:

- perfusion of the myocardium takes place during **diastole**
- the wall tension in the left ventricular myocardium is greater in the subendocardial zone than in the subepicardial region.

In a person with normal coronary arteries, the **perfusion drive** can be represented as the difference between the diastolic pressure in the aortic root and the intra-cavity pressure in the left ventricle (*Fig. 21.5*). The total perfusion during any single cardiac cycle is determined by the time during which the drive is allowed to act and, hence, by the length of diastole. Any circumstances which lessen the pressure difference between the aortic root pressure and the intra-cavity in the left ventricle, or which shorten the diastolic interval, may reduce myocardial perfusion sufficiently to produce ischaemic necrosis.

Complications of myocardial infarction. Each stage of the natural history of myocardial infarction may hold dangers for the patient (*Fig. 21.6*).

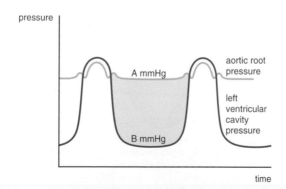

Fig. 21.5 Factors controlling perfusion of the subendocardial zone of the left ventricular wall.

Perfusion 'drive' = A mmHg – B mmHg. Total diastolic perfusion = (A–B) × length of diastole, and is represented by the shaded area. Any decrease in (A–B) or in the length of diastole may lead to subendocardial necrosis.

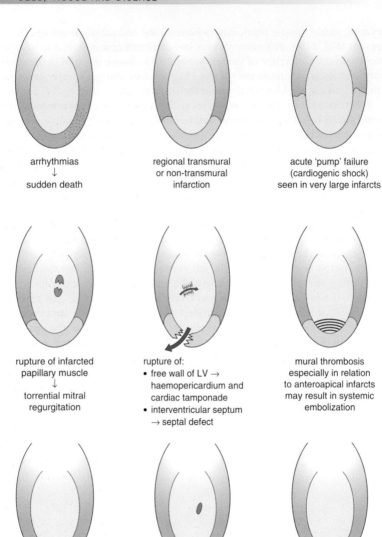

arrhythmias
↓
sudden death

regional transmural
or non-transmural
infarction

acute 'pump' failure
(cardiogenic shock)
seen in very large infarcts

rupture of infarcted
papillary muscle
↓
torrential mitral
regurgitation

rupture of:
• free wall of LV →
  haemopericardium and
  cardiac tamponade
• interventricular septum
  → septal defect

mural thrombosis
especially in relation
to anteroapical infarcts
may result in systemic
embolization

extensive post-ischaemic
scarring → chronic
pump failure

post-ischaemic
atrophy of papillary muscle
→ mitral regurgitation

stretching of scar
tissue → aneurysm

Fig. 21.6   Possible consequences of acute myocardial ischaemia.

LV, left ventricle.

In the early stages the chief danger is the possible development of ventricular fibrillation leading to asystole and sudden death.

As the coagulative necrosis develops and the dead muscle elicits a brisk acute inflammatory response, focal softening of necrotic muscle may occur. This can lead to rupture of the left ventricle; either the free wall may rupture into the pericardial cavity, death being due to the rapid accumulation of blood within the pericardial sac (**cardiac tamponade**), or the septum may rupture with the production of a defect in the interventricular septum.

Similar softening can affect the papillary muscles; if rupture of one or more of these occurs, the patient will develop a torrential regurgitant jet through the mitral valve. A somewhat less dramatic and not uncommon development of mitral valve incompetence may occur simply as a result of ischaemic necrosis and scarring of papillary muscles.

The abnormal haemodynamics that can occur within the left ventricular cavity following infarction may lead to the formation of mural thrombi. Portions of these can break off and embolize the systemic circulation.

Healing of the infarcted muscle can also be associated with circumstances unfavourable to the patient. If there has been extensive loss of cardiac muscle in the process of infarction, correspondingly large amounts of fibrous tissue are formed during healing. This tissue lacks the power of recoil possessed by muscle and becomes gradually stretched and thinned by the normal rise of intra-cavity pressure during ventricular systole. This may lead to a local dilatation or **ventricular aneurysm**, which can be a severe haemodynamic disadvantage to the patient. Extensive fibrosis following infarction of the anterior wall of the left ventricle may involve both bundle branches and lead to complete heart block.

The lung

Fewer than 10% of pulmonary emboli cause infarcts, a figure which emphasizes the importance of the state of the pulmonary circulation at the time when embolization occurs. In young people whose cardiac status is good, infarction is rare. This relative sparing is thought to be due, at least in part, to the double blood supply of the lung from the pulmonary and bronchial arteries.

Any rise in pressure in the pulmonary veins (as occurs in mitral stenosis or left ventricular failure) markedly increases the chances of infarction occurring if medium-sized branches of the pulmonary arteries become occluded. The vast majority of infarcts are due to emboli derived from thrombi in the leg veins; about 10% are derived from thrombi formed in the right side of the heart.

Pulmonary infarcts are generally described as wedge-shaped, the base of the wedge being situated towards the pleural aspect of the lung. In their early stages they are deep red in colour. At necropsy these infarcts are often more easily felt than seen. A fibrinous pleural reaction over the infarcted area is common and there may, on occasions, be small haemorrhagic effusions in the pleural cavity. Organization usually proceeds rapidly, perhaps because of the rich vascular network in the surrounding lung tissue. The infarcts are converted into inconspicuous scars and tend to be concealed by the surrounding lung tissue, which often shows compensatory overdistension.

The liver

True infarcts in the liver are rare, presumably because spontaneous occlusion of the hepatic artery is correspondingly rare. Also, like the lung, the liver has a double blood supply. However, accidental ligation of the hepatic artery in the course of surgery may produce true infarcts in the liver. Patchy hepatic infarction may also occur if the hepatic artery branches within the liver are involved in immune complex mediated diseases such as polyarteritis nodosa.

The intestine

The commonest causes of intestinal ischaemia are mechanical: **hernial strangulation**, **volvulus** (twisting of a segment of intestine) and **intussusception**. In the latter, excessive peristaltic contraction drives the affected segment of bowel forward, so that the segment of bowel immediately distal lies in a sleeve-like manner over it. Some of the mesentery is included in the portion of bowel which is pushed forward and the resulting local oedema leads to local ischaemia. Apart from such mechanical disasters, intestinal ischaemia can result from thrombotic or embolic occlusion of the mesenteric arteries or even from extensive mesenteric venous thrombosis. In this last instance the interference with venous drainage leads to a very marked degree of congestion affecting the mucosal and submucosal vessels, and the patient may pass fresh blood per rectum.

When the degree of intestinal ischaemia is sufficient to cause infarction, the bowel wall feels stiffer than normal and is a dark plum colour. The serosal surface is the site of a fibrinous inflammatory response; the normal shiny appearance of the serosa is dulled and slightly roughened. The necrotic bowel wall becomes colonized quite rapidly by the saprophytic organisms in the lumen and thus may show the features of true gangrene. Factors contributing to the death of such patients include intestinal paralysis (ileus) with loss of fluid and electrolytes into the gut lumen, haemorrhage, perforation, which causes generalized peritonitis, and bacteraemic shock.

Ischaemia of the gut need not lead in all cases to such a dramatic conclusion. It is now well recognized that periods of lowered arterial perfusion, affecting particularly the region of the splenic flexure, may lead to localized mucosal ulceration. Healing of these ulcers is accompanied by a very considerable degree of scar tissue formation, which may lead to localized narrowing of the gut lumen in the affected areas. During the healing phase these post-ischaemic ulcers show the presence of a broad band of granulation tissue extending into the submucosa and containing many macrophages laden with iron derived from broken-down red blood cells (haemosiderin).

SHOCK

Shock is a clinical syndrome characterized by systemic underperfusion of tissues due to prolonged, severe hypotension. The mechanisms capable of causing shock are:

- a significant decrease in the *volume of circulating blood* – **hypovolaemic shock**
- failure of the heart as a pump – **cardiogenic shock**
- a significant increase in the *capacity* of the circulatory system caused by an abnormal degree of vasodilatation – **redistributive shock**, seen most frequently in the context of bacterial sepsis.

HYPOVOLAEMIC SHOCK

Hypovolaemia occurs in:

- severe haemorrhage
- major loss of body fluids as in severe diarrhoea or vomiting or where there is extensive skin loss after burning.

The initial clinical picture reflects the compensatory mechanisms for the drop in cardiac output caused by the fall in blood or plasma volume. *The heart rate is increased and there is extensive peripheral vasoconstriction* brought about by vasoconstrictors such as catecholamines, vasopressin and the angiotensin system.

CARDIOGENIC SHOCK

This occurs when the cardiac output is insufficient to maintain normal tissue perfusion. It is most common in the context of acute myocardial infarction. Loss of 35% or more of ventricular muscle leads to a significant fall in cardiac output. Subendocardial myocardial necrosis occurs because of the low output, further worsening myocardial pump function.

REDISTRIBUTIVE (SEPTIC) SHOCK

Septic shock may occur as a result of systemic infections with a variety of pathogenic microorganisms including both Gram-negative and Gram-positive bacteria and, occasionally, viruses (dengue fever) and fungi (systemic candidiasis). The patients have severe hypotension and, *unlike cardiogenic or hypovolaemic shock, their skin is warm* due to **systemic vasodilatation**. This is a major factor in the pathogenesis of this syndrome and is difficult to reverse with commonly used vasopressors. Many of the lesions seen in fatal cases of septic shock are clearly ischaemic, e.g. renal changes causing acute renal failure and ischaemic colitis, but others are associated with certain features specific for septic shock:

- a **consumptive coagulopathy (disseminated intravascular coagulation)** manifest in a number of ways including purpura (e.g. meningococcal septicaemia)
- **adult respiratory distress syndrome (ARDS)**
- **reduction of the ventricular systolic ejection fraction and consequent ventricular dilatation**, possibly due to release of a molecule that depresses myocardial function.

Fully developed septic shock carries a mortality rate of 80–90%. Before it develops, however, there is a phase which should be recognized clinically; this is called the 'sepsis syndrome' and is characterized by fever, tachycardia and some evidence of inadequate tissue perfusion such as oliguria, alterations in mental status or hypoxaemia. At this stage, mortality rates are much lower (10–20%).

Pathogenesis

The role of endotoxin

Many of the features of septic shock depend on the action of bacterial endotoxin (lipopolysaccharide), a common component of the cell structure of many Gram-negative bacteria. Endotoxin consists of a lipid (lipid A), the 'toxic' portion of the molecule, linked with a complex polysaccharide. It is heat-stable and poorly immunogenic.

Endotoxin is directly cytotoxic under certain circumstances, most notably to endothelium, but it produces most of its effect by interacting with several different cell types and plasma protein cascade systems to cause the release of many other chemical signals. Some are vasoactive, causing vasodilatation and thus hypotension; others contribute to the pathogenesis of disseminated intravascular coagulation.

Endotoxin interactions and cytokine production

Compounds released from interactions between endotoxin, certain cells and plasma protein cascade systems result in the release of:

- cytokines such as TNF-1α, IL-1, IL-6 and IFN-γ
- nitric oxide (NO)
- products of arachidonic acid metabolism such as prostaglandins, leukotrienes and platelet-activating factor.

These are summarized in *Table 21.1*. One of the most important of the cytokines is TNF-α, which is responsible for many of the features of shock induced by both endo- and exotoxins. When injected in a purified form into small animals, TNF reproduces most of the features of septic shock. IL-1 and IFN-γ act in synergy with TNF.

Nitric oxide in septic shock Nitric oxide is a major, if not the principal, determinant of normal vascular tone. It is constitutively (normally) produced by vascular endothelium, and its production is upregulated by such

Table 21.1 Endotoxin interactions

Target for toxin interaction	Products released	Patho-physiological effects	Clinical effects
Macrophages	IL-1 TNF-α IFN-γ IL-6 Nitric oxide (NO) released via inducible NO synthase	Phagocytes activated Prostaglandin released in hypothalamus All inflammatory reactions upregulated NO causes abnormal systemic vasodilatation	Fever Drowsiness Increased capillary permeability, especially in lung
Complement	C3a C5a	Vasodilatation Increased capillary permeability Phagocyte activation	Hypotension Capillary leakage
Platelets	PAF Thromboxane A_2 Platelet factor 3	Upregulation of inflammatory processes Aggregation of platelets Procoagulant effect	Vasodilatation causing hypotension Intravascular coagulation
Neutrophils	Cationic proteins Kallikrein Lysosomal enzymes	Mast cell degranulation Kinins produced Complement activated	Hypotension Capillary leakage
Hageman factor	Kinin system activated Intrinsic clotting pathway activated Fibrinolytic pathway activated	Release of kallikrein and kinins Consumption of fibrinogen	Intravascular clotting Haemorrhage as a result of fibrinogen consumption Hypotension

compounds as acetylcholine and bradykinin which cause vasodilatation in normal arteries.

NO is derived from the amino acid L-arginine. Its production is catalysed by the enzyme NO synthase, the constitutive form of which is present in endothelial cells. NO can, however, be produced in cells which do not normally release NO, via an **inducible** form of the synthase. This type of NO production occurs in sepsis; major sources are macrophages, endothelial cells and vascular smooth muscle cells. *Induction can be brought about by endotoxin, certain exotoxins and cytokines.*

The inappropriately large amount of NO thus released causes marked vasodilatation, and the vessels are refractory to vasopressor agents. This refractory state can be overcome by administration of inhibitors of NO synthase.

Other bacterial toxins

The redistributive shock syndrome can occur also as a result of infections with certain Gram-positive organisms. The responsible molecules may be exotoxins such as staphylococcal enterotoxin, *exfoliatin* which cleaves the junctions between epidermal cells causing Lyell–Ritter's disease (scalded skin syndrome), or the toxic shock syndrome toxin 1 which is a product of some strains of *Staphylococcus aureus*. These exotoxins function as **super-antigens**, i.e. they can bind to and activate certain T cells without needing to be presented with an MHC class II protein. The T cells then release large quantities of cytokines such as TNF-1α and interferon-γ (IFN-γ).

It is believed that some cell wall components of Gram-positive organisms such as peptidoglycans and lipoteichoic acid may also exert a direct toxic effect.

Morphological features of shock

The pathological picture of shock is characterized by the results of poor perfusion due to ischaemia and by evidence of disseminated intravascular coagulation (microthrombi and haemorrhages). Virtually any tissue can be affected though some are clearly more vulnerable than others. The organs commonly affected are (in descending order of frequency) lungs, heart, kidneys, liver, pancreas, gut, brain, pituitary and adrenals.

ISCHAEMIA AND INFARCTION

- **Ischaemia** is a pathophysiological state where tissues are underperfused with blood in relation to their metabolic needs.
- **Infarction** is defined morphologically as an area of tissue necrosis caused by ischaemia.
- Ischaemia is rarely systemic, being caused by a drop in cardiac output. It is more commonly local when the most frequent cause is impairment of arterial perfusion, though occasionally venous occlusion (as in strangulated hernia) may cause ischaemia.
- Ischaemia may cause functional and/or structural changes. The former include angina pectoris and intermittent claudication. The latter range from 'drop-out' of a small number of cells to large areas of necrosis (infarction).
- The degree of ischaemia depends on the interaction of several important factors: the metabolic needs of the underperfused tissue, the speed of decline of perfusion, and the anatomy of the local blood supply.
- Infarcts are normally the expression of coagulative necrosis, except in the brain where the necrosis is usually liquefactive.

22 Abnormal accumulations of fluid and disturbances of blood distribution

A normal physiological state requires an appropriate relationship between **intravascular** and **extravascular** fluid. Gross increases in extravascular fluid volume in certain anatomical situations, notably the lung and brain, may kill. There may also be alterations in the distribution of blood in various tissue beds leading, for one reason or another, to local increases in the amount of blood present in a given organ or tissue.

OEDEMA

Clinical oedema is an abnormal accumulation of fluid in the extracellular space. (This, therefore, excludes the increases in cytoplasmic sodium and water considered in the section on cell injury.) From a simple clinical point of view, the recognition of oedema depends on the identification of this excess fluid within the interstitial tissues and is exemplified by the pitting that finger pressure causes in the lower part of the legs in cardiac failure.

Factors controlling distribution of extracellular body water

Total body water is approximately 49 litres. The intracellular component accounts for about 35 litres, and varies very little. The intravascular compartment contains about 3 litres, and a further 11 litres are present in the extravascular compartment. *The maintenance of a relatively constant relationship between intravascular and extravascular water depends on several factors.*

Factors that tend to cause fluid to leave the vascular compartment
Increased intravascular hydrostatic pressure may produce profound changes in fluid distribution. For instance, severe mitral stenosis causes a chronic rise

in pulmonary venous pressure and hence increased pulmonary capillary pressure. If such a patient takes severe exercise, the resulting increase in pulmonary artery pressure may be sufficient to overcome all other relevant homeostatic mechanisms; fluid will then leak from the pulmonary alveolar capillaries, first into the alveolar walls and then into the air spaces themselves.

Increased colloid osmotic pressure in the extravascular compartment also causes more fluid to leave the microvasculature.

Factors that, under normal circumstances, tend to keep fluid within the vascular compartment

The osmotic pressure of the plasma proteins. Albumin, with its relatively low molecular weight and high concentration relative to other plasma proteins, is the most important. A fall in the plasma concentration of albumin, due either to **reduced synthesis** as in chronic liver disease, or to **excessive loss** as in certain forms of kidney disease, may be associated with quite severe oedema.

Selective permeability function of endothelium. Normally albumin does not leave the vascular compartment in significant amounts. Should the permeability barrier function of the capillary wall become impaired, there will be a decline in the plasma concentration of albumin and a corresponding increase in the protein content of the fluid in the interstitial tissues.

Tissue tension in the interstitial tissue. This tends to limit the egress of fluid from the microvasculature. Normally this tension is low (less than 1 kPa).

All these physical factors can be summed up in the following mathematical expression:

$$J_v = k[(P_c - P_i) - \pi_c - \pi_i]$$

where J_v is the local rate of fluid flux along the length of a capillary; k is the capillary hydraulic permeability; P_c is the capillary hydraulic pressure; P_i is the hydraulic pressure; π_c is the capillary osmotic pressure; and π_i is the colloid osmotic pressure in the interstitial fluid.

Normally there is a **net loss** of fluid from the vascular compartment to the interstitial tissue but no oedema develops. This is because excess fluid drains away via the lymphatics from the site where it might otherwise accumulate, eventually returning to the blood via the thoracic duct. Should the normal flow of lymph be obstructed, oedema fluid will collect.

Some of the most striking examples of local oedema occur in the context of lymphatic obstruction, this being known as **lymphoedema**. Examples include the severe chronic swelling of the upper limb seen in some women following removal of the breast and axillary contents for carcinoma of the breast (radical mastectomy) and the spectacular oedema that may occur in the tropics in individuals infected with the helminth *Wuchereria bancrofti* (so-called **elephantiasis**).

Table 20.1 The characteristics of exudates and transudates

Characteristics	Exudate	Transudate
Total protein	High	Low (1 g/100 ml)
Protein pattern	As in plasma	Albumin only
Fibrinogen	++ (and clots)	Nil
Specific gravity	1.020	1.012
Cells	++	Few mesothelial cells

Types of oedema fluid: transudate and exudate

Oedema may be either **local** or **systemic**. The characteristics of the oedema fluid depend on the mechanisms predominantly involved in its formation (see *Table 22.1*). If the collection of fluid in the interstitial tissues is due to increased **vascular permeability** then the fluid will contain large amounts of macromolecular proteins including fibrinogen; this is termed an **exudate**. If the mechanisms involved are predominantly **hydrostatic** then the protein content of the fluid will be low; such fluid is spoken of as being a **transudate**.

In practical terms the three most important factors causing oedema are:

1) raised intracapillary pressure
2) low plasma oncotic pressure
3) retention of salt and water.

Coexistence of any two of these is likely to be associated with oedema of considerable severity.

SYSTEMIC OEDEMA

Cardiac oedema

Although systemic oedema caused by congestive cardiac failure has been recognized for many centuries, the mechanisms involved are by no means simple or easy to understand. There is not only a redistribution but a general retention of fluid, this being shown by an increase in body weight of the patient. The distribution of the excess fluid is determined largely by gravity. When the patient is ambulant, the legs are first involved; swelling of the ankles at the end of the day is often the first sign reported. When the patient is confined to bed, the oedema appears in the sacral or, less commonly, in the genital region. The oedematous areas pit readily on finger pressure.

It would be tempting to ascribe this oedema purely to failure of the pumping function of the ventricles, leading to an increase in venous pressure and a consequent increase in capillary hydrostatic pressure with the formation of a transudate. However, this would be not only a gross oversimplification, but also wrong, although this mechanism does contribute to the development of cardiac oedema.

Doubt about the significance of the role of back pressure in cardiac oedema arises from three observations:

1) There is often an increased **plasma volume** in heart failure, which may occur before there is any rise in central venous pressure.
2) Oedema frequently occurs **before the rise in central venous pressure**.
3) The **degree of oedema is not proportional to the height of the central venous pressure**.

The most important mechanism in causing the oedema of cardiac failure is **excess retention of sodium and water by the renal tubules**. Failure of the heart as a pump leads initially to a fall in mean capillary pressure. This will in turn lead to a reduction in renal perfusion, aggravated by vaso-constriction mediated by the sympathetic nervous system. This relative renal ischaemia causes an increase in the production of renin and thus of angiotensin I. The rise in angiotensin levels causes an increased release of aldosterone from the zona glomerulosa of the adrenal cortex and retention of sodium and water. At first, such retention has a good effect because it allows the mean filling pressure in the circulation to be increased. The increased filling of the heart stretches the heart muscle fibres and thus leads, in terms of Starling's law, to increased force of contraction. In due time, however, any advantage arising from sodium and water retention is lost.

Once cardiac filling pressure and hence stretching of muscle fibres exceeds a certain point, there is no further increase in cardiac output; indeed there is a decline in the work output of the cardiac muscle. Excess accu-mulation of fluid in the lung (pulmonary oedema) may ensue and this may interfere with gas exchange in the alveoli.

Renal oedema

Oedema related to renal disorders occurs under two different sets of circum-stances, in association with the nephritic and the nephrotic syndrome.

Oedema associated with acute glomerulonephritis (the nephritic syndrome)

Oedema is often a presenting feature in this disease, although it is usually not severe. The face and eyelids are affected predominantly, although some-times the ankles and genitalia may be involved as well. There is no entirely satisfactory explanation for either the cause of the oedema or its distribution. However, it is likely that the control of sodium excretion in the urine is multifactorial and that states of sodium retention may exist in which there is no associated disturbance of plasma volume. In most examples of systemic oedema the kidney behaves as if it were responding to a low plasma volume stimulus. There are other vasoactive stimuli, however, including circulating catecholamines, aldosterone and intrarenal hormones such as prostaglandins or kinins, that may influence renal tubular handling of sodium. It has been suggested that the primary mechanism responsible for **nephritic oedema** is a fall in glomerular filtration rate, tubular reabsorption of sodium remaining more or less normal. The resulting increase in extracellular fluid volume would normally be followed promptly by excretion of sodium in the urine but this response appears to be blunted in acute glomerulonephritis. The oedema fluid in acute glomerulonephritis has the characteristics of a transudate, indicating that no significant change has occurred in the permeability of the microcirculation.

Oedema associated with the nephrotic syndrome

The nephrotic syndrome encompasses a group of features that most notably includes **heavy proteinuria** (in excess of the ability of the liver to synthesize albumin) leading to **hypoalbuminaemia** and a resulting **decrease in plasma oncotic pressure**. While this loss of plasma protein certainly plays a part in the genesis of the systemic oedema encountered in this syndrome, other mechanisms also operate, including excess retention of sodium by the renal tubules. This is partly due to increased aldosterone production by the adrenal cortex, but some workers believe that non-systemic intrarenal mechanisms related to sodium reabsorption are also of importance.

Nutritional oedema

Oedema is a well-recognized feature of prolonged starvation. There is no correlation between the degree of oedema and the concentrations within the blood of albumin and other plasma proteins; indeed, oedema associated with starvation may be seen in the presence of normal concentrations of plasma protein. It has been suggested that the explanation for this variety of oedema lies in the loss of subcutaneous adipose tissue. The subcutaneous connective tissue is therefore of much looser texture than normal and there is an associated decline in the tissue tension within it. Bed rest is usually followed by a brisk diuresis and consequent lessening of the degree of oedema.

An important and, regrettably, common variant of nutritional oedema occurs in **kwashiorkor**. This is the result of protein and calorie undernutrition in young children in economically deprived communities in Africa, Asia, and Central and South America. The children fail to grow normally, are anaemic and have grossly fatty livers. They often exhibit a curious combination of **oedema** (associated with hypoalbuminaemia), **mucocutaneous ulceration** (the skin of the inner thighs often looks as if it has been scalded), and **depigmentation of the hair**. Adequate nutrition in terms of the protein content of the diet can produce a complete return to normal.

Oedema due to chronic liver disease

In liver disease oedema often appears as **ascites** (excess free fluid in the peritoneal cavity). Its pathogenesis is complex and involves such factors as:

- raised intracapillary pressure in the splanchnic bed
- decreased plasma albumin leading to a lowered plasma oncotic pressure

- increased formation of hepatic lymph
- in cirrhosis, increased sodium retention.

Pulmonary oedema

As elsewhere, distribution of fluid between intravascular and extravascular compartments in the lung is governed by:

- intracapillary hydrostatic pressure
- capillary permeability.

An increase in either or both will lead to pulmonary oedema, which is defined as more than 4–5 ml of fluid per gram of dry, blood-free lung.
   High pressure oedema (the commonest variety) occurs in:

- left ventricular failure from any cause
- ventricular and supraventricular tachycardias
- high pulmonary vein pressure as seen in mitral valve disease.

High capillary pressure is also a major contributor in:

- intravenous fluid overload
- severe anaemia
- brain injury including subarachnoid and intracerebral bleeding
- renal failure
- high altitude.

Severe oedema due to increased permeability of the pulmonary capillaries occurs in adult respiratory distress syndrome (ARDS). The commonest conditions associated with ARDS are:

- aspiration of gastric contents into the lung
- disseminated intravascular coagulation
- pneumonia
- severe trauma
- bacteraemia.

In terms of risk of dying, the most dangerous are aspiration of gastric contents, bacteraemia and pneumonia.

Local oedema

Local oedema may be due to three types of disturbance.

  1. A **local increase in the hydrostatic pressure within the micro-circulation**. This can occur in pregnancy, in patients with occlusive venous thrombosis, and in those with varicose veins where the valves are incompetent and give rise to increased pressure in the superficial plexus of draining veins.

2. **Increased local vascular permeability** as in acute inflammation and type I hypersensitivity reactions such as urticaria and angioneurotic oedema.
3. Lymphoedema.

Any obstruction to the normal lymph flow from surgery or inflammation may cause quite severe local oedema. For example, some patients undergoing radical surgery with axillary clearance for carcinoma of the breast develop severe, intractable oedema of the arm on the side of the operation. The inflammatory disease classically associated with lymphatic obstruction is infestation by the nematode worm *Wuchereria bancrofti* (filariasis). Adult worms inhabit the groin lymphatics. While alive, the parasite produces little disability; when it dies, however, there is brisk local inflammation which leads eventually to lymphatic obstruction. The resulting oedema of the lower limbs and the genitalia is severe and chronic, so severe that the condition is sometimes spoken of as **elephantiasis**. Sometimes lymphoedema may develop as a result of congenital malformations in the lymphatic drainage; an autosomal dominant variety of this is known as Milroy's disease.

HYPERAEMIA AND CONGESTION

These two terms mean that there is a **greater amount of blood than normal** in a given organ or tissue. Clearly there can be only two mechanisms for this: an **increased inflow** or a **diminished outflow** of blood (*Fig. 22.1*).

Increased blood inflow must be due to arteriolar dilatation (**active hyperaemia**). It occurs in inflamed areas, with excess heat, in flushing, and at the margins of areas of ischaemic necrosis.

Diminished outflow is essentially **obstructive**. The obstruction may be functional rather than structural. An example of this occurs in chronic bronchitis: hypoxia causes reflex constriction of the pulmonary arteriole, which leads to pulmonary hypertension, increased right ventricular afterload and hence, in due time, to congestive cardiac failure. Because of the basically obstructive nature of the phenomenon, congestion of this type is generally spoken of as **passive**. As in the case of oedema, passive congestion can be generalized or local.

Generalized venous congestion

Acute generalized venous congestion may be seen in many patients dying suddenly from a variety of causes. It represents the sudden accumulation of blood behind a failing ventricle with resulting engorgement of the affected organs or tissues. However, in clinical practice, generalized venous congestion is most often chronic, the basic cause being, again, a failing ventricle. Congestion results partly from increased pulmonary and systemic venous pressure, and partly (in so far as the pulmonary circulation is concerned)

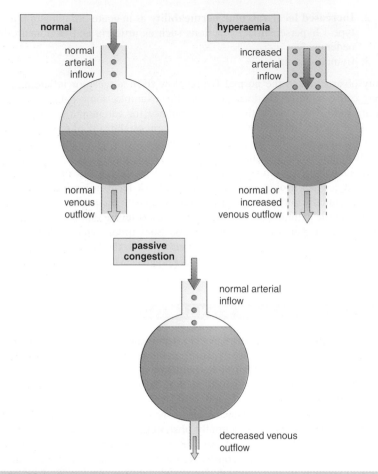

Fig. 22.1   Hyperaemia and congestion.

Abnormal accumulations of blood in vascular beds arise either because of increased arterial inflow (hyperaemia) or because of diminished venous outflow (passive congestion).

from the shift of blood from the systemic to the pulmonary circulation as a result of peripheral vasoconstriction.

Generalized venous congestion also occurs in pulmonary disorders associated with pulmonary hypertension. This form of cardiac failure is known as **cor pulmonale**; it may be the result of disorders affecting the bronchioles and alveoli, thoracic movements or pulmonary vasculature.

Morphological changes of chronic venous congestion

Generally speaking, chronically congested organs are swollen, darker in colour, and firmer in consistency than normal.

The lung

Marked engorgement of the alveolar capillaries is seen on microscopic examination, each capillary being stuffed with blood. This capillary distension gives the alveolar septa a beaded appearance. Quite often small intra-alveolar haemorrhages occur due to rupture of the overdistended capillaries. This may be so marked (especially in patients with severe pulmonary venous hypertension, as in mitral stenosis) that the patient coughs up blood-stained sputum (**haemoptysis**). The red blood cells break down and the iron-containing moiety of haemoglobin becomes converted to a yellow-brown crystalline pigment known as haemosiderin. This pigment is engulfed by alveolar macrophages, which are then known as **siderophages** or 'heart failure cells'. With time the congested alveolar septa become thicker than normal. In the early stages of chronic pulmonary venous congestion this is due largely to the presence of oedema fluid within the interstitial tissue of the septa. Later, fibrosis occurs within the septa and the lung tissue becomes much firmer than normal. The combination of a significant degree of iron pigmentation and interstitial fibrosis in long-standing pulmonary congestion is known as **brown induration**.

The liver

The structural changes seen in the chronically congested liver of a patient suffering from cardiac failure result from a combination of two processes. Firstly, there is a rise in pressure in the hepatic veins, central veins and sinusoids; secondly, that part of the hepatic lobule which is furthest from its arterial supply is poorly perfused.

Terminal hepatic venules and sinusoids in this part of the liver are dilated and packed with red blood cells. The surrounding hepatocytes show fatty change. Macroscopically, the liver shows a variegated red and yellow appearance likened, by some, to a nutmeg.

The spleen

The congested spleen is moderately enlarged (up to 250 g) and is firmer than normal. The cut surface is smooth and firm and the red pulp is a dark, purplish colour. On microscopic examination congestion is shown by distension of the sinusoids, which are packed with red blood cells. There is some increase in the amount of reticulin in the walls of the sinusoids and also in the connective tissue in the trabeculae.

Local venous congestion

This results from obstruction to venous return from any part of an organ or tissue. It is usually due either to venous thrombosis or to external pressure on veins as, for example, when a large tumour mass is present. The consequences will depend largely on the speed with which the obstruction develops and the effectiveness of any collateral draining systems.

If venous obstruction is **acute**, the presence of an effective collateral drainage system is vital if local oedema and, in some instances, haemorrhage are to be avoided. For example, if large veins in relation to the brain become obstructed, their tributaries will become severely engorged; because collateral draining systems are absent, haemorrhage from the swollen tributary veins is not uncommon. A similar sequence of events may occur when a hernia becomes impacted. The venous drainage from a segment of the intestine may be obstructed completely; the bowel wall then becomes engorged with blood and may become necrotic.

In chronic local venous obstruction, collateral veins usually become markedly distended and may, under certain circumstances, rupture. This is seen in **portal hypertension**, which may occur as a result of disturbances in hepatic lobular architecture brought about by the processes involved in cirrhosis, as a result of pathological changes in the portal tracts, or as a result of obstruction to the portal vein itself. The rise in portal vein blood pressure leads to distension of the short gastric veins and of the anastomotic veins at the lower end of the oesophagus; this confers a risk of serious haemorrhage.

ABNORMAL ACCUMULATIONS OF FLUID AND DISTURBANCES OF BLOOD DISTRIBUTION

- Clinically, **oedema** is defined as the accumulation of excess fluid in the extracellular and extravascular space.
- Factors promoting oedema formation include increased intravascular hydrostatic pressure and decreased colloid osmotic pressure. The latter is caused by decreased synthesis or increased loss of plasma proteins or an increase in the permeability of micro-vessels to plasma proteins.
- Systemic oedema is associated with a number of clinical syndromes: cardiac failure, a variety of pathological states affecting the renal glomeruli, and under- and malnutrition, especially in children (kwashiorkor).
- Maintenance of normal fluid volumes in the extracellular and extravascular space depends on normal lymphatic drainage. If this is obstructed, severe intractable local oedema (lymphoedema) develops.
- The terms **hyperaemia** and **congestion** equate with a greater than normal amount of blood within an organ or tissue. The former implies an increased **inflow** of blood; the latter a decreased **outflow**.

23 Pigmentation and heterotopic calcification

Abnormalities in endogenous pigmentation involve the following groups:

- melanin
- pigments derived from haemoglobin
- pigments associated with fats.

Melanin gives hair, skin and eyes their colour. It also occurs normally in leptomeninges, nerve cells in the substantia nigra and the adrenal medulla. Some melanin pigmentation may also occur in the mucous membranes of the vulva and mouth where they adjoin the skin. Melanin-producing cells may also be found in small numbers in the ovary, gastrointestinal tract and urinary bladder.

As anyone with moles and freckles knows, melanin usually produces a yellow-brown colour. If the pigment is present in very large amounts, the local tissue area may appear black. On histological examination melanin appears as brown intracellular granules. It can reduce solutions of ammoniacal silver with the consequent deposition of black granules of silver on the melanin granules. Substances that can do this are spoken of as '**argentaffin**'. Where pigmentation is very heavy the melanin can be removed from the tissue sections by bleaching with oxidizing agents such as hydrogen peroxide.

Melanin is produced by specialized cells, **melanocytes**, which are concentrated in the basal layer of the epidermis. They originate in the neural crest and migrate to various permanent locations during embryonic life. The average number of skin melanocytes is 1500 per mm^2, the number varying from 2000 per mm^2 in the forehead and cheeks to 800 per mm^2 in the skin of the abdomen. This number is relatively constant regardless of race. *The darker skin of Afro-Caribbeans is due to increased activity of the melanocytes, not to increased numbers.*

403

Melanin is synthesized in small membrane-bound bodies known as melanosomes in the Golgi apparatus. The melanin granules are transferred to neighbouring epidermal cells. At the point of contact between the dendritic process of the melanocyte and the plasma membrane of the epidermal cell, there is considerable excitation of the latter; clumps of pigment are taken into the epidermal cell and come to lie in a perinuclear position.

The basic starting point for the synthesis of melanin is the amino acid tyrosine. The melanocyte is distinctive for its complement of tyrosinase. Absence of this enzyme results in complete inability to synthesize melanin. The resulting syndrome is **albinism** (absence of pigmentation in skin, hair and conjunctiva). All normal melanocytes contain tyrosinase but not all are actively engaged in producing melanin. For this reason it is sometimes necessary to employ special means for the identification of melanocytes. This may be done by incubating the tissue sections in a solution of either dopa or tyrosine. If tyrosinase is present within the cells, melanin will be produced.

The activity of melanocytes appears to be related to certain hormones of the pituitary and, to a lesser extent, the gonads. The pituitary secretes **melanocyte-stimulating hormone** (**MSH**), which shares part of its amino acid sequence with adrenocorticotrophic hormone. In Addison's disease, where there is destruction of adrenal tissue due to either autoimmune processes or tuberculosis, there is loss of normal feedback mechanisms because of the fall in adrenal activity. Additional MSH is secreted by the pituitary; skin and mucosal pigmentation is thus a common feature of Addison's disease.

ABNORMALITIES IN MELANIN PIGMENTATION

Generalized hyperpigmentation

Hyperpigmentation occurs in:

- Addison's disease
- acromegaly
- chronic arsenical poisoning
- haemochromatosis, in which excess storage of iron in parenchymal cells occurs
- chlorpromazine administration; a curious violet-grey pigmentation occasionally develops after treatment with this drug and may affect the eyes and parts of the skin exposed to sunlight.

Large doses of **oestrogens** given for treatment of prostatic cancer also sometimes cause generalized hyperpigmentation. In addition, the effects of oestrogen may be the reason for the hyperpigmentation that sometimes occurs in chronic liver disease, in which it is alleged that there is inadequate hepatic breakdown of oestrogen. In pregnancy, the nipples and genitalia become darker and there is sometimes a blotchy hyperpigmentation in the butterfly area of the face. This is known as **chloasma**.

Focal hyperpigmentation

This may occur in a number of situations.

Freckles are probably genetically determined.

Café au lait spots are large hyperpigmented macules. Unlike common freckles, these show an increase in the number of melanocytes. They are found in two rare systemic conditions:

- **neurofibromatosis**, a condition characterized by the presence of multiple tumours derived from the fibrous element of the nerve sheath
- **Albright's syndrome**, which consists of a triad of polyostotic fibrous dysplasia, hyperpigmentation, and sexual and skeletal precocity.

Peutz–Jeghers syndrome is a rare syndrome inherited as an autosomal dominant. It has two main characteristics: a curious focal hyperpigmentation involving the lips and the skin around the mouth, and multiple polyps in the gastrointestinal tract, which may cause acute or subacute intestinal obstruction.

Lentiginosis is the presence of multiple hyperpigmented spots characterized by an increase in the number of melanocytes. This has been reported to be associated with hypertrophic cardiomyopathy in a few cases.

Tumours arising from melanocytes are most commonly seen in the skin but may occur at any of the sites in which melanocytes have been described. Most of these are benign – the 'moles' of various kinds – but a small proportion are malignant (mostly *ab initio*). These are termed 'malignant melanomas'. Other skin tumours may accumulate melanin, and this may cause some concern as to their nature. This type of pigmentation is common in seborrhoeic warts and basal cell carcinoma.

Focal hyperpigmentation can also result from exposure to ionizing radiation, ultraviolet light, heat (*erythema ab igne*) and chronic irritation (as in itchy dermatoses).

Hypopigmentation

Albinism

Albinism is due to a **deficiency of tyrosinase**. In classical cases the skin is very white, the hair pale, the irides transparent and the pupils pink. Such extreme cases are fortunately rare among humans. These patients tend to suffer from the skin tumours believed to be associated with exposure to sunlight, thus emphasizing the importance of melanin as a protective agent against the effects of ultraviolet light.

Focal hypopigmentation (**vitiligo**) is very common and is characterized by the presence of well-demarcated areas of depigmentation. Histological examination shows either paucity or absence of melanocytes.

IRON-CONTAINING PIGMENTS

Excess iron is initially stored in the form of **ferritin**. This is a micelle about

5.4 nm in diameter which consists of a ferric core surrounded by a shell of protein subunits. Ferritin cannot be seen under the light microscope and does not give positive reactions with the staining methods commonly employed for recognition of iron. It may, however, be seen fairly easily with the electron microscope.

With further increases in intracellular iron accumulation, ferritin molecules aggregate to produce a coarse crystalline yellow-brown pigment that is easily seen on light microscopy. This is known as **haemosiderin**. These crystals are about 36% iron and can be identified with certainty by the Prussian blue method (also known as Perls' or Turnbull's reaction). This involves treating either tissues or tissue sections with a mixture of hydrochloric acid and potassium ferrocyanide. The tissue iron is present in a trivalent form and a blue precipitate of ferric ferrocyanide is produced. This method is both easy and sensitive.

Localized deposition of haemosiderin is due to haemorrhage at the site of pigmentation. Haemosiderin pigmentation is therefore frequently seen in relation to bruises, organizing haematomas, fracture sites and haemorrhagic infarcts. It may also be seen in certain tumour-like lesions such as sclerosing haemangioma in the dermis and pigmented villonodular synovitis in the large joints.

The cells of the renal tubules can convert haemoglobin to haemosiderin, and haemosiderinuria may sometimes follow haemoglobinuria.

Pulmonary haemosiderosis is usually associated with high pulmonary venous pressure as in 'tight' mitral stenosis or left ventricular failure. Sometimes severe pulmonary haemosiderosis will be caused by immune injury of the Gell and Coombes type 2 variety. This is accompanied by acute immune-mediated injury to the glomerular basement membranes and is known as Goodpasture's syndrome.

If the body is overloaded with iron, haemosiderin is formed in excessive amounts and deposited in a wide range of tissues. The total quantity of iron normally present in the body is 4–5 g; this level appears to be controlled by powerful homeostatic mechanisms. Normal Western-style diets contain 10–15 mg of iron per day; only about 10% of this is absorbed. There is a normal loss of about 1 mg per day through shedding of cells from the gastrointestinal tract, skin, etc. Females lose about 200–300 mg per year as a result of menstruation.

There are two basic morphological patterns for the deposition of the excess haemosiderin:

1) parenchymatous deposition
2) deposition in the cells of the reticuloendothelial system; this pattern is seen following parenteral iron administration or repeated blood transfusion.

Possible mechanisms for the accumulation of excess iron in the body are:

- increased absorption of iron
- decreased excretion (although there is no evidence for this as yet)

- impaired utilization
- excess breakdown of haemoglobin with release of iron.

Haemochromatosis is associated with an increase in total body iron due to inappropriately high levels of iron absorption. Iron is deposited in the parenchymal cells of the liver and in many other organs, causing cell damage, scarring and, eventually, organ dysfunction. The classic clinical picture is one of liver enlargement, skin pigmentation and diabetes mellitus (so-called 'bronzed diabetes'). It is one of the commonest genetically determined diseases in the West and is inherited in an autosomal recessive fashion. The defective gene is linked to the A genes of the major histo-compatibility complex.

PIGMENTS ASSOCIATED WITH FATS

Endogenous pigments, **lipofuscins** (L. *fuscus*, dark or sombre), are often termed 'wear-and-tear' pigments because they increase with ageing. Lipo-fuscins are yellowish-brown granular pigments within atrophic parenchymal cells, particularly in the liver and heart of old people. In large amounts, they impart a brown colour to the affected organ or tissue, called **brown atrophy**. Lipofuscins represent the breakdown products of membranes of 'worn out' organelles. With ageing of cells, autophagic vacuoles (vacuoles containing particles of cell debris) are formed in increasing number as active metabolic organelles become 'redundant'. With these autophagic vacuoles, the lipid portions of the membranes tend to resist lysosomal digestion and undergo auto-oxidation to form lipoperoxides and aldehydes with a yellow colour. The pigment remains within lysosomes and produces no ill effects on the tissues.

HETEROTOPIC CALCIFICATION

Heterotopic calcification is deposition of calcium salts in tissues other than osteoid and enamel. There are two main varieties: **dystrophic** and **metastatic calcification**.

Dystrophic calcification
In dystrophic calcification, serum calcium levels are normal and calcium salts are deposited in dead or degenerate tissues. This occurs in the following sets of circumstances:

- caseous necrosis (calcification is the hallmark of old caseation)
- fat necrosis
- thrombosis
- haematomas (e.g. subdural haematoma or myositis ossificans)
- atherosclerotic plaques
- chronic inflammatory granulation tissue (e.g. constrictive pericarditis)

- Mönckeberg's sclerosis of the medial coat of muscular arteries
- degenerate colloid goitres
- cysts of various kinds
- degenerate tumours (e.g. uterine leiomyomas).

Metastatic calcification

In metastatic calcification there is a raised blood calcium level. This may result from bone resorption, as for example in hyperparathyroidism, or from excess calcium absorption from the gut. Occasionally, as in renal osteo-dystrophy, the precipitating factor appears to be a high blood phosphate concentration. This type of calcium deposition occurs at a variety of sites:

The kidney. Calcium is deposited round the tubules and damages them. Ultimately this may lead to renal failure. These patients often can not acidify the urine. Stone formation in the renal pelvis and ureter is often associated with nephrocalcinosis.

The lung. Calcium is deposited in the alveolar walls.

The stomach. The calcium is deposited around the fundal glands. It has been suggested that because these glands secrete hydrochloric acid, the tissues are left relatively alkaline; this is said to favour calcium deposition.

Blood vessels. The coronary arteries are most affected.

The cornea.

There are five common causes of metastatic calcification:

Primary hyperparathyroidism. Here the parathyroid is overactive and does not respond to normal negative feedback control. It is most commonly associated with a benign neoplasm (adenoma) but also occurs when the glands are hyperplastic. Very rarely it occurs in association with malignant tumours of the parathyroid. The excess secretion of parathyroid hormone upregulates osteoclastic resorption of bone leading to hypercalcaemia.

Excessive absorption of calcium from the bowel. This may be due to hyper-vitaminosis D or vitamin D-sensitive states such as idiopathic hyper-calcaemia of infancy. It may even occur through excessive milk drinking.

Hypophosphatasia.

Destructive bone lesions. Hypercalcaemia in this context is usually associated with osteolytic secondary deposits of malignant neoplasms. It is worth remembering that hypercalcaemia may be associated with malignancy in the absence of bone deposits. This is known as humoral hypercalcaemia of malignancy; in many instances, it is due to the synthesis and release from the tumour cells of a parathyroid hormone-related peptide.

Renal tubular acidosis.

On microscopic examination calcium salts appear as granules staining a deep blue colour with haematoxylin. They typically form encrustations on structures such as elastic fibres in the lung or arteries.

Calcium stained with alizarin red shows a magenta colour. More commonly the von Kossa method is used, in which silver impregnation forms the basis of the stain. What it shows is, in fact, phosphate and carbonate; however, because these are almost always associated with calcium in its particulate and insoluble form, the method is fairly effective in the demonstration of calcium.

PIGMENTATION AND HETEROTOPIC CALCIFICATION

- Endogenous and exogenous pigments may accumulate in human tissues.
- There are three types of endogenous pigment: melanin, and those derived from haemoglobin or lipids.
- Melanin normally colours the hair, skin and eyes. It is derived from tyrosine and appears as brown granules within cells. It is identified by its ability to reduce solutions of ammoniacal silver.
- Absence of the enzyme tyrosinase inhibits melanin formation; this leads to **albinism** where there is no pigment in the skin, hair or iris. Such individuals are more at risk of sun-related skin cancer.
- Generalized hyperpigmentation occurs in association with Addison's disease, acromegaly and occasionally, when large doses of oestrogen have been used to treat prostatic cancer.
- The principal pigment derived from haemoglobin is **haemosiderin**; its presence within tissue is most commonly associated with haemorrhage, not infrequently from capillaries.
- Pigments derived from lipids (**lipofuscins**) accumulate in the tissues of the elderly, especially in the heart and liver.

24 Neoplasia: disorders of cell proliferation and differentiation

In developed countries neoplasia comes second only to cardiovascular disease as a cause of death. In the UK it will kill over 100 000 people in the next 12 months. The commonest malignant neoplasms in men and women respectively are shown in *Figs 24.1* and *24.2*.

DEFINITIONS

The term **neoplasia** is derived from two Greek words: *neos* meaning 'new' and *plassein* meaning 'to mould'. This is usually translated as **new growth**, although this phrase begs certain important questions as to the essential nature of neoplasia.

Neoplasia is, in fact, not easy to define. Some regard the best available definition as being:

> '*an abnormal mass of tissue, the growth of which exceeds and is uncoordinated with that of normal tissues, and which persists in the same excessive manner after cessation of the stimulus evoking the change.*'

In operational terms there are at least three types of disturbance of cell behaviour inherent in neoplasia. Thus we can redefine neoplasia as a set of disorders showing a disturbance in:

- **cell proliferation**
- **cell differentiation**
- **the relationship between cells and their surrounding stroma.**

Cell proliferation

Neoplasia involves defects in the mechanisms that normally maintain a cell population within relatively narrow limits. This escape from normal control

411

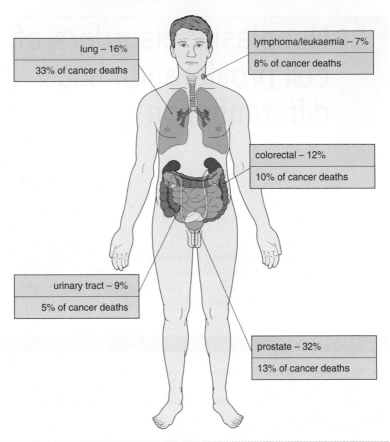

Fig. 24.1 Excluding skin tumours, five tumours account for 75% of cases of malignancy in males.

gives rise to a population of dividing cells which, in a sense, is **immortal** in that cell division occurs a far greater number of times than in a normal cell line. The end result is a focus made up, in most instances, of a single type of cell in numbers totally inappropriate for the anatomical location. This leads to the formation of a mass or tumour.

Cell differentiation

Differentiation is the sum of the processes by which the cells in a developing multicellular organism achieve their **specific set of functional and morphological characteristics**. Cells sharing a set of such characteristics become organized into tissues, and these in turn may be arranged as organs.

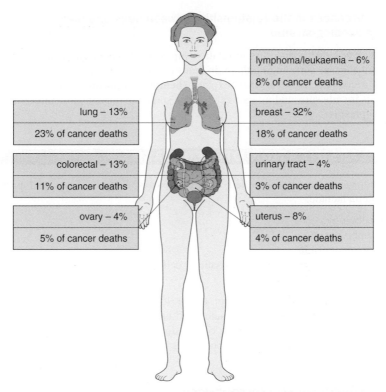

Fig. 24.2 **Excluding skin tumours, seven tumours account for 80% of cases of malignancy in females.**

A fertilized ovum contains all the genetic information required for that organism and is, thus, totipotent in terms of future structure and function. A differentiated cell such as a liver cell expresses only a small part of the genetic information; thus differentiation must involve a progressive **restriction of genomic expression**.

Impairment of differentiation of the cell line involved is extremely common in the formation of a neoplasm. Its degree may, in many instances, give useful information as to the likely natural history of the disease. *In general terms, the poorer the degree of differentiation, the worse the behaviour of the neoplasm is likely to be.* Loss of the ability to differentiate fully may lead to the expression of functional characteristics foreign to those of the mature differentiated cell. This is seen when neoplastic cells secrete fetal proteins or hormones inappropriate for that particular cell type (**ectopic hormone production**) (see pp. 467–470).

Disturbances in the relationship between cells and their surrounding stroma

There is a disturbance in the relationship between neoplastic cells and the normal tissue surrounding them. In many cases the cells of a neoplasm grow as a compact mass as they expand (**benign neoplasms**); in others the cells **invade** surrounding tissues and may spread to distant sites (**malignant neoplasms**).

CLASSIFICATION OF NEOPLASMS

Neoplasms may be classified in several ways. Some current, and past, criteria include:

- aetiology
- embryogenesis
- organ of origin
- histogenesis or cytogenesis (tissue or cell of origin)
- biological behaviour.

On a practical day-to-day level, the most useful of these are the cell type from which the neoplasm originated and biological behaviour, as the latter largely determines the outcome of the disease in an individual. Analysis of the morphological features contributes significantly to the prediction of biological behaviour.

HISTOGENESIS AND CYTOGENESIS

The cell and tissue types from which neoplasms arise constitute the basis of the most commonly used classifications (*Table 24.1*). At the simplest level these tissues of origin can be divided into two categories: **epithelium** and **connective tissues**. However, a much greater degree of subdivision is both possible and desirable. Even at this basic level of grouping, difficulties may arise in correctly attributing a neoplasm to one or other of these categories. For instance, neoplasms arising from mesothelial cells that line serosal cavities may show morphological characteristics suggestive of both epithelium and connective tissue. A more frequent problem in practice is that the cell population of a neoplasm may be so poorly differentiated as to make it very difficult or even impossible for the pathologist to identify the original cell type. In this situation, the use of immunological methods to identify either specific antigens or specific cell products may be helpful.

BIOLOGICAL BEHAVIOUR

Clinically, the most important characteristic of a neoplasm is its behaviour. All neoplasms, with only a few exceptions, are divided on this basis into two main groups: **benign** and **malignant**.

Table 24.1 A classification of tumours

Tissue of origin	Benign	Behaviour Intermediate	Malignant
Epithelium			
Covering and protective epithelium	Squamous, transitional and columnar cell papilloma		Squamous and transitional cell carcinoma; adenocarcinoma
Compact secreting epithelium	Adenoma: if cystic, cystadenoma; if papillary and cystic, papillary cystadenoma		Adenocarcinoma: if cystic, cystadenocarcinoma
Other epithelial neoplasms		Basal cell carcinomas; salivary and mucous gland neoplasms; carcinoid tumours (argentaffinoma)	
Connective tissue			
Fibrous	Fibroma		Fibrosarcoma
Nerve sheath	Neurilemmoma Neurofibroma		Neurofibrosarcoma
Adipose	Lipoma		Liposarcoma
Smooth muscle	Leiomyoma		Leiomyosarcoma
Striated muscle	Rhabdomyoma		Rhabdomyosarcoma
Synovium	Synovioma		Synoviosarcoma
Cartilage	Chondroma		Chondrosarcoma
Bone			
Osteoblast	Osteoma		Osteosarcoma
Unknown		⟵ Giant cell tumour ⟶	
Mesothelium	Benign mesothelioma		Malignant mesothelioma
Blood vessels and lymphatics			Angiosarcoma
Meninges	Meningioma		Malignant meningioma
Specialized connective tissue			
Neuroglia and ependyma		⟵ Astrocytoma, oligodendroglioma ⟶ Ependymoma	
Chromaffin tissue	Carotid body tumour; phaeochromocytoma		Malignant variants
Lymphoid and haemopoietic tissue		Myeloproliferative disorders	Malignant lymphoma of varying degrees of differentiation, Hodgkin's disease; plasmacytoma; multiple myeloma syndrome; Waldenström's macroglobulinaemia; leukaemias
Melanocytes			Malignant melanoma
Fetal trophoblast	Hydatidiform mole		Choriocarcinoma
Embryonic tissue			
Totipotential or pluripotential cell	Benign teratoma		Malignant teratoma
Kidney			Nephroblastoma
Liver			Hepatoblastoma
Unipotential cell	Ganglioneuroma		
Retina			Retinoblastoma
Hindbrain			Medulloblastoma
Sympathetic ganglia and adrenal medulla			Neuroblastoma
Unipotential embryonic cells in pelvic organs			Juvenile rhabdomyosarcoma (botryoid sarcoma)
Embryonic vestiges			
Notochord			Chordoma
Enamel organ		Ameloblastoma	
Parapituitary residues		Craniopharyngioma	

Malignant neoplasms arising from **epithelium** are called **carcinomas**; those that have their origin in **connective tissue elements** are called **sarcomas**. These behavioural characteristics are reflected to a considerable extent in the morphological appearances of the lesion.

Benign neoplasms

The word 'benign' does not imply that such neoplasms may not be clinically important or dangerous. In the context of neoplasia, benign means that the cells making up the neoplasm **show no tendency to invade the surrounding tissue** and, by the same token, **never spread to distant sites (metastasis)**. The growth pattern of a benign neoplasm is an **expansile** one, often associated with the formation of a capsule derived from the surrounding connective tissue (*Fig. 24.3*) and with some pressure atrophy of surrounding parenchyma. The growth rate is often low; few, if any, cells undergoing mitosis are seen.

Malignant neoplasms

The absolute criterion of malignancy is **invasiveness**. Malignant cells characteristically separate from one another and grow out in an irregular pattern into the surrounding tissue (*Fig. 24.3*). In many instances the cells gain access to vascular channels – either lymphatics, blood vessels or both. Once such vascular invasion has occurred, groups of malignant cells can be carried in the blood or lymph until they impact at some distance from the primary growth. From the site of impaction the malignant cells emigrate into the extravascular compartment and may form new deposits of neoplastic

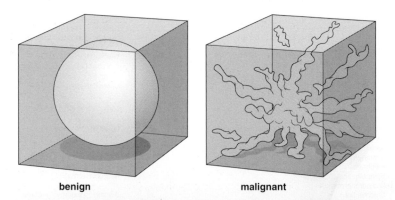

benign   malignant

Fig. 24.3   Benign and malignant neoplasms.

Benign and malignant neoplasms are, in general, distinguished from each other by their growth patterns. Benign tumours have an expansile growth pattern whereas malignant ones are infiltrative.

tissue (**secondary deposits** or **metastases**). The mechanisms involved in tumour spread are discussed in Chapter 27.

Morphologically, malignant cells and the structures they form tend to show evidence of increased cell proliferation and incomplete differentiation.

Increased cell proliferation is expressed by an increased number of **mitoses**. Not infrequently these mitoses are abnormal in appearance, with tripolar, quadripolar or annular spindles.

Incomplete differentiation shows itself both at the level of individual cells and in the relationship of cells to each other.

- Malignant cells tend to be larger than their normal counterparts and to show a much greater degree of **variation in size and shape** than normal cells of the same origin.
- The nuclei occupy a much greater proportion of the total cell volume than is normal; this is termed an increase in the **nuclear:cytoplasmic ratio**. The DNA content of the nuclei of malignant cells may be much greater than normal, and chromosomal analysis not infrequently shows loss of normal ploidy.

Loss of differentiation involves cell arrangement as well as individual cell morphology. The normal orderly relationships between cells tend to disappear and structures, such as ductules or glands, formed by malignant cells may differ considerably from their normal counterparts. In other instances the neoplasm may be so poorly differentiated that no recognizable structures are formed and the malignant cells grow in disorganized sheets or islands.

DYSPLASIA

Cell changes characteristic of malignancy may be found, especially in epithelium, at a stage when **no invasion of the surrounding tissue is evident**. This is termed **dysplasia** (Gk. *dys*, bad). Dysplastic epithelium correlates with some irreversible and heritable change in the genome of affected cells. However, a fully malignant phenotype shown by invasiveness has not yet occurred. Finding dysplasia sounds a warning note to the clinician that full-blown malignancy may develop in the future at the dysplastic site and that careful surveillance is required.

Dysplasia is particularly common in squamous and transitional epithelia, such as those of the uterine cervix, the skin, urinary bladder and larynx. Dysplasia (intraepithelial neoplasia – CIN) of the **uterine cervix** is diagnosed by microscopic examination of cells exfoliated from the epithelial surface and collected on a spatula ('cervical smear cytology'). Such cytological diagnoses can be confirmed histologically by taking very small biopsies under direct vision (colposcopic biopsy). If the dysplastic process is severe and widespread within the cervix, the patient may be treated by a wide cone-shaped excision of cervical tissue in which, it is hoped, all the dysplastic epithelium is removed. Freedom from epithelial dysplasia in the lines of excision is checked by histological examination.

In some cases of epithelial dysplasia, the whole thickness of the epithelial covering shows dysplastic change; for these situations, the term **carcinoma in situ** (CIN-3) is often used. Dysplasia represents a continuum of change which, as already stated, may end in frank malignancy.

Lesions that may be confused with true neoplasms

Hamartoma

This term is derived from the Greek *hamartanein* meaning 'to make an error'. Hamartomas are tumour-like masses which may grow to a considerable size but which lack the autonomy and persistence of the excessive growth characteristic of true neoplasia. In hamartomas the tissue components are fully differentiated and are normally found in the organ or tissue in which the hamartoma occurs. However, the architectural pattern in these lesions differs considerably from that of normal tissues.

Hamartomas may occur in many sites and may consist of a wide variety of differentiated tissue elements. The lung is not an uncommon site; here the lesions occur as well-demarcated masses of cartilage measuring up to 2–3 cm in diameter. Microscopic examination shows small slits within the cartilage lined by bronchial-type epithelium. Thus the lesion consists of some of the elements of the normal bronchial wall. In easily inspected tissues such as the skin, where hamartomas are common, it is clear that a lesion may be present at birth but start to grow only much later.

The commonest hamartoma is vascular. Many types exist, ranging from the flat 'port-wine stain' to large, raised, complex masses of abnormal vascular spaces.

Hamartomas may form part of some inherited syndromes such as the Peutz–Jeghers syndrome which is characterized by multiple hamartomas involving glands and muscle of the intestinal wall and pigmentation around the mouth.

Heteroplasia

Heteroplasia means differentiation of part of an organ or tissue in a way that is quite foreign to the part. It differs from metaplasia in that there is no change from one fully differentiated form to another. Instead the anomalous differentiation occurs from the stem cell stage. For instance, gastric mucosa might be found within the wall of a Meckel's diverticulum in the distal part of the ileum or in the gallbladder wall. Similarly, anomalous masses of pancreatic tissue sometimes occur in the wall of the small intestine; it is of interest that these usually consist of ductal and acinar tissue only; islets of Langerhans are infrequent.

Occasionally heteroplasia occurs as large and complicated masses in which several differentiated tissues may be seen. For example, a large mass on a patient's face has been described containing ectopic liver, pancreatic tissue and gut epithelium. Such heterotopic masses have been termed **choristomas**.

STRUCTURAL FEATURES OF COMMON NEOPLASMS

Benign epithelial neoplasms

Benign epithelial neoplasms show two basic growth patterns which are largely, although not entirely, dictated by their anatomical situation.

1) Neoplastic epithelial cells tend to grow in sheets covering a surface. Very often this mass of cells has a wavy irregular outline and is called a **papilloma**.
2) Cells grow as solid islands or masses, separated from each other by stromal connective tissue. This growth pattern is seen most often in neoplasms derived from ductal or glandular epithelium and is known as an **adenoma**.

Three main types of papilloma are described, consonant with the three main varieties of covering epithelium: **squamous**, **transitional** and **columnar**.

Genesis of an adenoma

Benign neoplasms arising from gland or duct epithelium are termed adenomas. The basic structure of adenomas is based on the tendency of the proliferating cells to form small groups, which usually surround a lumen. In many instances this lumen is reduced to an inconspicuous slit and it may be impossible to see any lumen at all on light microscopy. This latter appearance is particularly common in adenomas arising within endocrine glands.

The neoplastic acini have no draining duct systems. If combined with active secretion by the cells of the tumour, this absence of drainage may lead to accumulation of the secretions, distension of the lumina and eventual **cyst** formation. Such a neoplastic cyst derived from acinar or ductal epithelium is called a **cystadenoma**. If cyst formation is accompanied by continued proliferation of the lining cells, the increase in the area of the lining will result in the appearance of papillary infoldings projecting into the lumen, a so-called **papillary cystadenoma**. Such neoplasms are frequently encountered in the ovary but may occur at many other sites.

A typical adenoma is usually a clearly demarcated and usually rounded mass, often with a thin fibrous tissue capsule and with some compressed normal tissue around it. If the acinar or ductal lumina are small, the adenoma appears solid when cut into, and is usually paler and more homogeneous in texture than surrounding tissue. If the gland or duct lumina are large and secretion has been a marked feature, this is usually easy to see when the lesion has been sectioned; either a single large cyst or many small ones may be present.

A common site for adenoma formation is the large bowel. Because of the peristaltic contractions, the localized islands of proliferated colonic glands may be pushed into the lumen. In the early stages of this process, the small mass of glands will appear as a small lump standing a little proud of the surrounding mucosal surface. With the passage of time, the adenoma may be pushed into the lumen, dragging with it a pedicle of subepithelial tissue containing blood vessels and connective tissue fibres. Such a lesion is called a **polyp**.

NEOPLASIA: DISORDERS OF CELL PROLIFERATION AND DIFFERENTIATION

- Neoplasia is the second most common cause of death in Western populations.
- Neoplasms are classified by their behaviour as either **benign** or **malignant**.
- The absolute criterion of malignancy is invasiveness, which may lead to dissemination of neoplastic cells to many other parts of the body (**metastasis**).
- Fundamental to the genesis of neoplasms are loss of normal control of cell proliferation (leading to principally monoclonal expansion of cell populations) and loss of normal differentiation.
- In general, the poorer the differentiation of neoplastic cell populations, the worse is the prognosis.
- The full phenotypic expression of neoplasia may be preceded by a phase known as **dysplasia**, in which affected cells show some of the morphological features of neoplasia. This indicates some irreversible and heritable change in these cells and an enhanced risk of full neoplastic transformation.
- **Hamartomas** should not be confused with neoplasms. Hamartomas are mass lesions in which elements normally present in the affected organ or tissue are arranged in an abnormal pattern.

25 Non-neoplastic disturbances in cell growth and proliferation

Increases or decreases in cell populations are not all neoplastic: **increases** (**hyperplasia**) and **decreases** (**involution**) in the cell number and size occur under both physiological and pathological circumstances. Hyperplasia is distinguished from the changes in cell proliferation occurring in neoplasia by the fact that in neoplasia normal mechanisms that control cell proliferation do not operate.

THE CELL CYCLE

Cells proliferate by undergoing **mitosis**. However, mitotic division itself occupies only a small part of the cell cycle. The length of the cell cycle determines, to an extent, the characteristics of a tissue in terms of its cell kinetics.

- After mitosis (**M phase**), which usually takes 1–2 hours, the daughter cells enter a gap phase known as **G1**. The length of G1 phase differs from cell type to cell type.
- The cell then enters a phase in which DNA is synthesized (**S phase**); during this, the content of DNA is doubled. This S phase lasts from 7 to 12 hours.
- After synthesis of DNA is complete, there is a second gap phase known as **G2**, which lasts as a rule, 1–6 hours.

In human tissues, the M, G2 and S phases are relatively constant in length. *The differences in cell cycle time that characterize different tissues are a function of variations in the length of G1, which may last for days or even years*. In cell culture models, arrest of the cell cycle occurs only in the G1 phase. This finding implies that, once past the G1 phase, the cell cycle proceeds to completion. In fact, the point of no return occurs late in the G1 phase; it is known as the **restriction point** and probably corresponds with the genetically programmed switching on of DNA polymerase synthesis.

421

Not all the cells in a tissue are actually within the cell cycle; after exiting the cell cycle most fully differentiated cells opt out, eventually to become obsolescent and die. For instance, a daughter cell arising from mitotic division in the basal layer of the epidermis migrates upwards into the malpighian layer where it begins to synthesize keratin. Eventually it moves to the horny layer of the epidermis and dies, being shed as a flake of keratin. There is, however, an alternative. Cells can leave the cycle temporarily and, under certain circumstances, re-enter it much later. 'Resting' cells are said to be in G0, although clearly it is not easy to distinguish between these cells and those in which there is a very long G1 phase.

That part of the cell population which remains within the cell cycle is known as the **growth fraction (stem cell compartment)**. The proliferative activity in any tissue is a function of the length of the cycle and the size of the growth fraction.

HYPERTROPHY AND HYPERPLASIA

Excess growth with *no* escape from normal control mechanisms may be expressed in two ways (*Fig. 25.1*):

1) In **hypertrophy** the increase in the bulk of a tissue or organ results solely from an **increase in the size of the constituent cells**.
2) In **hyperplasia** there is an **increase in the number of cells**, often associated with an increase in cell size.

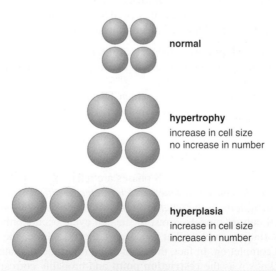

normal

hypertrophy
increase in cell size
no increase in number

hyperplasia
increase in cell size
increase in number

Fig. 25.1 Hypertrophy and hyperplasia.

Hypertrophy and hyperplasia can, in most instances, be recognized as being caused by some specific stimulus and can be regarded as adaptation phenomena. Once the stimulus is removed, the tissue reverts to normal. This stimulus is often a physiological one, such as an increased demand for a function that will lead to an increase in cell number, cell size or both.

HYPERPLASIA

In many instances, hyperplasia is a **demand-led physiological event**, being the response to an increased functional need. This occurs, for example, in such tissues as the breast and thyroid at the time of puberty or pregnancy. The negative feedback mechanisms that appear to control these phenomena will act in a wide range of circumstances, even when the circumstances themselves are pathological.

Operation of this negative feedback is seen quite commonly in **endocrine hyperplasia**. Some examples are given below.

Congenital adrenal hyperplasia

Congenital adrenal hyperplasia (*Fig. 25.2*) manifests clinically in infancy and early childhood. It is characterized by:

- masculinization in females
- precocious puberty in males
- occasionally a salt-losing state forms part of the syndrome.

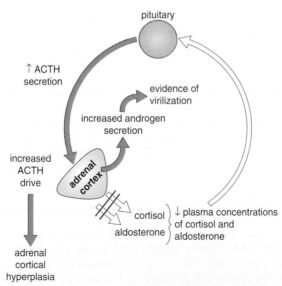

Fig. 25.2 Feedback mechanisms in congenital adrenal hyperplasia.
ACTH, adrenocorticotrophic hormone.

The basic defect is an enzyme deficiency in the cells of the adrenal cortex which synthesize cortisol and aldosterone. These cells lack either a C21 or a C11 hydroxylase, and thus pathways leading to the synthesis of cortisol and aldosterone from cholesterol are blocked. The abnormally low plasma concentrations of these hormones cause increased secretion of adreno-corticotrophic hormone by the pituitary; the adrenal cortex responds by increasing the number of functional cells. However, because the block in hormone synthesis persists, the dammed-back precursors are diverted to another metabolic pathway in the cortex, and large amounts of androgenic steroids (responsible for virilization) are formed.

Thyroid hyperplasia

This may be due to the operation of normal negative feedback mechanisms controlling the levels of **thyroid-stimulating hormone** (**TSH**), or the existence of **abnormal stimuli** (*Fig. 25.3*).

Many cases of hypothyroidism are associated with the structural changes of hyperplasia, irrespective of the mechanism causing the hypofunction. Abnormally low secretion of thyroid hormones may arise from a lack of:

- secreting tissue (as in cretinism)
- substrate (as in iodine-deficiency goitre)
- enzymes required for the various steps in hormone synthesis (dyshormonogenetic goitre).

In all these, low circulating levels of thyroxine lead to increased output of TSH from the pituitary and hence to hyperplasia of the thyroid tissue.

Similar morphological changes may occur in **hyperthyroid** patients being treated with thiouracil or carbimazole. These compounds block the synthesis of thyroxine, and the pituitary responds by secreting more TSH. The patient becomes clinically and biochemically euthyroid on this treatment, but the gland itself may become more hyperplastic.

Endocrine hyperplasia can occur also through the operation of abnormal drives. An example of this is primary hyperthyroidism (Graves' disease) in which the abnormal drive is a **thyroid-stimulating immunoglobulin** which binds to the TSH receptor on the surface of the thyroid acinar epithelium.

Pancreatic islet hyperplasia in infants with diabetic mothers

Maternal diabetes is a potent risk for perinatal mortality unless appropriate measures are taken. These infants tend to be fat, flabby and rather cushingoid in appearance. Microscopic examination of the pancreas shows a striking degree of islet cell hyperplasia. Interestingly, the islet cell hyperplasia seen in the infants of diabetic mothers is also seen in the stillborn infants of mothers who are destined to become diabetic, sometimes many years later, a state known as prediabetes.

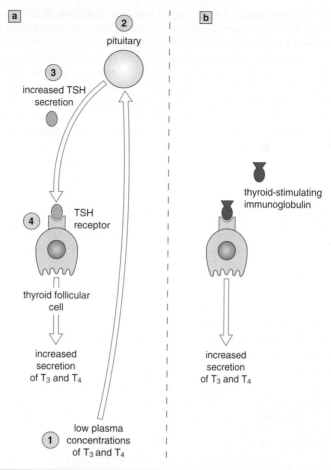

Fig. 25.3   Thyroid hyperplasia.

The hyperplasia is due **a** to increased drive controlled by negative feedback, and **b** to abnormal drive (in the form of thyroid-stimulating immunoglobulin). TSH, thyroid-stimulating hormone; T$_3$, tri-iodothyronine; T$_4$, thyroxine.

Hyperplasia in the target organs of hormones

Breast

An increase in the size of the breasts in the female is a normal feature of puberty and also occurs during pregnancy and lactation. These changes are hormone induced; both the epithelial elements and the rather specialized connective tissue elements that surround the breast ducts and demarcate the breast lobules from the interlobular connective tissue are affected. One of the most important factors in this change is oestrogen.

In clinical practice, breast hyperplasia of a rather different sort is common. This may manifest as a localized lump within the breast or as a generalized lumpiness in a fairly large area of the breast. It is not infrequently spoken of as 'chronic mastitis', a very poor term since the process is not inflammatory in nature. It is, instead, a mixture of hyperplastic and involuntionary changes, probably due to hormonal imbalance. The structural changes are basically an increase in the number of ducts within individual lobules (**adenosis**), in the number of cells lining individual ducts, with a consequent 'heaping up' of the epithelial cells ('**epitheliosis**'), and fibrosis. In any single case the appearances depend on the relative proportions of these three changes and the secondary effects (such as cystic change) resulting from them.

Prostate

Prostatic enlargement is extremely common in males past the age of 60 years. Both the fibromuscular and ductal elements are involved. It does not occur in the absence of intact testes and is almost certainly due to the effects of dihydrotestosterone.

Non-specific reactive hyperplasia

Lining epithelia of the skin, mouth, alimentary and respiratory tracts frequently become hyperplastic when any persistent irritant is applied to them. The irritant can be simple trauma, for example when a corn develops in response to the rubbing of ill-fitting shoes. Similarly, an incorrectly fitted denture can produce marked thickening of the squamous epithelium of the alveolar margin. Chronic inflammatory disease of the skin is often associated with thickening of the epidermis, and epidermal hyperplasia of a very marked degree can develop in response to the presence of certain intradermal lesions such as insect bites. At times this reactive epidermal hyperplasia may be so extreme as to raise suspicions that the process is neoplastic rather than reactive.

HYPERTROPHY

Isolated hypertrophy occurs only in muscle. The stimulus eliciting this response is an increased workload. Work-related hypertrophy occurs in **smooth muscle** in a number of pathological circumstances, particularly where there is partial obstruction to the normal outflow of the contents of any hollow muscular organ. Some examples are given below.

The urinary bladder

Any obstruction to urine outflow, as in post-inflammatory urethral strictures or with enlargement of the prostate, leads to an increase in size of the muscle fibres and a considerable degree of thickening of the bladder wall.

The orientation of the muscle in the bladder imparts a woven or trabeculated pattern, seen when the mucosal lining of the bladder is inspected at cystoscopy.

The gastrointestinal tract

The gut, an archetype of a muscular tube, shows muscle hypertrophy proximal to chronic obstructions arising from any cause. In the **oesophagus** this is seen in association with:

- post-inflammatory scarring
- carcinoma
- obstruction due to disorders of innervation (cardiac achalasia).

In the **stomach**, muscle hypertrophy may not only result from some obstructive lesion but may also cause obstruction. This is seen in **congenital hypertrophic pyloric stenosis**. In this condition affected infants, mostly males, present soon after birth with projectile vomiting shortly after feeding. On deep palpation of the abdomen, a small lump may be detected. At operation this is seen to be a thick ring of muscle around the pyloric opening. It is treated by dividing the muscle from the serosal aspect without damaging the mucosal lining. In this way the hypertrophied muscle ring is opened up and the obstruction is relieved.

The heart

Cardiac hypertrophy is common and is due to an increased workload. The workload may be of two types, each mirrored in the appearance of the heart. In **high pressure overload**, such as occurs in aortic valve stenosis, systemic hypertension or, much more rarely, coarctation of the aorta, there is a marked degree of left ventricular hypertrophy associated with a left ventricular cavity that is either normal in size or smaller than normal. In the case of **high volume overload**, the increased workload stems from an increase in end-diastolic volume (such as in aortic or mitral incompetence); this is inevitably associated with a left ventricular cavity of large capacity.

ATROPHY

Just as there may be an increase in tissue or organ size, so there may also be a decrease. If the diminution in bulk is acquired, it is spoken of as **atrophy**. As with hyperplasia and hypertrophy, atrophy may occur as a physiological phenomenon or in abnormal or pathological circumstances.

PHYSIOLOGICAL ATROPHY

This can occur at any age but is associated particularly with early life. In the fetus, many structures are formed during embryonic development which undergo regression during the later stages of gestation. These include the notochord, the branchial clefts and the thyroglossal duct. Persistence of these structures may occur to a greater or lesser degree, and patients may present (in the case of the latter two) with masses in the neck, whose true nature is revealed on histological examination after surgical removal.

In the neonatal period, the ductus arteriosus and umbilical vessels either disappear completely or remain merely as cords of fibrous tissue. Similarly, the fetal adrenal cortex undergoes a considerable degree of atrophy soon after birth.

Atrophy of the thymus occurs normally as adult life is entered, and in late middle and old age there is a significant decline in the amount of lymphoid tissue.

In the same way that increased functional demand can lead to hypertrophy and/or hyperplasia, a decrease in demand will lead to a degree of atrophy. This can be seen to a marked extent in voluntary muscle if a limb is immobilized as, for example, after a fracture. Muscle bulk decreases rapidly, and a considerable amount of exercise may be required to restore it to normal when the period of immobilization is over. Similarly, starvation is associated with some degree of atrophy of the gut, the epithelial lining being particularly affected.

Osteoporosis

A common and important example of atrophy is osteoporosis. This has been defined as a condition in which the mass of bone tissue per unit volume of 'anatomical' bone is reduced, with a decrease in the number and size of the trabeculae in cancellous bone. There is no defect in the mineralization of such osteoid matrix as is present, in contradistinction to **osteomalacia** where the bone tissue mass is normal but the degree of mineralization is subnormal. Osteoporosis is due to an increase in osteoclastic resorption of bone, decreased synthesis of bone matrix, or both of these.

LOCALIZED ATROPHY

Localized atrophy may occur in the following circumstances:

- ischaemia
- pressure
- denervation.

NON-NEOPLASTIC DISTURBANCES IN CELL GROWTH AND PROLIFERATION

- Non-neoplastic changes occur in cell populations and involve increases or decreases in cell size, cell number or both. Such changes may be pathological or physiological; physiological changes are the expression of alterations in the need for certain specialized functions.
- Increased cell size with no increase in cell number (**hypertrophy**) occurs only in muscle and indicates an increased workload. This may be due to a pressure overload, such as is seen in the heart in aortic valve disease or in high blood pressure, or a volume overload.
- Increased cell number (**hyperplasia**) is a response to an increased drive.
- Hyperplasia may be either demand-led (which is physiological) or associated with an abnormal drive such as in Graves' disease (thyrotoxicosis).
- Increased 'normal' drive leading to hyperplasia is common in endocrine organs and in bone marrow. In these situations it exemplifies the importance of negative feedback in controlling cell populations.

26 Cell proliferation and differentiation in relation to neoplasia

All non-neoplastic expansions of cell populations share one common feature: increased cell proliferation **ceases** following removal of the stimulus that has evoked it. In contrast, neoplastic cell proliferation appears to be **autonomous**; it is not demand-led, and a continuous application of an exogenous drive towards cell division is neither present nor necessary.

Much of our knowledge of the growth characteristics of neoplastic cells is derived from cell culture and one should not extrapolate too uncritically from this to the in vivo situation.

TRANSFORMATION

TRANSFORMED CELLS SHOW LOSS OF CONTACT INHIBITION

When normal cells are grown in a monolayer, their proliferation ceases once the cells are confluent. Thus, once each cell is in contact with a neighbour, cell division ceases (contact inhibition). In contrast, neoplastic cells lack this characteristic. Cell division continues even after the cells have reached confluence, and the cells heap up in a multilayered fashion.

It has been suggested that cells of any given line:

* **recognize** each other
* **exchange information** that regulates cell division
* **adhere to one another** (homotypic adhesion).

Transformed cells differ from normal cells in respect of their surface membranes

Neoplastic transformation appears to be commonly associated with changes in the surface membrane glycoproteins. One surface change can be detected by the use of a family of proteins known as **lectins**. These proteins, widely distributed through many phyla, are able to bind to different cell surface sugars with exquisite specificity. For example, wheatgerm lectin agglutinates neoplastic cells in suspension but not their normal homologues. It is believed that some component has been lost from the surface of the transformed cells with resulting exposure of the lectin-binding sugars.

The loss of contact inhibition shown by transformed cells in culture is an expression of disordered regulation of growth. So far as basic mechanisms are concerned there are two possibilities:

1) There may be a **failure in some inhibiting mechanism that normally restrains excessive cell proliferation**.
2) **Abnormal growth may represent a response to growth factors** encompassing:
   - excessive amounts of growth factor
   - overexpression of growth factor receptors
   - abnormal regulation of signal transduction following growth factor–receptor interaction.

'AUTOCRINE' GROWTH FACTORS AND AUTONOMOUS NEOPLASTIC CELL PROLIFERATION

Transformed cells in culture require **lower concentrations of growth factors for optimal growth and multiplication** than do their normal counterparts. Some portion of growth autonomy may be due to polypeptide growth factors acting on the cells that produce them by binding to appropriate surface receptors. This process – activation of cells by their own secretion products – has been called **autocrine secretion** (*Fig. 26.1*). It plays an important role in many tumours.

Many types of cultured tumour cells release polypeptide growth factors into the culture medium; these same tumour cells often possess specific receptors for the released peptide. Each type of growth factor acts on a specific membrane receptor, which in turn, through phosphorylation of proteins downstream, transduces the signal generated by binding between the peptide and its receptor into a mitogenic response.

Such a signalling system might be modulated in three ways: by the level of expression of:

1) growth factor
2) membrane receptor
3) post-receptor signalling pathway.

The peptides so far identified as functioning in this 'autocrine' fashion include:

- transforming growth factor α (TGF-α)
- platelet-derived growth factor (PDGF)
- bombesin (gastrin-releasing peptide).

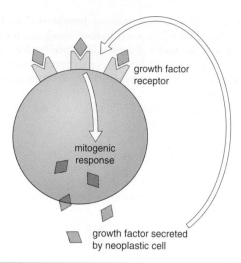

growth factor
receptor

mitogenic
response

growth factor secreted
by neoplastic cell

Fig. 26.1 'Autocrine' control of neoplastic cell proliferation.

Transformed cells secrete growth factors that bind to receptors on the surface membrane of the same cell. Binding to these specific receptors generates a mitogenic signal.

Autocrine activity in malignant cells was first described in rodent cells transformed by mouse sarcoma viruses. The peptide identified is structurally related to epidermal growth factor (EGF; see pp. 121–123) but distinct from it, and has been named **TGF-α**. It is released by several human neoplasms.

There is a very close relationship between TGF-α release and transformation. This can be demonstrated using a temperature-sensitive mutant of the mouse sarcoma virus as the transforming agent. If the target cells are not cultured at a temperature suitable for the mutant virus, transformation does not take place and there is no release of the TGF into the culture medium.

Molecules showing a considerable degree of homology with **PDGF** are released by a number of neoplasms. In humans these include:

- malignant connective tissue neoplasms of bone (osteosarcoma)
- malignant neoplasms of glial cells in the brain
- a cell line derived from human bladder cancer.

In animal cell lines, growth factors are released after transformation by a variety of RNA viruses. Many of these cell lines also possess receptors for PDGF, and such receptors may be targets for growth inhibition. For example, antibodies against PDGF block proliferation of the transformed cells. Cells secreting only small amounts of PDGF form small tumours when inoculated into immunosuppressed mice. In contrast, tumours secreting large amounts of the growth factor produce large masses in the mouse model.

Similar data relate to another growth factor, **bombesin**. This is a tetradeca-peptide produced and released by most human small-cell lung carcinomas ('oat cell carcinoma'). Monoclonal antibodies specific for the C-terminal end of bombesin prevent it from binding to its receptor and, in this way, inhibit the growth of small-cell lung cancer, both in culture and in xenografts in immunosuppressed mice.

An increase in effector peptide secretion may not be necessary for increased autocrine activity. An increase in the number or binding affinity of the **receptors** will have the same effect.

In some cases of human breast cancer, where transformation has involved activation of a cellular oncogene known as *her* or *neu*, the gene codes for a truncated version of the EGF receptor. This abnormal receptor cannot bind its ligand at the cell membrane but appears to be able to generate a mitogenic signal independent of ligand binding.

Other growth factor receptors also appear to be able to act as tyrosine kinases (and thus as initiators of mitosis) in the absence of their appropriate ligands.

Autocrine peptides can inhibit growth as well as stimulate it

Growth factors may be multifunctional. Some may downregulate or up-regulate cell growth and may also have effects on the immune system. For example, TGF-α has a suppressor effect on T lymphocytes that is ten times more powerful, on a molar basis, than that of the widely used immuno-suppressant cyclosporin A.

Transforming growth factor β

The TGF-β family includes at least three dimeric proteins secreted in an inactive form (TGF-β1–3). Either an acidic medium or cleavage by serine proteases is required for these peptides to become activated. They are related to a larger family of peptide signals, including factors responsible for bone morphogenesis, müllerian inhibiting factor and inhibin. TGF-β is widely distributed throughout adult tissues and binds to receptors on many different cell types. TGF-β1 is the most potent of the three types.

- TGF-β stimulates the growth of fibroblasts in culture in the presence of PDGF.
- If EGF is present, the TGF-β inhibits the growth of these same fibroblasts.
- Similarly TGF-β can stimulate the growth of osteoblasts but this mitogenic effect is reversed by other peptide growth factors such as EGF, PDGF and tumour necrosis factor α.

Thus the context in which a peptide signal operates may significantly modify its effect.

TGF-β inhibits the growth of most epithelial cell lines (including malig-nant cells) in culture. In other contexts (e.g. wound healing, atherogenesis) it promotes fibrous tissue growth.

DIFFERENTIATION

What kind of normal cells are transformed in the genesis of cancer? One of the cardinal features of neoplasia is autonomous growth, and so the cells from which the neoplasm arises must be able to respond to mitogenic signals (normal or abnormal) and divide. In most normal cell populations, such cells are found in the **stem cell compartment** and hence, by implication, are **undifferentiated cells**.

When a stem cell divides, one of its daughter cells may well retain the ability to divide. The other, by mechanisms that are not understood, becomes committed to differentiation and, ultimately, to death.

By definition, differentiation requires that, for each type of differentiated cell, a **heritable pattern of read-out of the genome** must exist. As all cells in the body possess the same genetic information, differentiation similarly implies that, in each type of cell, genes are expressed that are not expressed in other cell types.

If the stable differences between cell types depend on the expression of certain genes, then, clearly, there are several levels at which this control can be exercised. These include:

- **transcriptional control** (when and how often a gene is transcribed)
- **RNA processing control** (determining how the primary messenger RNA (mRNA) transcript is spliced)
- **RNA transport control** (determining which mRNAs are exported to the cytoplasm for translation)
- **translational control** (determining which mRNAs are translated by ribosomes)
- **degradation control** (the selective destabilization of some mRNA molecules in the cytoplasm)
- **control of protein activity** (some proteins may be sequestrated or inactivated after synthesis).

In most instances, it is the first of these – transcriptional control – that is most potent. Transcription is controlled by a series of gene regulatory proteins which recognize and bind to short, precisely defined, stretches of DNA. While there must be very many such regulatory proteins, a comparatively small number of structural motifs (e.g. zinc-finger motifs, leucine-zipper motifs and helix-loop motifs) is employed in the DNA recognition process.

In eukaryotes, gene regulatory proteins form large complexes which activate the promoter region of genes. One *Drosophila* gene, for example, has 20 000 nucleotide pairs in its controlling region and has binding sites for 20 different regulatory proteins.

Differentiation is also affected by the micro-environment of the cell

Genetic factors in the form of heritable patterns of gene transcription and translation undoubtedly play a major role in differentiation, but the process may be affected in other ways. For instance, **interaction between mesen-chymal and epithelial elements** is important in the development of many organ systems, including the pancreas, lung, kidney, salivary glands, breast, pituitary and liver.

Pancreatic epithelium alone, cultured from the developing rat pancreas, will not differentiate. If the same cells are seeded on to a filter, on the other side of which are mesenchymal cells in culture, then differentiation occurs. This suggests that a chemical differentiating signal is released from the mesenchymal cells. The effect of mesenchymal cell extracts is destroyed by trypsin and periodate oxidation, but not by ribonuclease or deoxyribo-nuclease. The signal is therefore presumably a glycoprotein. In cell culture systems, alteration of the medium may be sufficient to bring about profound changes in differentiation. A change in the medium may cause, for example, cartilage cells that synthesize type II collagen to revert to fibroblasts, which secrete type I collagen. The mechanism responsible for this switch is not known.

Cell–cell interactions also appear to play a role in differentiation. If mixed embryonic cells are cultured, cells of each type will segregate. It may well be that growth factors play a part in differentiation as well as in regulating the cell population size. For example, **EGF** causes granulosa cells from the ovary to differentiate into luteal cells.

METAPLASIA

Changes in differentiation patterns do not necessarily imply neoplastic transformation

A complete change in differentiation from one fully differentiated form to another, occurs often in cells subjected to chronic irritation or to changes in the hormonal milieu. This is known as **metaplasia**. One of the commonest forms is a change from cuboidal or columnar epithelium into squamous epithelium. Such metaplastic change may occur under the following circumstances:

The pseudostratified ciliated columnar epithelium of the bronchi may change into squamous epithelium. This occurs in cigarette smokers, patients with chronic bronchitis, and in chronic abscess cavities in the lung, which can become lined by epithelium.

Squamous metaplasia is common in chronic cervicitis. The metaplastic epithelium may spread down into the cervical glands and fill the lumina. This process is called 'epidermidalization' by some, and may be mistaken for invasion by squamous carcinoma by the inexperienced.

The transitional epithelium of the renal pelvis and urinary bladder may undergo squamous metaplasia in the presence of chronic infection. This is seen very often in Egypt where schistosomal cystitis is common. The presence of stones seems to increase the likelihood of metaplasia.

The columnar cell lining of the gallbladder sometimes undergoes squamous metaplasia in the presence of gallstones and chronic inflammation.

Prostatic ducts, which are normally lined by columnar epithelium, undergo squamous metaplasia in patients treated with oestrogens for prostatic carcinoma.

A deficiency of vitamin A may be associated with squamous metaplasia of the nose, bronchi and urinary tract. In addition, keratin formation is accelerated and increased in amount in the skin and conjunctiva.

Is there any identifiable mechanism causing metaplasia?

Recent experiments on cultured cell lines suggest that metaplasia can be caused by agents interfering with DNA methylation; this supports the idea that such methylation plays a part in keeping the state of expression of genes stable. If, for example, cells are grown for a few cycles in the synthetic nucleotide analogue 5-aza-cytosine, the analogue becomes incorporated into the DNA in place of some of the cytosine residues. The 5-aza-cytosine is incapable of being methylated and also inhibits the action of the methylating enzyme. This breaks the chain of events in which the pattern of DNA methylation of a gene is passed from one cell generation to the next. When cultured cells resembling fibroblasts are treated in this way they differentiate into a variety of cell types, including skeletal muscle cells, to which they would never give rise under normal circumstances.

Cellular differentiation in malignant neoplasms

Cancer cells are usually not fully differentiated. Because fully differentiated cells are unlikely to be able to 'regress' so far as differentiation is concerned, it is likely that the cancer cells are blocked at some stage in the maturation process. Unlike most normal cells that have progressed down the pathway toward full differentiation, these partly differentiated cells **still retain the capacity to divide**.

The degree of differentiation in neoplasms may be related to the precise point at which transformation occurs in the time-dependent sequence of events in which different genes are switched to the 'on' and 'off' positions after the stem cell has divided. This is particularly applicable to the liver, where there is marked heterogeneity in respect of differentiation in neoplasms induced by chemical carcinogens. Such neoplasms vary from very well differentiated lesions in which the constituent cells can be distinguished only with difficulty from those of normal liver, to highly malignant, very poorly differentiated, neoplasms in which the hepatic origin is difficult to determine.

KEY POINTS: CANCER

- Most cancers are monoclonal (derived from a single transformed cell).
- Most cancers are initiated by changes in the DNA of the target cell (genetic) rather than by changes in the expression of unaltered genes (epigenetic).
- The development of most cancers is a multistep process in which several mutations affect the target cell genome.
- The progression of cancer requires successive rounds of mutation and natural selection.
- Once cancer initiation has occurred, development of the tumour can be promoted by factors that do not affect the cellular DNA.
- Cancer incidence varies greatly from country to country: this may reflect different exposures to certain environmental factors.

The micro-environment in which malignant cells grow is involved in the maintenance of the malignant state

Malignant teratomas are neoplasms that arise from multipotent cells and can express a variety of differentiation patterns. The commonest site of origin is the gonads. Strains of mice exist in which malignant teratoma occurs in about 1% of the males. If cells from such a neoplasm are injected into the peritoneal cavity of unaffected mice of the parent strain, large cystic bodies develop. These so-called 'embryoid bodies' contain both cancer cells and differentiated cells, suggesting that both the differentiated and cancer cells arise from a single precursor.

If teratoma cells from mice with certain genetic markers are injected into 4.5-day-old embryos of mice with a different set of genetic markers, the embryos develop into **completely normal mice** which express the genetic markers of both the embryo and teratoma cells (a **chimaera**). None of these chimaeras develops teratocarcinoma. This shows that the micro-environment of the embryo is able to convert the neoplastic teratoma cells into fully differentiated normal cells.

If, on the other hand, single teratocarcinoma cells are injected subcutaneously into adult mice, large neoplasms regularly develop at the injection site. Thus the differentiation signals provided by the embryo are lacking in the adult subcutaneous tissue.

CELL PROLIFERATION AND DIFFERENTIATION IN NEOPLASIA

- Cell proliferation in neoplasia is autonomous: it is not demand-led, and continuous application of an exogenous stimulus is not needed.
- Cultured neoplastic cells show loss of contact inhibition (in contrast with their non-neoplastic counterparts) and a variety of changes in cell-surface molecules.
- Escape from normal control of proliferation may represent failure of inhibitory mechanisms or an abnormal response to growth factors.
- Abnormal responses to growth factors may represent excessive growth factor stimulation, over-expression of growth factor receptors and/or excessive transduction of growth factor signals.
- Some neoplastic cells release growth factors which stimulate their own growth (autocrine stimulation).
- Many cancer cells are not fully differentiated compared with their non-neoplastic counterparts; this may indicate a block in the normal maturation process.
- Changes in differentiation do not necessarily imply neoplastic transformation; change in differentiation from one fully differentiated form to another (**metaplasia**) occurs not infrequently in chronically irritated cells or cells in a new hormonal milieu.

27 Relationship of neoplastic cells with their environment: tumour spread

While a number of morphological and behavioural characteristics are used to differentiate between **benign** and **malignant** neoplasms, the only absolute criterion is **the ability of a malignant neoplasm to invade surrounding tissue and to colonize distant sites (metastasis)**.

ROUTES OF SPREAD

Malignant neoplasms can spread by the following routes:

- **directly** through the tissues adjacent to the primary growth
- via the **lymphatics**
- via the **bloodstream**
- through body cavities (**transcoelomic**).

Invasiveness is the prerequisite for spread to distant sites.

DIRECT SPREAD

This involves invasion of tissues adjacent to the original lesion; such spread occurs more or less in continuity with that lesion. It represents the coordination of a number of different processes – some favouring invasion and metastasis, and others inhibiting these events. Most of our knowledge in this field is derived from the study of tumour cell lines in culture and their use in certain animal models. Thus caution should be exercised in extrapolating too far from these laboratory findings to the human situation, although some supportive evidence from human studies has accrued.

The processes believed to be involved in invasion and metastasis are summarized in the box.

Adequate blood supply

Ingrowth of new blood vessels (**angiogenesis**) is required for sufficient expansion of the primary mass of tumour cells. If angiogenesis does not occur, the tumour will be unable to expand more than a few millimetres in any direction (*Fig. 27.1*).

The greater the new blood supply acquired by a tumour, the greater the risk of metastatic spread. For example, in excised breast cancers each increase of 10 in the total number of microvessels identified in 200 microscopic fields was found to be associated with a 1.59-fold increase in the risk of metastases.

The new blood vessels are derived from adjacent venules and capillaries and not from arterioles, arteries or veins. Their ingrowth is stimulated by chemical signals such as basic fibroblast growth factor, transforming growth factor α and a polypeptide known as angiogenin, first isolated from cultured tumour cells and known to show considerable homology with tumour necrosis factor α. The process is inhibited by transforming growth factor $\beta 1$.

The stimulated endothelial cells in capillaries and venules adjacent to the tumour:

- degrade their own basement membranes
- migrate into and through the extravascular stroma
- form capillary sprouts which become luminated.

The processes involved in the formation of these new blood vessels (**proliferation, motility, proteolysis**) are functionally indistinguishable from those occurring in invasion by malignant cells. The great difference, however, is that angiogenesis is not autonomous and ceases when the angiogenic stimuli are removed, the endothelial cells then reverting to their resting state. Proteolysis, a pivotal process in the migration of both tumour and endothelial cells, is also important in relation to the acquisition of lumina by the new blood vessels. Agents that inhibit proteolysis, such as some of the **tissue inhibitors of metalloproteases** (**TIMPs**) block angiogenesis.

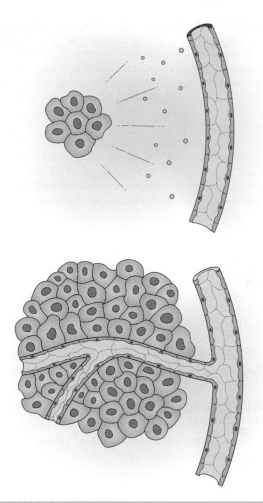

Fig. 27.1 Angiogenesis.

Angiogenesis is necessary for tumour progression. The colony of tumour cells at the top has secreted angiogenic factors which cause new blood vessels derived from neighbouring venules to grow into the tumour cell mass. The acquisition of this new blood supply permits a much greater degree of tumour cell proliferation.

Loss of homotypic cell adhesion

Infiltrating malignant cells are shed from the original primary. *This implies that cell-to-cell adhesiveness in malignant neoplasms is reduced in comparison with that of normal cells of the same type.* Several mechanisms are normally involved in such homotypic adhesion:

Normal epithelial cells develop well-established points for anchorage with each other (desmosomes), but these appear to be either totally lacking or partially deficient in malignant cells.

It has been suggested that reduced adhesiveness of malignant cells may be due to an increase in the net negative surface charge of tumour cells. This could result from synthesis of abnormal amounts of a negatively charged sialomucopeptide or of normal amounts of a strongly negatively charged molecule of the same type.

Cadherins in relation to malignancy. Cadherins are calcium-dependent cell–cell adhesion molecules which are most important in homotypic adhesion. They occur in a number of subclasses, of which the most relevant to tumour invasiveness are the **E-cadherins** (epithelial cadherins). The degree of expression of these molecules correlates inversely with the invasiveness of tumour cells (*Fig. 27.2*). Thus:

- If DNA coding for E-cadherin is inserted into highly invasive cells, the cells revert to a non-invasive form.
- Treatment of cells with antisense RNA specific for E-cadherin increases invasiveness.
- Treatment of cells with antibody raised against E-cadherin increases invasiveness.
- Carcinoma cell lines that show loss of E-cadherin expression are highly invasive.
- There is an inverse relationship between E-cadherin expression and both loss of differentiation and invasiveness in some human tumours.

Adhesion of malignant cells to basement membranes and extracellular matrices

Invasiveness involves malignant cells crossing certain connective tissue barriers that normally separate the epithelial and stromal tissue compart-

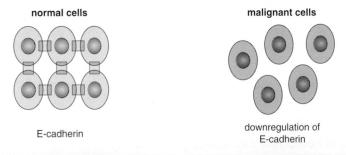

normal cells   malignant cells

E-cadherin   downregulation of
                                E-cadherin

Fig. 27.2 Homotypic adhesion.

Non-malignant epithelial cells adhere to one another partly through the agency of epithelial cadherins (red squares). In many tumours, E- cadherin expression is markedly downregulated, causing a reduction in the adhesiveness of cells one to another.

ments from each other. One of the most important of these is the **basement membrane**. On one side of the basement membrane are attached the epithelial cells. On the opposite side is the interstitial stroma, which consists of fibrillar and non-fibrillar connective tissue proteins and glycoproteins, and contains stromal cells of various types.

In benign tissue remodelling, non-neoplastic proliferative disorders and intraepithelial neoplasia (carcinoma *in situ*), *no* breaching of the basement membrane occurs. *The transition from* in situ *to invasive carcinoma is, however, marked by malignant cells crossing the basement membrane and reaching the stromal compartment.*

The basement membrane is a dense matrix of proteins and glycoproteins, and its pore size is not large enough for tumour cells to penetrate. Thus breaches in the basement membrane must be accomplished by focal destruction of the matrix.

Tumour cell–basement membrane interaction involves three steps:

1) **attachment** of tumour cells to basement membrane components
2) **lysis** of the basement membrane matrix
3) **movement** of tumour cells through the breach created in the basement membrane.

Attachment of tumour cells to basement membrane involves adhesion to matrix components such as **collagen, fibronectin and laminin** (*Fig. 27.3*). Binding to these requires appropriate receptors on the tumour cells. **Integrins** have a role of fundamental importance in this binding process, as they do in inflammation and wound healing (see pp. 61–62). Some tumour cell integrins and their binding matrices are shown in *Table 27.1*. The

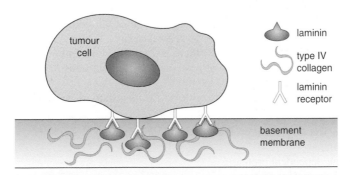

Fig. 27.3   Penetration through basement membranes by tumour cells is preceded by adhesion to basement membrane components.

Tumour cells express receptors for the basement membrane protein laminin, and the ligand receptor interaction between laminin and its receptor on tumour cells is an important mechanism mediating binding.

Table 27.1 Interaction between matrix proteins and tumour cell integrins

Binding molecule on cell	Matrix protein or glycoprotein
VLA-2 ($\alpha_2\beta_2$)	Collagen and laminin
VLA-4 ($\alpha_4\beta_1$)	A variant of fibronectin
VLA-5 ($\alpha_5\beta_1$)	Fibronectin
VLA-6 ($\alpha_6\beta_1$)	Laminin
$\alpha_6\beta_4$	Laminin
$\alpha_v\beta_3$	Vitronectin

VLA, very late activation antigen.

integrins bind to their respective adhesion molecules by recognizing the specific RGD (Arg–Gly–Asp) sequence.

Laminin is a cross-shaped glycoprotein present in both the basement membrane and the interstitial stroma. In normal cells laminin receptors occur on the aspect of the cell apposed to the basement membrane and are occupied by basement membrane laminin. Invasive cells, however, have laminin receptors diffusely distributed over the entire cell surface and these are often unoccupied. If such tumour cells are treated with the receptor binding fragment of laminin, their invasiveness is greatly reduced.

Proteolysis of basement membrane and interstitial stromal matrices

Penetration by malignant cells of the basement membrane and interstitial stromal matrix requires proteolysis by degradative enzymes secreted by the tumour cells (Figs 27.4 and 27.5).

This proteolysis is carried out in a highly organized manner in both space and time; cell migration during invasiveness requires attachment and de-attachment to the matrix as the cell moves forward. The importance of proteolysis can be demonstrated by the use of antibodies raised against the enzymes or of inhibitors of protease activity (TIMPs). *In both cases, invasion is blocked.* Conversely, there is a positive correlation between the expression of several classes of proteinase by tumour cells and aggressive behaviour by the tumour.

The classes of proteolytic enzyme so far identified as being responsible for connective tissue lysis include:

• metal ion-dependent proteases (metalloproteinases)
• heparanases
• serine-dependent proteases
• thiol-dependent proteases.

In connection with invasiveness, the metalloproteinases have been studied most extensively. There are three main groups of these, the division being based on substrate preference:

• interstitial collagenases

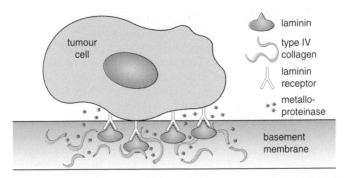

Fig. 27.4

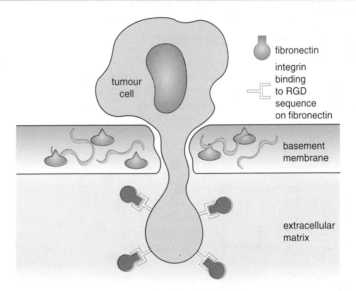

Fig. 27.5

Figs 27.4 and 27.5   Proteolysis of basement membrane and matrix.

Binding to connective tissue matrix proteins is followed by proteolytic breakdown of these matrices and deattachment of tumour cells, which can then move through the breaches created by matrix protein breakdown.

- gelatinases
- stromelysins.

All the metalloproteinases are secreted in an inactive form and their activation is an important control step but how this occurs in vivo is still unknown.

Other tumour-associated proteolytic enzymes

It has been known for 60 years that extracts from virally induced tumours in chickens can lyse plasma clots; human sarcomas have been shown to have similar fibrinolytic properties. This activity is due to production by the tumour cells of **plasminogen activator**, a phenomenon which occurs in many cell lines following malignant transformation. There is some evidence to suggest that acquisition of the ability to produce plasminogen activator is associated with the ability to invade extracellular matrix. In this connection it must be remembered that some normal cells also produce plasminogen activator. Some of these cells (such as macrophages, neutrophils and trophoblastic cells) travel through the connective tissue matrix, whereas others (such as breast epithelium, Sertoli cells in the testis, thyroid and parathyroid epithelium, and β cells in the islets of Langerhans) are fixed.

Active movement of malignant cells

Invasion and metastasis by tumour cells require active movement. Whether the movement involved in invasion is random (**kinesis**) or directed (**taxis**), or both of these, is not clear. Several factors increase one or other of these forms of movement (*Fig. 27.6*). These include:

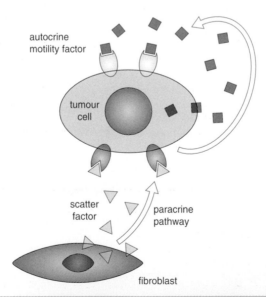

Fig. 27.6   Chemical signals stimulating active movement of tumour cells.

Movement of tumour cells through connective tissues is mediated *inter alia* by an autocrine motility factor and a paracrine signal, in the form of 'scatter factor' derived from fibroblasts. The scatter factor binds to a receptor encoded by the proto-oncogene c-*met*.

Intact and fragmented molecules of the extracellular matrix such as collagen or fibronectin.

Tumour autocrine motility factor (AMF).   This is a 64 kD protein secreted by certain tumour cell lines. It binds to a glycoprotein receptor on the tumour cells, binding is then followed by activation of a G protein-mediated signalling system. *Movement of the tumour cells appears to be associated with phosphorylation of the receptor.* The action of AMF can be simulated by treating tumour cells with monoclonal antibodies that bind to the AMF receptor.

'Scatter factor'.   This protein, synthesized and secreted by fibroblasts, exerts a scattering effect on many epithelial cells in culture. This effect, which appears to be exerted in a paracrine fashion, occurs at picomolar concentrations. Scatter factor is a molecule that resembles plasminogen in some respects and is identical to **hepatocyte growth factor**. It is multi-functional, being able to induce motility in tumour cells, to induce proliferation in epithelial cells and also to act as a morphogen in that it can induce tubule formation in some epithelial cell lines cultured in collagen gels. This suggests that scatter factor binds either to separate receptors on different target cells or to a single receptor that is linked to multiple signalling pathways.

A ligand for scatter factor is the gene product of a proto-oncogene, *c-met*. This is a transmembrane heterodimer with tyrosine kinase activity; it is widely expressed in normal epithelial tissues.

A role for mechanical pressure in direct spread of malignant tumours

Invading cells tend to follow the paths of least resistance and thus spread along natural clefts or within tissue planes. This occurs in cancer of the alimentary tract: the invading cells reach the main muscle layers and then tend to avoid the muscle itself and pass instead through connective tissue septa separating muscle bundles. On naked-eye examination the muscle has a curiously segmented appearance as if the muscle fibres were bricks and the intervening tumour-infiltrated septa, the mortar.

Changes associated with neoplasia in the extracellular matrix

Malignant cells can alter the extracellular matrix in three ways:

1) by destroying the matrix of tumour cells
2) by increasing production of matrix by the host ('desmoplasia')
3) by synthesizing matrix.

The first of these has already been discussed in the previous section.

Desmoplastic response

The amount of stroma associated with malignant neoplasms determines their consistency to a considerable extent. The extreme hardness and 'gritty' feel of some tumours is due to the high proportion of fibrous tissue within them. The ancient Greek physicians recognized this phenomenon and coined the term **scirrhous** (rock-like) for such lesions. The biological purpose of desmoplasia is not clear. Its presence is certainly not necessary for invasion to occur; some invasive tumours have very little desmoplasia, whereas others, notably those of the breast, stomach and bile duct, show a marked desmoplastic reaction.

Synthesis of matrix
The origin of the fibrous tissue related to malignant tumours is controversial. Some maintain that the new collagen is synthesized and secreted by the invading tumour cells. The results of other studies support a role for the host cells. Recently, myofibroblasts, which are not normally present in breast connective tissue, have been identified in the stroma of some breast cancers. It has been suggested that malignant cells may, in some unknown way, either recruit or stimulate the formation of myofibroblasts, which then produce the excess connective tissue matrix found in tumours with a marked desmoplastic response.

Other phenotypic characteristics of malignant cells that may contribute to invasiveness

Loss of anchorage dependence
With the exception of lymphocytes and haemopoietic cells, normal cells, when cultured, grow only on a firm surface such as glass, plastic or solid agar. This characteristic is termed 'anchorage dependence'. Many cell lines derived from malignant neoplasms or from cells that have undergone malignant transformation in culture can grow **in suspension or in semi-solid soft agar**. This growth feature in cell culture systems, more than any other, correlates with the ability of the cultured cells to produce malignant tumours when injected into animals of the appropriate species ('tumorigenicity').

Loss of fibronectin from the cell surface
Fibronectin is a glycoprotein identified as a component of the extracellular matrix of many cells in culture. It is also found in basement membranes and interstitial stroma in many animals and human tissues, and circulates in the blood (where it was originally called cold-insoluble globulin). Fibronectin occurs on the external surface of many cells, forming a fibrillary meshwork around and between them. It acts as an adhesive protein in cell–cell binding and in the binding of cells to their substratum. Malignant transformation is accompanied by a loss or marked reduction of cell surface fibronectin. The loss of this surface protein (and presumably the decreased adhesiveness that follows) may be an expression either of an increase in degradative enzymes on the surface of the malignant cells (see pp. 446–448), or of a disturbance in the cytoskeleton, more particularly the microfilaments beneath the cell surface.

LYMPHATIC SPREAD

The invasion of lymphatic channels at an early stage of infiltration is characteristic of **carcinoma** (malignant epithelial neoplasm). Malignant tumours derived from connective tissue cells (**sarcomas**) show a much greater tendency to invade the small blood vessels.

Invasion of the lymphatics may be made easier by the fact that their basement membranes contain neither type IV collagen nor laminin. This difference makes it possible, with the use of appropriate antibodies, to determine whether small vascular channels in tissue sections showing invasion by tumour are lymphatics or venules.

Little is known about the actual mechanics of lymphatic invasion. In certain experimental models, tumour cells have been seen to line up alongside the lymphatic channels and to enter the lymphatic by first pushing cytoplasmic processes between the endothelial cells and then travelling through the interendothelial gap, in a reverse direction to that seen when leucocyte emigration occurs in inflammation. Such invasion is likely to make use of the mechanisms previously discussed in relation to direct spread.

Once malignant cells have gained access to the lymphatic vessel, they can grow along the lumen as a continuous cord, permeating the lymphatic drainage in that area and extending quite widely. Such intralymphatic tumour seen in a tissue section is, of course, an indicator of possible spread to regional lymph nodes. However, in some cases the presence of intralymphatic tumour in the absence of lymph node deposits may have an even more ominous prognostic significance, because it has been reported that patients with breast cancer in whom there is evidence of lymphatic permeation by tumour but no regional node deposits have an increased risk of developing distant metastases.

Lymphatic permeation is a particularly prominent feature of **carcinoma of the breast**, in which lymphatic blockage occurs quite frequently. This results in diversion of lymph flow and may be accompanied by a similar diversion of groups of tumour cells. These cells may impact within the lymphatic drainage of the breast, producing satellite tumour nodules. Lymphatic blockage also causes lymphoedema of the tissues caudal to the block. In patients with carcinoma of the breast this produces an appearance of the skin which has been aptly termed **peau d'orange**. In the lung, extensive lymphatic permeation by tumour, often from a breast or gastric primary, produces the condition known as **lymphangitis carcinomatosa**. On chest radiography the lung shows a curious reticulated appearance. This is mirrored by the outlining of the subpleural lymphatic channels seen when the lung is removed at post mortem examination.

Malignant melanoma is another neoplasm that tends to permeate along the local lymphatic drainage. If the tumour cells are producing melanin, the cord of cells permeating the lymphatics may be seen as a black streak in the subcutaneous tissue.

Tumour cells enter the regional lymph nodes and gain access to the subcapsular peripheral sinus in the first instance. From here, the cells extend to involve the sinuses in the node centre. Within the node, tumour cells may be destroyed, remain dormant for long periods, or establish a growing focus with partial or total replacement of the node. For the last of these, acquisition of an adequate blood supply is important. Normal nodes have a dual blood supply, partly from hilar vessels and partly from transcapsular anastomoses. If the tumour nodules invade intranodal vessels, haemorrhage and necrosis may occur within the secondary deposit.

Tumour cells within lymph nodes may gain access to the bloodstream in a number of ways. These include:

- invasion of small intranodal blood vessels
- invasion of extranodal blood vessels by nodal deposits that have breached the lymph node capsule
- opening up of small lymphaticovenous communications
- via the thoracic duct.

Connections between the lymphatic channels and the bloodstream work in both directions. If radioactively labelled tumour cells are injected into a peripheral vein of a rat, tumour cells can be recovered from lymphatics within one hour. Thus, malignant cells within the bloodstream are not always trapped in the first capillary bed they encounter, but can escape into the lymphatic system.

BLOOD SPREAD

Apart from the connections between the lymphatic system and the blood vessels mentioned above, malignant cells may enter the bloodstream by invading either small new vessels within the substance of the tumour itself or the host blood vessels near the growing edge of the tumour. This is made easy in newly formed vessels by their defective basement membranes and lack of normal perivascular connective tissue. Sarcomas often contain large, irregular, blood-filled channels, the linings of which consist partly or entirely of malignant tumour cells; these lining cells can, of course, be shed directly into the bloodstream. This may, in part, account for the predilection shown by sarcomas for spread via the bloodstream.

Permeation in continuity along invaded venous channels occurs in certain malignant tumours. These include carcinomas arising from renal tubular epithelium (so-called **hypernephroma**) and carcinoma of the bronchus. In the case of renal adenocarcinoma, venous invasion may occur quite early and the tumour cells extend as a solid mass along the course of the renal vein. In rare instances, the inferior vena cava may be involved, and cases have been recorded where tumour has grown up into the right atrium. When the left renal vein is involved in this way, the first clinical evidence may be the appearance of a left-sided scrotal mass consisting of dilated spermatic veins (**varicocele**). This is said to be due to the fact that the spermatic veins of the left side drain directly into the left renal vein. If the latter becomes blocked by tumour, hydrostatic pressure rises in the spermatic veins and they become distended.

METASTASIS

A growing colony of malignant cells that becomes established at a point distant from the original or primary lesion and with **no continuity between the primary lesion and the new deposit** is termed a **metastasis** or **secondary deposit**. The majority of metastases arise as a result of invasion of lymphatics or blood vessels, but in some instances they owe their existence to 'seeding out' of malignant cells across serosa-lined spaces such as the pleural and peritoneal cavities.

Metastasis is, fundamentally, an **embolic process**. It may be viewed as a series of events occurring sequentially (*Fig. 27.7*) and including:

- **liberation** of cells from the primary tumour mass
- **invasion** of blood vessels or lymphatics
- **transfer** of tumour cells as tumour emboli to distant sites
- **adhesion to endothelium** in the vascular bed of some distant organ or tissue; the expression of appropriate adhesion molecules may be one of the important determinants for the localization patterns of metastasis seen in association with certain tumours
- **migration** from the vessels in which the emboli have impacted
- **survival** at the new site, which probably involves angiogenesis
- **multiplication** and **growth** to form secondary tumours.

Determination of the extent of spread (staging) of tumours gives useful prognostic information

In patients with carcinoma, deposits of tumour in the regional nodes are a common occurrence. If the lymphatics draining lymph from these nodes are invaded by the tumour cells, the stage is set for further extension to the next set of nodes, which may also become wholly or partly replaced by tumour. The extent of such nodal invasion is important in assessing the prognosis of patients with cancer. Despite the introduction of a number of new criteria in recent years, the presence or absence of lymph node metastasis remains one of the more reliable indicators of the natural history of an individual patient with cancer. For instance, in one of the commonest malignant neoplasms encountered in clinical practice – carcinoma of the breast – absence of lymph node metastases after a careful search of the axillary contents is associated with a 5-year survival rate of 75–80%. The presence of lymph node deposits reduces this figure considerably, perhaps to approximately 50%.

A combination of assessment of direct spread and lymph node metastasis gives valuable prognostic information in carcinoma of the colon and rectum, and forms the basis of the Dukes' staging scheme for these tumours.

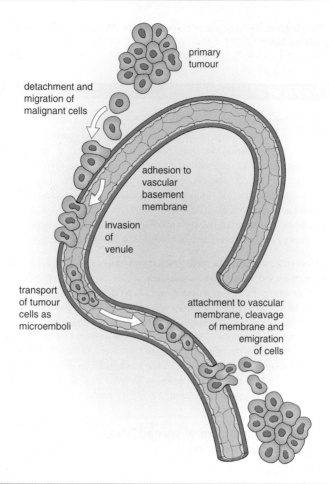

primary
tumour

detachment and
migration of
malignant cells

adhesion to
vascular
basement
membrane

invasion
of
venule

transport
of tumour
cells as
microemboli

attachment to vascular
membrane, cleavage
of membrane and
emigration
of cells

Fig. 27.7   Outline of the operational steps involved in metastasis.

- If a colonic and rectal carcinoma penetrates the bowel wall no further than the main muscle coat (Dukes' stage A), the 5-year survival rate should be 80–90%.
- Penetration of the bowel wall by tumour through the muscle to reach the subserosa (Dukes' stage B) reduces the 5-year survival rate to approximately 50%.
- If the tumour is associated with lymph node deposits (Dukes' stage C) the 5-year survival rate is reduced to about 30%.

Blood-borne metastases are the feature of malignant disease that is responsible for death in most fatal cases. When an accessible tumour such as carcinoma of the breast can be apparently completely excised with relative ease, it is obvious that it is the presence of **occult** metastases at the time of primary excision that determines the outcome for the patient.

Much of our knowledge of the metastatic process comes from experimental systems such as transplantable breast cancers or malignant melanomas in mice. Once a transplantable tumour has grown to a few grams in weight, it starts to release several million malignant cells into the blood every day. Fortunately the presence of malignant cells in the blood (or lymph) does not mean that metastases will inevitably develop. An overwhelming majority of tumour cells released in the blood die very quickly. In studies carried out using radioactively labelled malignant melanoma cells, it was found that only 1% of injected cells survive for 24 hours. After 2 weeks, only 0.1% survive. However, at this stage deposits of secondary tumour could be seen in the lungs.

The metastatic process

While in the bloodstream the malignant cells may adhere to each other and form clumps. They may adhere to platelets or lymphocytes, and when they enter the capillary bed in which they may impact, they can adhere to the capillary endothelium. The greater the degree of clumping of tumour cells, the more likely is impaction and the greater the chances that a secondary deposit will form.

After impaction in a small vessel, some tumour cells stimulate the production of fibrin; it has been suggested that this fibrin tends to protect the clump of malignant cells and enables them to proliferate. In animal models of the metastatic process, administration both of plasmin and anticoagulants has been shown to reduce the number of metastases after intravenous injection of malignant cells.

After impaction in small vessels, the malignant cells must emigrate from the vascular compartment into the perivascular tissues. It has been shown in experimental tumours that endothelial cells retract, leaving cell-free spaces through which the tumour cells can escape, using the same mechanisms to attach to basement membranes and penetrate them as have been described in the section dealing with invasiveness.

Within the extravascular tissues, a new and suitable micro-environment must be established if the colony of tumour cells is to grow and flourish. If the colony is to grow to a significant size, a new blood supply must become available both for nutrition of the tumour cells and for carrying away cellular waste products. The new blood vessels, as mentioned earlier, are derived from the host vasculature. The effect of this neovascularization can be shown in a number of animal models. For example, if tumours are implanted into the cornea of animals, initially tumour growth is slow. After about 1 week small capillaries begin to grow out from the iris into the cornea and, when these vessels reach the tumour, a marked spurt of tumour growth occurs. Implantation of normal tissues does not have this effect. Extracts from tumours applied to the chorioallantoic membrane of a fertilized chicken egg also show a considerable angiogenic effect.

Are malignant cells homogeneous in respect of their tendency to metastasize?

Only a small fraction of the malignant cells released into the circulation from a primary tumour survive to establish secondary deposits. Does this mean that the successful cells have some special properties not shared by the other cells of the tumour?

This hypothesis has been tested in the mouse melanoma model. Malignant melanoma in humans frequently develops lymphatic and blood-borne metastases; non-human melanomas behave in much the same way. Murine B16 melanoma, arising spontaneously in a certain strain of black mice, can be transplanted from one animal of the strain to another, and tumour cells can be cultured with relative ease. When B16 cells are implanted into the subcutaneous tissue of mice, the melanoma metastasizes at a low or moderate rate. To quantify this phenomenon it is customary to inject a known number of tumour cells into the mouse tail vein and then to count the number of lung metastases. If the metastatic deposits are harvested and cultured, and these cultured cells are then injected into mouse tail veins, the yield of metastases is greater. After, say, 10 cycles a cell line will have been established which has a much greater metastatic potential than cells from the original tumour line. *These data suggest that the original tumour cell population was not homogeneous in respect of the qualities needed to establish metastases.*

This model may also throw some light on the common clinical observation that particular primary tumours metastasize preferentially to certain sites. For example, breast cancers commonly spread to lung, liver, bone and brain; lung tumours often spread to the brain and adrenals; and prostatic cancers frequently spread to bone. About 90 years ago, Ewing and Paget suggested that different patterns of metastasis were due to the fact that different tumour cells would thrive in certain 'biological soils' but not in others. More recently the use of experimental models has suggested that properties of the malignant cells themselves also influence the pattern of their metastasis.

For instance, is the pattern of metastasis due solely to anatomical factors such as the vascular bed first encountered by tumour emboli?

If radioactively labelled B16 melanoma cells are injected into the tail veins of a batch of mice and also into the left ventricles of other mice, the initial distribution of the radioactivity suggests that the cells have indeed impacted in different sites in the two groups of mice. Within 24 hours, however, the distribution and number of surviving cells is the same, irrespective of the site of injection, and after 2 weeks the number of metastases in the lungs is the same in both cases. These results suggest that tumour cells destined to form secondary deposits in a particular organ detach themselves from their initial impaction site and 'home' on to the favoured tissue. By cell selection procedures similar to those described previously, it has been possible to isolate a subpopulation of B16 cells that metastasizes only to one area of the brain, and another that preferentially colonizes the ovaries. Although the nature of this 'homing' mechanism is unknown, it appears to be related to the nature of the surface membrane of the malignant cell. Each tumour cell line that produces metastases at preferred sites has been shown to have a specific pattern of cell surface proteins.

How far these observations relate to the behaviour of malignant tumours in humans is unknown, although there is increasing evidence that human tumours are heterogeneous with respect to several features.

Are there genes that determine metastatic phenotype?

The NM23 gene

It is clear that cell populations derived from a single tumour contain clones whose potential to form metastases varies. The screening of complementary DNA 'libraries' derived from tumours of 'high' and 'low' metastatic potential has shown that certain messenger RNAs (mRNAs) are present in different concentrations in these two classes of cell. The genes encoding these have been investigated as possible regulators of metastasis.

Currently, the most interesting of these is a suppressor gene for metastasis which has been called *NM23*. It was recognized in the first instance by the fact that, in mouse melanoma cell lines, mRNA for this gene was reduced in amount in cells of high as opposed to low metastatic potential. *In human breast cancer, poor survival is correlated with loss of expression of* NM23, *and increased expression is associated with a good prognosis.*

NM23 is coded for on the long arm of chromosome 17, a chromosome that is the site of a number of different genes involved in malignant disease. On the long arm are sited the loci for *NM23*, the retinoic acid receptor TIMP-2, and the gene involved in hereditary breast and ovarian cancer.

The gene product of *NM23* is almost identical with that of the *awd* gene product in the fruit fly *Drosophila*. Decrease in *awd* expression leads to maldevelopment of several tissues in postembryonic life. It has been suggested that loss of *NM23* may, in the same way, lead to a disordered state in which development may be abnormal or in which tumours may progress to become metastatic.

It is now known that the gene products of both *NM23* and *awd* are nucleoside diphosphate (NDP) kinases. NDP kinases play a part in two functions, either or both of which may be involved in malignancy. The first of these is the assembly and disassembly of microtubules. Microtubule assembly requires that GDP be changed to GTP by transphosphorylation, which is catalysed by a microtubule-associated NDP kinase. Lack of this kinase could lead to an aneuploid state, as is frequently observed in metastatic cells. The second is the fact that NDP kinases form complexes with a variety of G proteins which regulate many second-messenger pathways and may thus be involved in the regulation of a number of pathways that could be related to development, oncogenesis and metastasis.

Mutation or abnormal expression of oncogenes in relation to metastasis

In a variety of human malignancies, mutations or abnormal expression of the *ras* and *myc* oncogenes are associated with aggressive behaviour. When mutated *ras* oncogene sequences are transfected into an immortal line of mouse-derived fibroblasts, the resulting cells produce metastases when injected into athymic mice.

Some common patterns of metastasis in human tumours

The liver

The liver is the commonest site for blood-borne metastases. Gastrointestinal and pancreatic tumours regularly metastasize there, which is not surprising in view of their venous drainage via the portal system. Other primary tumours commonly metastasizing to the liver are carcinomas of the lung, breast and genitourinary system, malignant melanoma and various sarcomas. Rare examples of transplacental metastases have also been recorded in the liver.

The lung

Tumours that commonly metastasize to the lung are carcinoma of the breast, carcinoma of the stomach, and sarcomas. Blood-borne metastases in this tissue may be single or multiple and tend to occur as well-demarcated rounded masses. Sometimes it may be difficult to distinguish between a single secondary deposit and a peripherally situated primary carcinoma of the lung. In a city-dweller, whose lung tissue is usually laden with carbon pigment, the absence of pigment from the centre of the tumour may be helpful in differentiating a secondary deposit.

The skeleton

After the liver and lungs, the skeleton is the most frequent site for metastases. Common sites of origin are breast, prostate, kidney and thyroid. Bony metastases may either elicit the production of new bone (**osteoblastic**) or destroy bone (**osteolytic**). In the former, the secondary deposits are very hard as a result of the abundant new bone formation and appear as radio-opaque shadows on radiography. Plasma alkaline phosphatase levels are high, reflecting active osteogenesis. Serum calcium and phosphate concentrations are usually normal. Such osteosclerotic secondaries are commonly seen in association with carcinoma of the prostate. When this is the case, plasma concentrations of acid phosphatase (of tumour cell origin) are also much raised. Osteolysis shows itself on radiological examination by the presence of zones of radiolucency. Clinically, it draws attention to itself by pain or because of pathological fractures (fractures that occur after only slight trauma). If bone destruction has been extensive, hypercalcaemia may be present.

The mechanisms of tumour-mediated bone destruction are not well understood. Many tumours contain collagenase, capable of degrading type I collagen. In organ culture systems where portions of breast cancer are incubated together with small pieces of mouse skull, osteolysis can be detected and can be inhibited by adding cyclo-oxygenase inhibitors such as aspirin. This suggests that prostaglandin release may play some part in mediating bone destruction.

The brain
Secondary deposits occur quite frequently in the brain; the lung is one of the commonest primary sites. Often neurological and/or psychiatric disturbances produced by the metastasis are the first indication of the presence of cancer in these patients.

The adrenal
Of all endocrine organs, the adrenal gland is most frequently involved by metastases. The medulla is the most favoured site but nodules of secondary tumour may also occur in the cortex. Common primary sites for adrenal secondaries include the lung and the breast.

TRANSCOELOMIC SPREAD

This term is applied to the sequence of events that follows invasion of the serosal lining of an organ by malignant cells. A local inflammatory response usually develops and the malignant cells may become incorporated into the inflammatory exudate on the serosal surface.

Small groups of cells become detached from the main colony of tumour cells and can be swept away by the fluid portion of the exudate and float out

KEY POINTS: TUMOUR SPREAD

- The fundamental functional attribute of malignancy is invasiveness.
- Invasive cells show loss of homotypic adhesion, probably due to decreased expression of cadherins.
- Invasion is mediated by the operation of a trio of linked processes:
  1) **adhesion** to connective tissue matrices
  2) **proteolysis** of matrix proteins
  3) **active movement** of tumour cells mediated by autocrine motility factor or 'scatter factor'.
- The extent of spread, as determined by clinical and pathological examination (staging), has important prognostic implications.
- Patterns of metastasis are probably determined by both the biological characteristics of the 'soil' (tissues in which deposits occur) and the 'seed' (tumour cells).
- Tumour cells are heterogeneous in their ability to metastasize. This may correlate with the expression of certain genes (e.g. NM23 and ras).

into the serosal cavity. They settle on the walls of the cavity, where some proliferate and set up small secondary deposits. These may elicit the formation of more exudation and the serosal cavity may, in time, come to contain a large volume of fluid.

This type of spread is most commonly seen in the peritoneal cavity of patients with gastric, colonic and ovarian carcinoma. The greater omentum may be so massively infiltrated that it becomes converted to a thick, firm, often rather gelatinous mass, which some, rather infelicitously, refer to as 'omental cake'. Deposits arising from gravitational seeding are especially common in the pouch of Douglas. From time to time, gastric or colonic carcinoma may be associated with a highly individual pattern of trans-coelomic spread in which the ovaries become involved preferentially. The ovaries become grossly enlarged and have smooth capsular surfaces and slightly mucoid cut surfaces. On microscopic examination much of the enlargement can be seen to be due to a desmoplastic response in the ovarian stroma to the presence of the relatively scanty cancer cells. The classical jargon for these ovarian deposits is 'Krukenberg' tumours.

TUMOUR SPREAD

- Malignant cells can spread directly through adjacent tissues, via lymphatic and blood vessels, or across serosa-lined cavities (*trans-coelomic* spread).
- **Invasion** requires:
  — acquisition of a new blood supply for the tumour
  — loss of homotypic cell adhesion
  — the ability of malignant cells to adhere to basement membranes and connective tissue matrix proteins
  — proteolysis
  — active movement of tumour cells.
- Molecules known as cadherins normally mediate homotypic cell adhesion; failure to express cadherins in sufficient numbers correlates with increased invasiveness.
- Binding of tumour cells to basement membranes and interstitial matrices depends on interaction between integrins on the tumour cell surface and collagen, fibronectin and laminin in connective tissue barriers.
- Malignant cells express several proteolytic enzymes which enable them to break down connective tissue barriers to invasion.
- Cell movement through tissues is facilitated by a number of factors that increase motility by binding to appropriate receptors on the malignant cells.

28 Effects of neoplasms on the host

Both benign and malignant neoplasms can produce a wide variety of effects on the host. While the term 'malignant' rightly has ominous prognostic overtones, 'benign' lesions that are not invasive and have no metastatic potential may, nevertheless, have serious or even fatal consequences.

LOCAL EFFECTS

MECHANICAL PRESSURE OR OBSTRUCTION

In many cases the effects of neoplasms on the host depend on the interaction between the **site** of the tumour and its **size**. A large number of such instances exists; only a few examples are given in the following section.

In the gastrointestinal tract, neoplasms may present clinically because they cause obstruction. This is usually, although not invariably, **chronic** and is expressed by a change in bowel habit. The obstruction may be caused by the actual bulk of the neoplasm itself, but is more often due to the fibrous tissue response elicited by the presence of cancer cells (desmoplasia). In a few cases, a polypoid tumour mass may lead to intussusception.

Obviously tumour site plays a major role in determining whether or not obstruction will occur. A small neoplasm in an unfavourable anatomical location produces significant obstruction. For instance, carcinoma in the common bile duct or head of the pancreas causes severe cholestatic jaundice, associated with marked dilatation of the biliary passages above the obstruction and, not infrequently, with dilatation of the gallbladder as well.

Mechanically, one of the most serious locations for neoplasms to occur is within the cranium. A common intracranial tumour arises from the meninges (**meningioma**). The overwhelming majority of meningiomas are benign, but they can cause serious or fatal consequences as a result of the rise in intracranial pressure that they produce and the distortion of normal anatomical relationships that follows.

In some cases the type of obstructive phenomenon is determined by the **pattern of spread** of the neoplasm. This is seen very strikingly in carcinoma of the uterine cervix. Here the direct spread of tumour within the pelvis often involves the lower portions of the ureters, which are encased in a rigid sleeve of tumour and associated fibrous tissue. The obvious sequel is ureteric obstruction; in due time, if the obstruction cannot be relieved, chronic renal failure ensues.

Another example of the role of anatomical location in determining the clinical picture may be seen, from time to time, in carcinoma of the lung occurring at the apices of the upper lobes. If the neoplasm extends beyond the anatomical confines of the lung, it may involve either the brachial plexus or the sympathetic chain. In either instance there may be striking local neurological consequences, with unilateral Horner's syndrome in the case of sympathetic involvement.

TISSUE DESTRUCTION

Destruction of tissue may occur as a result of:

- pressure
- aggressive invasive properties of the tumour.

Examples of the former may be seen in the erosive effects of a benign adenoma of the pituitary, which may be associated with destruction of part of the pituitary fossa, or in the mucosal ulceration that can occur over benign connective tissue tumours of the bowel wall such as smooth muscle tumours (leiomyomas) or tumours of nerve sheath (neurilemmomas).

Destruction of bone in association with local deposits of tumour is not infrequent and leads to a great deal of distress to the patient in the form of pain. In addition actual loss of tissue may lead to so-called '**pathological fractures**'. These are manifested in the vertebral column as collapse of infiltrated vertebrae. The presence of multiple bony deposits may be associated with extensive osteolysis, leading to hypercalcaemia. Skeletal metastases are responsible for many cases of hypercalcaemia, but hypercalcaemia can also occur in the presence of certain neoplasms **without secondary tumour being present within the skeleton**.

Non-metastatic hypercalcaemia

Hypercalcaemia is most commonly caused by upregulation of osteoclastic bone resorption. Some tumours (not of the parathyroid) have been found to secrete a parathyroid hormone-related peptide (PTHRP). This particular example of **ectopic hormone production**, considered in more detail later in this chapter, has been noted especially in tumours of the lung and kidney (*Fig. 28.1*). However, tumour-related hypercalcaemia can occur in the absence of both bony metastases and a raised PTHRP concentration.

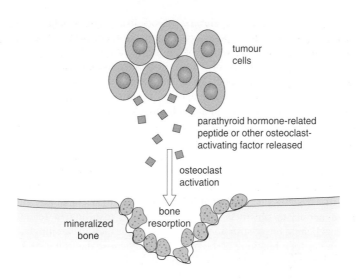

Fig. 28.1 Non-metastatic hypercalcaemia.

Humoral hypercalcaemia of malignancy is associated with the release of osteoclast-stimulating factors by tumour cells. This is exemplified by the action of parathyroid-hormone-related peptide, the release of which causes severe hypercalcaemia due to bone resorption.

Extracts of the tumours from these patients have an osteolytic effect in vitro. At least part of this effect is now thought to be due to prostaglandin (PG) production, either by the tumour cells or by cells associated with them. In a number of animal tumours, secretion of PGE_2 was noted and the hypercalcaemia could be prevented by the administration of a cyclo-oxygenase inhibitor such as indomethacin. PGE_2 can be shown to have a marked capacity for causing bone resorption in studies carried out in vitro. Several studies in humans have also indicated that increased secretion of PGE_2 is causally associated with hypercalcaemia.

Substances other than prostaglandins that are capable of inducing resorption of bone have also been found in association with certain tumours. Cultured cell lines of plasma cell tumour and from Burkitt's lymphoma (a B lymphocyte-derived tumour believed to be associated with infection by the Epstein–Barr virus) produce a non-prostaglandin, non-PTHRP, soluble factor which can stimulate osteoclasts to resorb bone in vitro. This has been identified as the cytokine, tumour necrosis factor (TNF) β.

HAEMORRHAGE

Epithelial surface neoplasms or those just beneath such surfaces often ulcerate and bleed. Mostly this bleeding is slow and unspectacular, although nonetheless dangerous. The chronic blood loss may produce a severe microcytic anaemia of the type associated with iron deficiency. Such 'occult bleeding' occurs often in cancers of the right side of the colon or of the caecum. Indeed, symptoms of vague ill-health associated with chronic anaemia may be the first and, for a long time, the only indication of a neoplasm. Occasionally, ulceration of a tumour may result in torrential haemorrhage, as for example in smooth muscle tumours of the stomach or intestine.

INFECTION

Infection in relation to malignancy is common and may determine the timing of a patient's death. **Local infection** tends to occur in any situation where a neoplasm obstructs a drainage system, resulting in retention of secretions behind the obstruction. This occurs in bronchial carcinoma, where narrowing or total blocking of the bronchus may cause damming back of the secretions derived from more distal parts of the bronchial tree. The retained secretions constitute a favourable medium for bacterial growth; this, coupled with the collapse of lung parenchyma distal to the obstruction, tends to lead to episodes of bronchopneumonia.

The role of malignant disease in promoting susceptibility to infection through immunosuppression has already been alluded to (see pp. 189–190) and will be considered further later in this chapter.

SYSTEMIC MANIFESTATIONS OF CANCER

FEVER

Febrile episodes are common in patients with malignant disease, even in the absence of recognizable evidence of infection. Fever is particularly common in malignant disease involving the lymphoid system such as malignant lymphomas, the leukaemias and Hodgkin's disease, although it also occurs in cases of disseminated, solid, epithelial tumours. This effect is likely to be mediated by the release of cytokines such as interleukin-1 or TNF-α, either from the tumour cells or from infiltrating macrophages.

Occasionally fever may be the presenting feature of neoplasm, most notably in renal adenocarcinoma (hypernephroma), a tumour particularly likely to produce non-metastatic systemic disturbances.

CACHEXIA

Marked weight loss and wasting of tissue, especially muscle, is well recognized in the later stages of the natural history of many malignant neoplasms. This state is known as cachexia; understanding of its pathogenesis is still far from complete. Processes canvassed as playing a role in the production of cachexia include:

Anorexia.   Loss of appetite is a conspicuous feature in certain malignant disorders and appears not to be related to tumour bulk or location. Many reasons have been advanced to account for this, but none can be shown to operate in all instances of tumour-related anorexia.

Malabsorption.   This may occur in association with neoplasms, such as medullary carcinoma of the thyroid, that secrete products that increase gastrointestinal motility. In most cases where malabsorption is present, the mechanism producing it is not known.

Release of some cachexia-inducing product liberated from the neoplasm.   The suggestion has been made that some toxic product liberated from the neoplasm could be responsible for the nutritional changes seen. Decreased hepatic catalase activity can be shown to occur both in certain patients with malignant disease and in animals with experimentally induced tumours; this decline in catalase activity can be reproduced in animals injected with a polypeptide extractable from human gastric or rectal carcinoma. This extracted material also produces changes in plasma iron concentrations, increases the levels of protoporphyrin in the liver, and may cause thymic involution.

Most of the changes of cachexia may be reproduced by injecting TNF-α into small laboratory animals. Indeed, one of the names given to TNF-α is **cachectin**. Patients with cancer do not as a rule show increases in the plasma concentration of TNF-α, but it is nevertheless possible that this peptide, perhaps working in concert with other cytokines, may play a significant role in cancer-related cachexia.

EFFECT OF NEOPLASMS ON THE IMMUNE SYSTEM

Patients with malignant disease, especially of the lymphoid system, may be immunocompromised and are thus more prone to infection. Depression of the defensive abilities of phagocytes is often present; patients, especially those with bone marrow involvement, quite commonly show a decline in the number of granulocytes.

Both humoral and cellular immune mechanisms may be depressed, a decline in the latter being associated with an increased liability to tuberculous, fungal and viral infections. It should not be forgotten that cancer treatment may also cause a decline in the efficiency of the host's defences against infection, as both chemotherapy and irradiation have an immunosuppressive effect.

An association with autoimmunity may also occur. Patients may develop non-organ-specific autoantibodies directed against such 'self' components as smooth muscle, nuclei and nuclear fractions. Immune complex formation may also occur, and some patients with malignant neoplasms present with an immune complex-mediated nephrotic syndrome (massive proteinuria, hypoalbuminaemia and oedema).

HAEMATOLOGICAL EFFECTS OF NEOPLASMS

Anaemia

Many patients with cancer are anaemic at some stage of their illness. A number of possible mechanisms may be invoked to explain the presence of such anaemia. **Iron deficiency anaemia** may result from occult blood loss associated with ulceration of a neoplasm involving an epithelial surface. A poor nutritional state may be associated with decreased folate intake; in the presence of malabsorption, such folate as is present may not be absorbed adequately, and **macrocytic anaemia** may result.

Excess red blood cell destruction may occur as a result of an **autoimmune haemolytic anaemia**, with autoantibodies directed against components of the patient's own red cells. This tends to occur in neoplasms of the lymphoreticular system such as Hodgkin's disease and non-Hodgkin's malignant lymphomas. Why such an autoimmune reaction should occur is not understood.

Lastly, anaemia may occur in association with malignant disease as a result of a **relatively decreased level of erythropoietin secretion**. Marrow cells from such patients appear to respond quite normally to erythropoietin in culture and the defect does not, therefore, appear to be a failure of response on the part of the red cell precursors.

Increased red cell production

An increased red cell mass is sometimes encountered in certain neoplasms, most notably in:

- **renal adenocarcinoma**
- **cerebellar haemangioblastoma**
- **uterine fibroleiomyoma**
- **liver cell carcinoma**
- less frequently, **ovarian carcinoma**, **adrenal tumours** and **carcinoma of the lung**.

The abnormal drive for red cell production seems to be due to the ectopic secretion of erythropoietic substances by the tumours.

Effects on platelets and clotting

In some patients with malignant disease there is a significant decrease in the number of circulating platelets, resulting in **thrombocytopenic purpura**.

In contrast, an increased clotting tendency is quite often seen. This, of course, may itself contribute to the decrease in platelet count. Evidence of continued intravascular coagulation may be found in some patients by determining the level of fibrinopeptide A in the plasma. In one recent study, 60% of a group of patients with advanced cancer showed such evidence of intravascular coagulation. In these patients serial determinations of fibrin degradation products revealed an upward trend, which appeared to be related to progression of the neoplastic disorder. This intravascular clotting is inhibited by giving oral anticoagulants such as warfarin.

In experimental tumour models, agents that promote clotting tend to promote tumour growth, whereas those that inhibit one or more aspects of the clotting process are associated with tumour regression.

Some malignant tumours are associated with a curious syndrome in which **recurrent migratory thrombophlebitis** occurs. Episodes of venous thrombosis involving both superficial and deep veins occur (see p. 359). Carcinomas of the bronchus, pancreas, stomach and female genital tract are most frequently implicated. In some instances, the thrombophlebitis may be the first indicator of occult malignancy.

ENDOCRINE EFFECTS OF NEOPLASMS

Hormonal effects associated with neoplasms fall into two main groups: **appropriate** and **ectopic** hormone production.

Appropriate hormone production

This applies to neoplasms occurring in endocrine glands; the hormones produced are appropriate to the location of the tumour. For example, the fact that an adenoma of the β cells of the islets of Langerhans in the pancreas produces large amounts of insulin surprises no one. *Such tumours retain the normal biosynthetic pathways for the production of hormones and differ from normal cells only in their escape from normal 'feedback' controls.* Examples of this type of endocrine disorder are given in *Table 28.1.*

Ectopic hormone production

Hormonal effects may be experienced by patients with various forms of neoplasm because hormones are secreted by cells of tumours arising in **tissues not normally associated with hormone production**. This is termed ectopic hormone production. It was first described in 1928 in a patient with a small-cell bronchial carcinoma who developed diabetes, hirsutism, high blood pressure and bilateral adrenal cortical hyperplasia (i.e. Cushing's syndrome). However, it was more than 30 years before it was proved that the cause of such syndromes in patients with tumours arising outside the endocrine system was secretion of adrenocorticotrophic hormone (ACTH) by the tumours.

Only a small proportion of patients with bronchial carcinoma of the small-cell variety show clinical evidence of excess ACTH secretion, but radioimmunoassay of extracts of such tumours shows ACTH to be present in many. The disparity between the number of tumours containing immunologically identifiable ACTH and those secreting 'active' ACTH arises

Table 28.1   Effects of appropriate hormone production by neoplasms

Tumour	Hormone	Effect
Acidophil adenoma of the pituitary	Growth hormone	Gigantism before puberty; acromegaly in adult life
Basophil adenoma of the pituitary	Adrenocorticotrophic hormone	Cushing's syndrome due to adrenal cortical hyperplasia and increased synthesis of cortisol
Chromophobe adenoma of the pituitary	Prolactin	Amenorrhoea Galactorrhoea Impotence
Adrenal cortical adenoma	Cortisol or aldosterone depending on cell type	Cushing's syndrome (cortisol) Conn's syndrome (aldosterone)
Parathyroid adenoma	Parathyroid hormone	Hypercalcaemia
Islet cell tumours of pancreas	Wide variety: commonest insulin and gastrin	Episodes of hypoglycaemia (insulin) Intractable peptic ulceration (Zollinger–Ellison syndrome in gastrin-secreting lesions)

because, in most cases, the hormone exists in the form of an inactive precursor or 'big' ACTH, which has less than 5% of the biological activity of ACTH secreted by the pituitary.

A wide variety of '**paraendocrine**' syndromes has now been described. Some examples are given in *Table 28.2.*

Why are ectopic hormones produced by 'non-endocrine' tumours?

One hypothesis suggests that the tumour cells involved in ectopic hormone secretion are derived from cells with potential endocrine functions that are normally present in many tissues and that would normally secrete amines such as serotonin and catecholamines.

Two groups of cells might fill this role:

- neuroendocrine cells
- the APUD series.

Neuroendocrine cells are widely distributed in many tissues. The argentaffin cells in the gut, which can secrete serotonin and from which **carcinoid** tumours can arise, might be taken as an example.

The APUD series.   The acronym APUD stands for amine precursor uptake and decarboxylation, describing some of the outstanding characteristics of these cells. Associated with these is the ability to produce biologically active amines and peptide hormones. Such cells are present in small numbers in many individual locations and could produce the 'ectopic' substance continuously. Clonal expansion of such a cell population, as occurs in

Table 28.2   Ectopic hormone production by tumours

Hormone	Principal tumours	Chief effects
Adrenocorticotrophic hormone	Bronchus Pancreas Thymoma Thyroid Ovary	Hypokalaemic alkalosis, weakness, thirst, polyuria
Antidiuretic hormone	Bronchus Duodenum Lymphoma Prostate Thymoma Ewing's tumour	Dilutional hyponatraemia
Thyroid-stimulating hormone	Lung Breast Choriocarcinoma	Hyperthyroidism
Melanocyte-stimulating hormone	Bronchus	Abnormal pigmentation
Parathyroid hormone	Bronchus (squamous) Kidney Liver Adrenal	Hypercalcaemia, vomiting, constipation, psychotic behaviour
Human chorionic gonadotrophin	Breast Bronchus Testis Stomach Pancreas Liver Ovary	Gynaecomastia; precocious puberty
Luteinizing hormone	Trophoblastic Malignant teratoma Bronchus	Gynaecomastia
Growth hormone	Lung Stomach Ovary Breast	Acromegaly; hypertrophic pulmonary osteoarthropathy
Glucagon	Kidney	Hyperglycaemia, etc.
Prolactin	Bronchus Breast	Galactorrhoea

tumour formation, would obviously be associated with an increase in the total amount of hormone produced. This is sufficient in some instances to produce a recognizable biological effect.

It has been suggested that APUD cells are derived originally from the neural crest and migrate from there, principally to organs formed during development of the foregut. Support for this neural origin comes from the fact that:

- A number of the active substances secreted by so-called APUDomas are also secreted within the brain.
- Many APUD cells and the tumours arising from them express markers such as **neurone-specific enolase**.

This neural origin is no longer believed to apply to all cells and tumours in this group, some of which are thought to have an endodermal origin.

An acceptable example of an APUD cell is the parafollicular or C cell of the thyroid. This cell secretes the calcium-mobilizing hormone, **calcitonin**. The tumour arising from these C cells is known as a **medullary carcinoma**. It may occur as one of the genetically determined syndromes that can affect more than one endocrine organ simultaneously or as an isolated phenomenon. Most medullary carcinomas have amyloid in the stroma, the amyloid protein containing amino acids 9–19 of calcitonin (see p. 288).

The 'oat cell carcinoma' of the lung is an archetype of APUD tumours. It is one of the small-cell tumours occurring in the bronchi; the cells are arranged in a ribbon-like pattern in close relation to sinusoidal blood vessels. Electron microscopy shows the presence of dense-cored neurosecretory granules. These tumours are associated not only with a number of para-endocrine syndromes (see *Table 28.2*) but with some other systemic manifestations.

NON-METASTATIC OSSEOUS AND SOFT TISSUE CHANGES

Clubbing

Clubbing of the fingers was first described more than 2000 years ago by Hippocrates. The angle between nail and cuticle becomes filled and the nail appears to 'float' on the nail bed. The curvature of the nail itself is altered, the nail being curved from front to back and having a rather 'beaked' appearance. In more severe instances, the periosteum over the terminal phalanges, wrists and ankles becomes thickened and new bone is formed from stem cells within the periosteum. In its most severe form, the complex of soft tissue and bony changes is termed **hypertrophic pulmonary osteo-arthropathy (HPO)**.

Clubbing and HPO occur in association with a number of disease states. These include:

- the cyanotic forms of congenital heart disease
- chronic pulmonary sepsis
- infective endocarditis
- mesothelioma of the pleura
- carcinoma of the bronchus.

The pathogenesis of this curious change is still far from clear. Some studies suggest that in affected patients the blood flow to the limbs is increased. Dividing the vagus nerve from the hilum of the affected lung relieves the condition in some instances, and is certainly associated with a reduction in blood flow to the affected part. Other studies suggest that there may be ectopic secretion of growth hormone in some cases of tumour-related HPO.

Interestingly enough, in view of the many systemic manifestations of small-cell carcinoma of the bronchus, HPO shows a strong negative correlation with this tumour. The commonest thoracic neoplasm to be associated with HPO is pleural mesothelioma. However HPO occurs also in both squamous carcinoma and adenocarcinoma of the bronchus.

NON-METASTATIC CHANGES IN NERVE AND MUSCLE

Nerve and muscle changes associated with neoplastic disorders have been separated into three groups:

1) **encephalomyeloneuropathy**, where degeneration of ganglion cells in the central nervous system is the dominant pathological feature
2) **myopathies**, with or without features of myasthenia
3) **demyelinating** disorders.

In the first two there is no constant relation between progress of the neoplasm and that of the neurological condition. Indeed, neurological abnormalities may precede the diagnosis of tumour by up to 3 years or, at the other end of the spectrum, may appear after the tumour has been removed. The primary tumours most frequently implicated are carcinomas of the bronchus, breast, ovary, uterine cervix and colon.

The cause of these neurological conditions is unknown. They are not uncommon: an overall prevalence of neurological change of this type has been recorded in 14% of patients with carcinoma of the bronchus (chiefly of the small-cell variety).

CUTANEOUS MANIFESTATIONS OF MALIGNANCY

Polymyositis and dermatomyositis

This rather uncommon condition, encountered chiefly in the fifth and sixth decades of life, is associated with malignancy in 25–30% of cases. Muscular symptoms include pain and weakness, especially of proximal muscles such as those of the shoulder and hip girdles. Joint pain and stiffness are quite common. If the disorder is confined to muscle it is termed **polymyositis**, but the full clinical picture may include a striking rash as well, ranging from a barely perceptible flush to a red or violaceous eruption, usually over the malar areas and the flush areas of the chest, back of neck and extensor surfaces of the arms and legs. Fine telangiectases (dilated small blood vessels) are almost always present on the cuticles.

If the disease appears when the patient is more than 40 years old, there is a 50% chance that it is associated with malignancy. Neoplasms associated with dermatomyositis are often those of the gastrointestinal tract, but carcinomas of the bladder, the bronchus and other endodermally derived tumours are not rare in this context. In cases associated with tumour, complete eradication of the tumour, where this is possible, cures the dermatomyositis.

Acanthosis nigricans

In this condition there is increased pigmentation of the skin, especially of the axilla, the back of the neck, and the periareolar region of the breast. In the early stages, despite the name **acanthosis**, there is little or no thickening of the skin, although itching is often present. Later the skin becomes thick, velvety and pigmented. The process may extend to involve quite large areas of skin. Acanthosis nigricans associated with malignancy appears most often in middle age when the age-related incidence of tumours is rising. About two-thirds of tumours associated with this skin lesion are carcinomas of the stomach.

Erythema gyratum repens

This is a rare but highly characteristic dermal accompaniment of malignancy. It appears as wavy irregular bands of large red papules which coalesce to form a 'snake-skin' or 'wood-grain' pattern across the affected area of skin. This condition has been reported in patients with adenocarcinoma of the bronchus, small-cell carcinoma of the bronchus, and carcinomas of the breast, uterine cervix, tongue and gastrointestinal tract. In some cases, such as 'oat cell' carcinoma of the bronchus, the eruption usually occurs after obvious metastases have been diagnosed.

BIOLOGICAL MARKERS OF MALIGNANCY

The alterations in gene expression, whether qualitative, quantitative or both, that occur in malignant transformation may be associated with either the secretion of inappropriate substances or the expression of new antigens. Such biological markers can be helpful in diagnosis or in monitoring the progress of certain neoplasms.

These 'tumour markers' fall into three main groups:

1) hormones
2) isoenzymes
3) tumour-associated antigens.

The first of these categories has already been described (see pp. 467–470).

ISOENZYMES

Acid phosphatase

An association between raised acid phosphatase concentrations in the plasma and **carcinoma of the prostate** has been known for many years. High plasma concentrations are particularly likely in patients whose carcinomas have already metastasized, especially where secondary deposits are present in the skeleton.

Carcinoplacental alkaline phosphatase (PLAP)

This enzyme was discovered in the blood of a patient named Regan who had carcinoma of the bronchus, and so some workers term it the **Regan isoenzyme**. It is similar to the alkaline phosphatase found in the human placenta.

PLAP may appear in the blood of 3–15% of patients with malignant neoplasms. Primary tumours that can express PLAP include carcinomas of the bronchus, colon, pancreas and liver. Germ cell tumours may also express this enzyme.

The use of PLAP as a diagnostic test for the presence of malignant disease has proved disappointing. An increase in its concentration tends to occur late in the natural history of malignancy. False-positive results have been recorded in patients suffering from certain chronic inflammatory bowel diseases such as ulcerative colitis and also in those with cirrhosis of the liver. Low levels of the enzyme can be found in the plasma of some normal subjects. Nevertheless, as is the case with some other tumour markers, measurement of PLAP may give useful information about the natural history of certain tumours, most notably response to treatment and the appearance of recurrence or secondary deposits.

TUMOUR-ASSOCIATED ANTIGENS

Alterations in the antigenic state of transformed cells are discussed further in Chapter 29. In some instances transformation and tumour growth may be associated with the appearance of certain antigens on tumour cells; these antigens are characteristic of fetal development and are not present in fully differentiated adult cells. Such antigens are spoken of as **oncofetal antigens**.

α-Fetoprotein

α-Fetoprotein (AFP) is an α_1-globulin secreted in embryonic life, first by the **yolk sac** and later by the **fetal liver**. Secretion in the liver is established by the sixth week of embryonic life and reaches a peak of 3–4 mg/ml in the plasma by week 13 of intrauterine life. From this point, AFP concentrations fall rapidly: in normal adults the amount detectable in the plasma by immunoassay is only about one-millionth of that present in fetal plasma.

In 1963 it was discovered that adult mice with transplantable liver cell tumours had high plasma concentrations of AFP. This observation was extended to humans with liver cell cancer 2 years later, and the presence of raised plasma concentrations of AFP has proven to be a fairly useful marker for this tumour. Subsequent studies have shown that AFP may appear also in the plasma of up to 50% of patients with **malignant germ cell tumours**. There is a strong correlation between the presence of raised concentrations of AFP in the plasma and teratomas containing elements that show **yolk sac** differentiation.

Carcinoembryonic antigen (CEA)

This substance was discovered in 1965 to be present in fairly large amounts in malignant tumours of the large bowel. It is normally found in the gastrointestinal tract, liver and pancreas during the first 6 months of embryonic life. CEA is a water-soluble glycoprotein intimately associated with the glycocalyx on cell surface membranes. It can be localized to the luminal surface of the neoplastic cells that express it. Early studies suggested that the presence of raised plasma concentrations of CEA was specific for neoplasms derived from the endoderm. However, this is not correct.

Increased levels of CEA can be found in association with neoplasms arising in different tissues; they may also occur in association with some non-neoplastic conditions. This last factor clearly limits the usefulness of CEA as a diagnostic marker. A further disadvantage is that CEA levels tend to be correlated with the extent of spread in certain neoplasms; CEA concentrations may not be raised significantly until such spread has occurred. For example, in carcinoma of the colon or rectum, localized (Dukes' stage A) tumours are associated with increased CEA levels in only 40% of cases. In those cases of colorectal carcinoma where metastasis has occurred, 80–95% of patients have increased CEA levels.

The main application for the determination of CEA levels in the plasma is in the follow-up of patients with cancer after surgery and in monitoring the effects of therapy. After successful removal of a tumour associated with raised CEA concentrations in the plasma, the CEA concentration tends to fall to normal over a period of 2–4 weeks. If there is no tumour recurrence, these normal levels persist. A subsequent rise in the plasma concentration of CEA probably indicates either the presence of metastases or local recurrence of tumour. Such a rise of plasma CEA concentration may precede clinical evidence of metastatic or recurrent disease by several months.

EFFECTS OF NEOPLASMS ON THE HOST

- The effects produced by neoplasms may be local or systemic.
- **Local effects** are caused by the presence of a neoplasm within a given tissue and may be related to:
  — mechanical factors, such as obstruction
  — the intrinsic destructive powers of the neoplasm, as seen in osteolytic deposits
  — the local effects of tumour secretions
  — the neoplasm undergoing complications such as haemorrhage.
- **Systemic effects** are due, in the main, to secretion products of the tumour cells; for example, calcium may be released from bone in the absence of skeletal metastases because some tumours release a peptide with the same functional effects as parathyroid hormone.
- Systemic effects may occur in many physiological systems (e.g. blood clotting abnormalities and the endocrine system).
- Ectopic hormone production occurs in some neoplasms arising in non-endocrine organs and tissues. Thus small cell carcinomas of the lung may secrete a wide range of hormones.

29 Effect of the host on neoplasms

The effect of the host on the neoplasm must reside in the interaction between the host's immune system and the tumour; it is difficult to think of any other mechanism through which resistance to the progression of malignant disease might be mediated. This question might be examined in a number of ways:

- Is there direct evidence that immune mechanisms modulate the behaviour of human neoplasms and cause them to regress?
- Is there histological evidence that human neoplasms excite an immune response?
- Is there any increase in the frequency of neoplastic disease in patients with immune deficiency states?

Tumour regression

Tumour regression is extremely difficult to prove. It is true that in some instances malignant neoplasms regress; this has been noted most frequently in neuroblastoma and malignant melanoma. However, there is no direct evidence that such tumour regression is caused by immune mechanisms, although in some cases of malignant melanoma that remain localized for a long time there may be antibodies in the plasma that are cytopathic for the patient's tumour cells in culture.

Other clinicopathological oddities such as the prolonged survival of some patients with malignant disease, the frequency of clinically occult tumours found at necropsy, and the occasional regression of metastases after removal of the primary tumour have all been cited as possible expressions of an immune response. However, proof is lacking.

Histological features suggesting an immune response to the presence of tumour

On microscopic examination, some tumours are seen to be infiltrated by lymphocytes, macrophages and plasma cells. This is especially common in carcinomas of the breast. A marked degree of hyperplasia of the macrophages lining the sinuses of lymph nodes draining a tumour may also be seen, as well as epithelioid cell granulomas. There is some evidence from prospective studies that these histological features may correlate positively with an improved prognosis, particularly in the case of breast cancer.

Immune deficiency states and malignancy in humans

If host immune reactions play a significant part in inhibiting the development and growth of malignant neoplasms, then one would expect an **increased frequency of malignant disease** in patients with immune deficiency. Up to a point, this is true: patients with inborn deficiency syndromes such as **ataxia telangiectasia**, the **Wiskott–Aldrich syndrome** and the **Chediak–Higashi syndrome** all show an increased frequency of malignant disease compared with their peers. However, most of these neoplasms primarily involve the lymphoid system.

There is also an increase in the frequency of malignant disease in cases of iatrogenic immunosuppression, such as in patients who have received renal allografts. The vast majority of these neoplasms are of the lymphoid system. There have been occasional reports, however, where recipients have received kidneys from patients dying with malignant disease. Although the donor kidneys were macroscopically free from tumour, tumours with histological characteristics of the donor's primary are said to have grown in some of these kidneys. In two cases the withdrawal of immunosuppressive drugs on which the patient had been maintained was reported to have led to regression of the tumour. These observations, scanty as they are, suggest that immunosuppression creates a favourable milieu for tumour progression.

Tumours can be rejected by animal hosts

The possible role of cell-mediated immunity in controlling tumour growth can be studied most easily in relation to animal tumours induced by certain viruses. The most fully studied example is **polyomavirus**, a small DNA virus that infects many laboratory and wild mouse colonies. When large doses of the virus are injected into **adult** mice, no tumours result. Inoculation of the virus into **newborn** mice of the same susceptible strain produces large numbers of tumours. If, however, newborn mice are thymectomized and are inoculated with the polyomavirus when they have grown to adulthood, tumours occur in fairly large numbers.

Such experiments provide good evidence that adult mice are protected against the oncogenic effect of the polyomavirus because they can mount an effective cell-mediated response. The same sort of events are seen when mice of the C57BL strain, which are resistant to the oncogenic effect of the polyomavirus, are studied. Neonatal thymectomy or the use of repeated injection of antilymphocyte serum can make young mice of this strain develop polyoma-induced tumours.

While there is some evidence that cell-mediated rejection of some virally induced tumours can occur, the picture is by no means a simple one. If T cell-mediated immunity plays a major role in **immune surveillance** against tumour development, a high frequency of spontaneous tumour development would be expected in the '**nude mouse**', which is athymic. This is not the case, although this mouse has been used with some success in the study of transplantable tumours.

Tumour-associated transplantation antigens

A number of experiments in inbred strains of mouse indicate that **tumour rejection can occur as a result of the expression of certain antigenic determinants on the surface of the tumour cells** which have nothing to do with the histocompatibility antigens coded for by the major histocompatibility complex.

In general, tumours that have been induced by irradiation or chemicals have unique antigenic determinants on the cell surface which function as **transplantation antigens** (TATA – tumour-associated transplantation antigen) and can thus elicit rejection. Even two tumours produced by the same carcinogen in a single animal will have distinct transplantation antigens.

Tumours caused by viruses, however, show new antigens on the cell surface which cross-react with those on other tumours induced by the same virus. These virally induced TATAs appear not to be typical viral structural proteins.

Unfortunately, spontaneous tumours arising in both animals and humans show much less tendency to develop transplantation antigens on their cell surfaces. Some neoplasms, however, appear to elicit a cell-mediated immune response which cannot be ascribed to allogeneic rejection mediated through the major histocompatibility complex. Tumours of this class include malignant melanoma, renal carcinoma and astrocytomas in the brain.

In melanoma, which has been studied in most detail, three classes of cell surface antigen have been identified.

1) antigen distinctive for the particular patient's tumour
2) antigen specific for malignant melanoma cells, but which may be shared with cells of other malignant melanomas
3) antigens found on both tumour cells and some normal cells.

MECHANISMS BY WHICH THE IMMUNE SYSTEM CAN COMBAT TUMOUR GROWTH

A number of possible effector arms of the immune system may play a role in destroying tumour cells. These include:

- the macrophage system
- effector T cells

- antibodies that can promote antibody-dependent cell-mediated cytotoxicity
- natural killer (NK) cells.

Macrophages

In culture systems, macrophages can destroy tumour cells. The precise mechanism is not clear, but does appear to involve cell–cell contact. The macrophages can be activated in two ways:

1) by contact with tumour antigen
2) as a result of the release of activating factors from T cells that have been stimulated by contact with tumour antigens.

Activation is associated with an increase in the number of Fc receptors on the surface of the macrophage. It is possible that coating of tumour cells by antibodies may help, through the binding of Fc to Fc receptors, to bring the macrophage into close contact with the tumour cell.

Effector T cells

Cell killing by the T-cell arm is presumably carried out by cytotoxic T cells. The helper T cell may also play a part through its stimulatory effect on the cytotoxic subgroup.

The relative proportions of T helper and T suppressor cells may have some influence on the immune status of the host in respect of tumour cells. In certain transplantable tumours in animals, tumour growth is increased if there is a large population of T suppressor cells. It has been suggested that this comes about through an autoimmune reaction against the specific clone of cytotoxic T cells that bind to the tumour cells. This reaction is mediated by T suppressor cells, which recognize surface markers of a certain idiotype on the cytotoxic T cells and are themselves specifically cytotoxic for cells bearing that idiotype. In this way, the cytotoxic T cells are prevented from destroying the tumour cells.

Antibodies

Theoretically, as outlined earlier, humoral immune mechanisms could act in two possible ways in the destruction of tumour cells:

1) They could bind to tumour cells and initiate complement-mediated cell lysis. Such evidence as we possess suggests that this is not a significant mechanism in tumour control.
2) They may adhere to the surface of tumour cells and thus attract potentially cytotoxic cells that have Fc receptors on their surface. These include macrophages, T lymphocytes and **NK cells**.

Natural killer cells

NK cells constitute a subset of the lymphocyte population. They are believed by some workers to be derived from clones of immature pre-T lymphocytes. They are non-adherent, non-phagocytic and have Fc receptors on their surface. Their ability to kill tumour cells does not depend on the host being immunized against determinants on the tumour cells. It has been suggested that the NK cell can itself recognize several different types of determinant on cells that may exhibit cross-reactivity, and that this may explain its broad range of cytotoxic activity. The activity of NK cells is stimulated by interferon γ, released in this context by T cells and by NK cells themselves, the latter constituting a positive amplification loop.

DOES IMMUNE SURVEILLANCE EXIST?

The original concept of immune surveillance was that malignant transformation of cells occurs frequently and these cells are being eliminated by immune mechanisms before clonal expansion can take place. In respect of 'spontaneously arising' neoplasms, this mechanism has failed in every case where a clinically or pathologically apparent neoplasm arises. However, in chemically or virally induced tumours in experimental animals, immune protection can be shown to be reasonably effective. It is possible that, in humans, immune mechanisms may be responsible for the fact that most people infected with the Epstein–Barr virus develop a self-limiting illness (infectious mononucleosis) and not a malignant lymphoma.

If immune protection is not effective in spontaneously arising neoplasms, how is it that the malignant cells survive and form tumour masses, evading the potential cytotoxicity inherent in immune effector mechanisms? It may be that many malignant cells are **poor immunogens**; natural selection processes would favour the survival of such cells in an antigenically heterogeneous tumour cell population. It is known, however, that it is possible for the host to develop an immune response to malignant cells but be unable to kill them. This 'blocking effect' appears to be associated with the presence of tumour-specific antibodies in the host plasma. It has been suggested that in such instances the tumour cells constantly shed surface antigens which form circulating complexes with the tumour antibody. These complexes can bind to any killer cells with Fc receptors for the tumour antibody and thus prevent them from having a cytotoxic effect on the tumour cells themselves.

Another factor determining the effectiveness or otherwise of an antitumour immune response appears to be the actual **physical bulk** of the tumour. Small tumours are much more likely to yield to efforts to improve a host's immune response. The removal of much of a host's tumour load, either by surgery or by other means, appears to be associated with an improvement in the effectiveness of the antitumour response.

EFFECT OF THE HOST ON NEOPLASMS

- The single most important effect of the host on neoplasms is **regression**.
- In those instances where tumour regression occurs, it is most likely to be mediated by the immune system.
- In regressing tumours there are morphological features (such as a lymphocytic infiltrate) that suggest an immune response.
- An increase in the risk of certain neoplasms occurs in patients with immune deficiencies. The neoplasms occurring under these circumstances are principally of the lymphoid system.
- Effector mechanisms in the host that may be involved include macrophages, natural killer cells, T lymphocytes and antibodies.

30 Oncogenesis and the molecular biology of cancer

Cancer may be defined as a set of disorders with three pivotal disturbances in cell behaviour:

1) **in the mechanisms that control cell proliferation**
2) **in cell differentiation**
3) **in the normal relationship between the proliferating cells and the surrounding connective tissue stroma**; this is expressed by **invasiveness** and ultimately metastasis and is, therefore, a fundamental part of the malignant phenotype.

Many epidemiological data relate the risk of malignancy to a variety of environmental factors, and there are clearly many different causes of cancer (see pp. 513–540). Despite this, it is likely that the number of mechanisms operating at the cellular level is small and that these are mediated through abnormalities affecting **three classes of gene**: oncogenes, tumour suppressor genes and mutator genes.

ONCOGENES, SUPPRESSOR GENES AND MUTATOR GENES

Homeostatic control of growth and differentiation in cell populations is the resultant of interactions between growth-promoting and growth-restraining forces. These are the expression of transcription of **growth-promoting genes, known as proto-oncogenes**, and **growth-inhibiting genes, known as tumour suppressor genes** (*Fig. 30.1*). When cell populations need to expand in order to meet increased functional demands, then upregulation of growth-promoting genes occurs.

More than 100 proto-oncogenes have been identified, although not all of these have been found to be mutated in human neoplasms.

The number of tumour suppressor genes so far identified is much smaller.

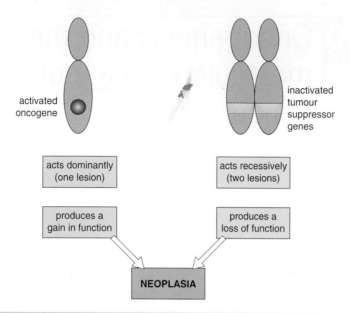

acts dominantly
(one lesion)

acts recessively
(two lesions)

produces a
gain in function

produces a
loss of function

NEOPLASIA

Fig. 30.1   Some basic properties of oncogenes and tumour suppressor genes.

The existence of certain inherited neoplasms has provided much help in the recognition of suppressor genes. Mutation or deletion of suppressor genes is clearly also a common feature of many neoplasms that are not inherited.

DOMINANTLY ACTING ONCOGENES

As already stated, neoplastic transformation arises from a disturbance in the dynamic equilibrium that normally exists between growth-promoting and growth-inhibiting forces. Just as the speed of a motor car may be increased either because the driver presses on the accelerator or because the brakes have failed, so, in the cancer model, the gene products of the dominantly acting oncogenes represent the accelerator and those of the tumour suppressor genes represent the brakes. In this section some aspects of dominantly acting oncogenes are considered.

Proto-oncogenes form part of the normal genome; they contribute to neoplastic transformation only if they are qualitatively or quantitatively altered. When they are not abnormally activated, the term **cellular proto-oncogene** is applied; when they are altered, the term **oncogene** is more appropriate. Such alteration (*Fig. 30.2*) may result in encoding of abnormal gene products, overexpression of unaltered proto-oncogenes and the formation of novel genes.

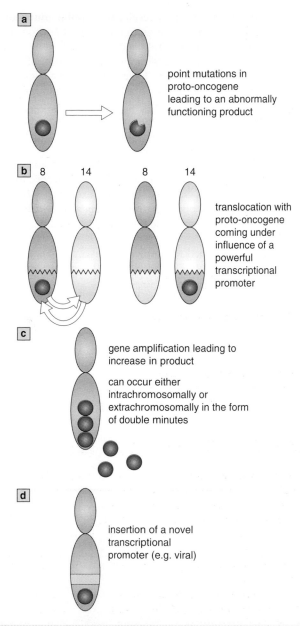

Fig. 30.2   Mechanisms of cellular proto-oncogene activation.

Encoding of abnormal gene products results from **point mutations** in the proto-oncogene. This is seen in relation to the *ras* proto-oncogenes, which are mutated in 10–15% of human solid tumours.

Overexpression of unaltered proto-oncogenes is due to a variety of mechanisms including the presence of abnormally large numbers of copies of the gene (**amplification**), and **translocation** of a proto-oncogene to a region where its transcription is significantly increased. The latter occurs in **Burkitt's lymphoma** where the c-*myc* proto-oncogene on the long arm of chromosome 8 is translocated to chromosome 14 and comes to lie adjacent to the gene encoding the heavy chain of immunoglobulin.

Formation of novel genes and the expression of chimaeric gene products as a result of the fusion of proto-oncogenes with parts of other genes. This occurs as a result of translocation of portions of chromosomes. It is exemplified by the formation of the *bcr–abl* gene in chronic myeloid leukaemia in the course of translocation of *abl* from chromosome 9 to chromosome 22.

Proto-oncogenes are concerned with processes involved in cell division and proliferation (see *Table 30.1*, *Figs 30.3* and *30.4*). Thus different proto-oncogenes encode:

- growth factors (*sis*, *int-2*, *IGF-1*)
- growth factor receptors with protein kinase activity (*erb-2*, *fms*, *met*, *trk*, *ret*)
- abnormally functioning growth factor receptors (*neu*)
- factors that act in the transduction of signals arising from ligand–receptor interactions:
  a) G proteins (*ras*)
  b) guanosine 5′-triphosphatase activators (GTPase) (*gap*, *krev*)

Table 30.1 Functions of some oncogenes

Oncogene	Growth factor	Normal growth factor receptor	Abnormal growth factor receptor	Signal transducer	DNA-binding protein concerned with transcription
sis	+				
erbB1		+			
fms		+			
erbB2			+		
ras				+	
src				+	
myc					+
fos					+
jun					+

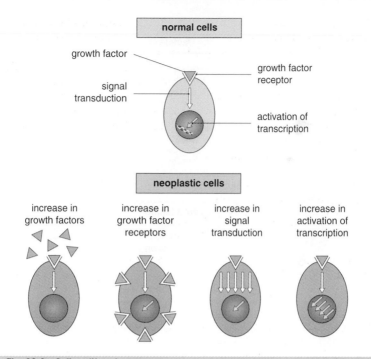

Fig. 30.3   Cell proliferation.

Proliferation of normal cell populations results from a sequence of operations involving the binding of growth factors to receptors, transcription of the growth-promoting signal and activation of DNA transcription. The abnormal degree of proliferation in neoplastic cell populations results from the upregulation of one or more than one of these steps.

  c) membrane-associated cytoplasmic kinases (*src, yes, fgr*)
  d) non-membrane-associated cytoplasmic kinases (*raf, mos, pim-1, fps*)
- DNA-binding proteins concerned in transcription:
  a) heterodimeric transcription factors (*fos–jun, myc–max*)
  b) transcription factors (*myb, rel, ets*)
- cell cycle proteins.

The cell cycle is driven by enzymes – **cyclin-dependent kinases** (**CDK**). **Cyclins** are proteins whose function is to 'turn on' the cyclin-dependent kinases. Cyclin production in excess or at inappropriate times stimulates inappropriate cell division by switching on CDK when they should be switched off. An example is the gene encoding cyclin, D1 (active during the G1 phase of the cycle), which is now regarded as a proto-oncogene. The D1 gene is amplified in about 33% of oesophageal cancers and in 15% of breast cancers. It is also implicated in the genesis of benign neoplasms of the parathyroid gland.

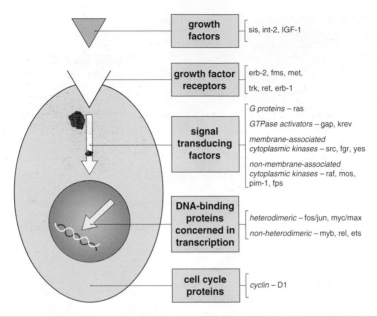

Fig. 30.4 The relation between the gene products of several proto-oncogenes and the operational steps involved in cell division.

The role of oncogenes and suppressor genes in the molecular basis for cancer

Most malignant neoplasms are **monoclonal** – the cells of an individual neoplasm are all descended from a single 'ancestor'. This ancestor cell was once normal but at some point must have changed fundamentally so that the cell line acquired 'immortality' and release from normal constraints on cell proliferation. Just like normal cells, the progeny of malignant cells inherit the characteristics of their parents; this suggests that the alterations mentioned above must have occurred in the genome of the 'ancestor' cell.

Recognition that a relatively small number of molecular determinants may be active in malignant transformation comes from the convergence of two lines of investigation. The first of these relates to malignant transformation effected by a variety of animal retroviruses. The second focuses on the effects, largely in cell culture systems, of gene transfer from the cells of human malignant tumours that are not obviously viral in origin. These studies support the view that there is a group of functionally heterogeneous genes that can be altered by mutation, amplified, made to overexpress their protein products, or physically moved within the genome by chromosome translocations. These **cellular oncogenes** may act individually or, more likely, in cooperation with one another, to cause malignant transformation of cells.

Lessons from oncogenic retroviruses

RNA viruses capable of producing tumours in their host species and of transforming certain cells in culture are known as **oncornaviruses** or **oncogenic retroviruses**. Their genome is composed of RNA enclosed within a capsid wrapped in a glycoprotein envelope. Once this virus infects a cell, the envelope and capsid are removed and the viral RNA is copied by the viral enzyme **reverse transcriptase** into a portion of DNA called **provirus**. The provirus is incorporated into the DNA of the infected cell and, by the normal processes of transcription, emerges as RNA molecules identical with the original viral RNA. This new RNA can act both as messenger RNA (mRNA) for virus-coded proteins or as RNA for the genomes of new viruses. The viral components thus synthesized can be assembled into new complete viruses, which bud off from the surface of infected cells.

Oncogenic retroviruses can be divided into two groups
One group of retroviruses induces tumours very slowly and irregularly but replicates well (*Fig. 30.5*). It has three encoding genes:

* *gag*, encoding a group-specific antigen
* *pol*, encoding reverse transcriptase
* *env*, encoding envelope glycoproteins.

Non-coding sequences at either end (**long terminal repeats**) promote gene replication and expression.

These three encoding genes contain all the information necessary for new viral synthesis within the infected cell. This viral group includes natural, 'wild' viruses that typically produce malignancies of the lymphoma–leukaemia group in poultry, mice and cats.

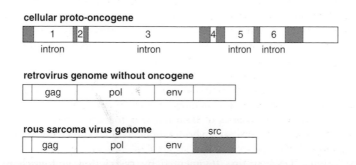

Fig. 30.5 Comparison between the arrangement of coding sequences (exons) in mammalian DNA and in the genome of oncogenic retroviruses.

The differences support the view that retroviral oncogenes originated from cellular proto-oncogenes.

The second group of oncogenic retroviruses can produce tumours in the appropriate host very quickly – in days or weeks. These are uncommon in the 'wild' state, most having been isolated from animal tumours. In contrast to the first group, inoculation is usually required because the viruses do not infect animals via natural pathways. Most lack the full complement of genes necessary for viral replication with one noteworthy exception, the **Rous sarcoma virus**.

The Rous sarcoma virus genome has two distinct portions. The first contains the genes necessary for replication (*gag*, *pol* and *env*), the second a gene called *src*. The *src* gene is both *necessary* and *sufficient* for the virus:

- To cause sarcomas in appropriate hosts (poultry).
- To transform fibroblasts cultured in a monolayer (*Fig. 30.6*). On infection with the *src* gene, the normal orderly monolayer is lost and groups of cells pile up forming colonies many layers thick. This transforming gene codes for the production of a tyrosine kinase called pp60src.

The viral gene (v-*src*) belongs to a family of about 20 transforming genes, **viral oncogenes** (**v-oncs**); each is characteristic of a rapidly transforming oncornavirus. Several v-oncs encode kinases that phosphorylate tyrosine in certain proteins. An oncogene from the avian erythroblastosis virus (*erbB*) encodes a protein homologous with a portion of the cellular receptor for epidermal growth factor. Another oncogene, *sis* from the simian sarcoma virus, encodes a protein homologous with one chain of platelet-derived growth factor.

Homology between viral oncogenes and cellular proto-oncogenes in other species and phyla

With cloned DNA copied from v-onc RNA, one can scan the genome of any eukaryotic cell for the presence of matching sequences. This is known as **DNA hybridization** and depends on the base-pairing relationship in double-stranded DNA. Adenine in one strand always pairs with thymine, and cytosine with guanine, so the sequence of bases in one strand dictates the sequence in the other. It is thus possible to use a radioactively labelled sample of DNA as a tracer to see whether other samples of DNA contain matching sequences. *If the tracer used is the DNA copy of the whole or part of a v-onc RNA, one can investigate whether DNA from normal cells contains sequences that match with those in the v-onc.*

Southern blotting. Finding matching sequences in DNA, which may contain hundreds of thousands of base pairs, is made much easier by the application of a very sensitive hybridization method known as Southern blotting (*Fig. 30.7*).

The cellular DNA is first fragmented by **restriction endonucleases**, enzymes that cleave DNA at specific sites defined by base sequences recognized by the enzyme. These DNA fragments can be separated by electrophoresis in an agarose gel. This may produce more than 100 000 such fragments from human DNA. The DNA fragments are then transferred from

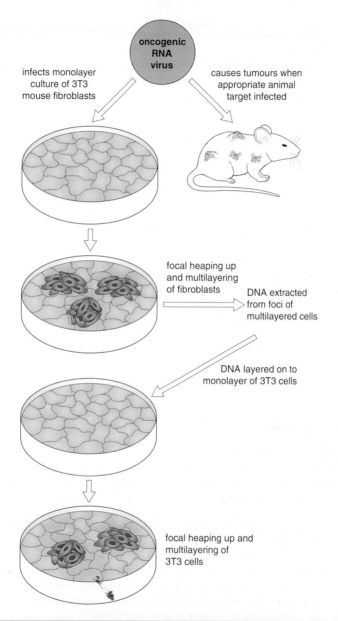

oncogenic RNA virus

infects monolayer culture of 3T3 mouse fibroblasts

causes tumours when appropriate animal target infected

focal heaping up and multilayering of fibroblasts

DNA extracted from foci of multilayered cells

DNA layered on to monolayer of 3T3 cells

focal heaping up and multilayering of 3T3 cells

Fig. 30.6 Transformation of fibroblasts by Rous sarcoma virus.

The existence of actively transforming sequences in oncogenic retroviruses can be demonstrated either in the course of infection of the appropriate animal targets or by showing that infection of 3T3 murine fibroblasts in culture is followed by permanent and heritable changes in growth characteristics of the cells.

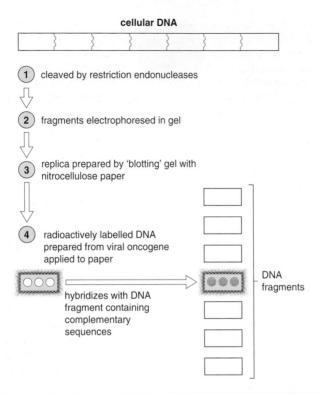

Fig. 30.7 Hybridization between single-stranded DNA copies of retroviral oncogenes and mammalian DNA shows homologies that serve to identify cellular proto-oncogenes.

the gel to a sheet of nitrocellulose paper (hence the term 'blotting'). A radioactively labelled sample of DNA (the **probe**) derived from the viral oncogene is applied to the paper and small fragments of cellular DNA containing complementary base sequences can be identified.

Southern blotting shows complementary sequences to all retroviral v-oncs in restriction fragments prepared from DNA derived from widely disparate species (e.g. human, yeast, fruit fly). These normal genes that show homology with v-oncs are the **proto-oncogenes** referred to in the previous section.

The term 'proto-oncogene' implies correctly that these constituents of the genome of normal cells have the potential to be converted into active genes capable of contributing to malignant transformation.

Viral oncogenes originate from cellular proto-oncogenes

Two possible explanations exist for the homology between v-oncs and cellular proto-oncogenes: either v-oncs derive from cellular genes, or the reverse holds true. Several facts suggest that the former is correct. First, there is a very high degree of **conservation** of the cellular proto-oncogenes during evolution (from yeasts to humans). Second, the **structure** of proto-oncogenes differs in some respects from their v-onc homologues. In v-oncs the nucleotide sequences coding for certain proteins usually occur in a solid block. In the proto-oncogene the information is split up, portions of the protein-coding sequences (exons) alternating with intervening sequences (introns). This is the characteristic structure of a vertebrate gene. Following transcription of the proto-oncogene, the mRNA corresponding to the introns is stripped away, leaving mRNA that is almost identical with the viral mRNA. Lastly, the fact that cellular proto-oncogenes code for growth factors, growth factor receptors or enzymes concerned with the modulation of these receptors suggests a physiological role for the proto-oncogenes in normal cells in relation to growth regulation, and hence a cellular rather than a viral origin.

Thus we believe that v-oncs arose as a result of transcription from cellular proto-oncogenes, and that this genetic material has been incorporated into the viral genome (see *Fig. 30.5*).

DNA from chemically transformed cells and from some 'spontaneous' human tumours can also transform cells in culture

When DNA extracted from transformed cells is introduced into cultures of untransformed mouse fibroblasts (**transfection**), foci of piled up transformed cells appear and these foci grow into tumours after inoculation into young mice. Thus certain varieties of chemically transformed cells carry oncogenic sequences in their DNA.

Even more interesting is the discovery that transfected DNA from biopsies of some human tumours produces exactly the same effect. Many types of human tumour cells develop transforming sequences in their DNA during progression from the normal to the malignant state. They include carcinomas of the bowel, lung, bladder, pancreas, skin and breast, fibrosarcomas and rhabdomyosarcomas, glioblastomas, neuroblastomas and various haemopoietic neoplasms. In all these studies we must remember that the recipient cell (the 3T3 mouse fibroblast) differs significantly from the donor tumour cell, and it may well be that tumour-derived DNA samples that do not transform these fibroblasts may possibly do so in other cell lines.

Some active oncogenes from human tumours have been isolated and cloned. In each case, as with the retroviruses, the transforming oncogene has been found to be closely related to a DNA sequence present in the normal cell genome (a proto-oncogene).

Successful transfection and transformation of cultured cells by the oncogenes listed in *Table 30.2* has been reported.

How do cellular proto-oncogenes become activated?

Five separate mechanisms of cellular proto-oncogene (c-onc) activation have been discovered so far (see *Fig. 30.2*).

Table 30.2   Oncogenes that can transform cell lines following transfection

Oncogene	Human tumour
Ki-ras	Carcinoma of thyroid, melanoma, acute myeloid leukaemia
Ha-ras	Carcinoma of colon, pancreas, lung
N-ras	Carcinoma of thyroid and genitourinary tract, melanoma
fos	Carcinoma of kidney, colon, lung, ovary
met	Osteosarcoma
mos	Carcinoma of breast
myc	Burkitt's lymphoma, carcinoma of breast, colon, lung, ovary
sis	Glial tumours
ret	Carcinoma of thyroid
raf	Carcinoma of lung
int-1	Carcinoma of breast
trk	Carcinoma of thyroid
db1–mcf2	Carcinoma of breast, some B-cell lymphomas

Over-expression of the c-onc following the acquisition of a novel transcriptional promoter

Some proto-oncogenes are activated by the addition of a strong transcriptional promoter. For instance, avian leucosis virus (ALV) does not normally cause tumours but may occasionally do so after long incubation periods. When the DNA of such rare tumours is analysed by Southern blotting, the ALV provirus sequence is found to hybridize to the same fragment as the v-onc, **v-myc**. This suggests that the ALV provirus must have been inserted into the host cell genome very near the proto-oncogene **c-myc** and that this proximity of the normally active ALV activates the c-*myc*, the ALV acting as a strong transcriptional promoter. This sequence of events is termed **insertional mutagenesis**.

Amplification of either proto-oncogene or oncogene

A second activation mechanism involves amplification of a proto-oncogene or oncogene. In human promyelocytic leukaemia the *myc* proto-oncogene is amplified between 30 and 50 times. Such amplifications occur in relation to a number of c-oncs in several different human tumour cell lines. Once there is an increased number of copies of the gene in a single genome, it is assumed that there is a significant increase in the amount of gene product; this can be demonstrated using the Northern blotting method. In neuroblastoma, a malignant neoplasm of childhood, the aggressiveness of the tumour correlates with the degree of amplification of the oncogene n-*myc*.

Alteration in the structure of the oncogene protein

Point mutations in the oncogene proteins occur in relation to the products encoded by the *ras* genes. In the case of a cell line derived from a human bladder carcinoma, a single point mutation converts the **Ha-*ras*** proto-oncogene into a potent oncogene. This mutation causes the 12th amino acid in the 21 kD protein coded for by *ras* to be changed from glycine to valine. Studies carried out with oncogenes of the **Ki-*ras*** group have also shown that alteration of the gene product at position 12 leads to oncogenic activation. A human lung carcinoma oncogene of the Ha-*ras* group carries a mutation that alters the gene product at residue 61. It has been suggested that the codons specifying residues 12 and 61 of the gene product are critical sites which, when mutated, will often produce oncogenic alleles.

'Enhancer sequences' can increase the activity of transcriptional promoters

The level of transcription, and hence the amount of gene product, can be increased by '**enhancer sequences**' which increase the utilization of transcriptional promoters. The linked promoter may be a considerable distance from the enhancer sequence, which may be situated either upstream or downstream of the promoters.

Chromosome translocation

Chromosome translocation can be associated with movement of a proto-oncogene to a different site in the genome. This change in position may cause a c-onc to become activated. This is believed to occur in Burkitt's lymphoma, in which translocations of material from chromosome 8 to chromosomes 2, 14 or 22 occur very commonly (the 8:14 translocation is the most frequent). The c-*myc* proto-oncogene has been located on chromosome 8 near the breakpoint, and in chromosomes 2, 14 and 22 the genes that encode immunoglobulin chains are also present near the breakpoint. When translocation occurs, the c-*myc* gene derived from chromosome 8 and the immunoglobulin genes that are being actively transcribed in B cells become juxtaposed. This appears in some cases to result in deregulation of the c-*myc* gene, possibly through the action of enhancer sequences contained within the immunoglobulin gene.

Translocation may also cause the formation of novel genes when proto-oncogenes fuse with the genes on the chromosome to which they are translocated. A classic example is the formation of a fused gene by the translocation of c-*abl* (which has tyrosine kinase activity) on chromosome 9 and a gene termed *bcr* (breakpoint cluster region) on chromosome 22. This occurs in chronic myeloid leukaemia and in some lymphoblastic leukaemias of childhood. The altered chromosome 22 is known as the **Philadelphia chromosome**.

Oncogenes and multistep carcinogenesis

Spontaneous and chemically induced tumours are believed to arise as a result of several steps, although the transformation of cultured fibroblasts on the 3T3 line by an oncogene such as Ha-*ras* appears to be a **single event**.

This discrepancy arises from the nature of the 3T3 cells, which have been 'immortalized' as a line. If the oncogene is applied to a line not far removed from the ordinary rat fibroblast, the complete phenotypic picture of malignant transformation does not develop, although one phenotypic change, **loss of anchorage dependence**, does occur. This implies that if the recipient cell line is normal, the *ras* oncogene requires cooperation from some other factor or factors before transformation can occur.

ras *can cooperate with other viral oncogenes*

The changes occurring in 'immortalization' of a cell are poorly understood. However, they can be mimicked by the action of certain DNA tumour viruses, notably polyomaviruses and adenoviruses, which contain true viral genes capable of inducing cells to grow continuously in culture. *The polyomavirus genome encodes three proteins (the small, middle and large T antigens).* The middle T antigen induces morphological changes in cultured cells and also loss of anchorage dependence. The large T antigen increases the lifespan of the cultured cells and also alters the dependence of these cells on certain serum factors.

When large T and the *ras* gene are transfected into a cell line that does not transform when the *ras* gene alone is used, a dramatic degree of transformation occurs. Inoculation of transformed foci into nude mice produces rapidly growing tumours. Thus cooperation between a viral gene and cellular genes can convert normal cells into tumour cells.

Other cellular oncogenes can cooperate with ras

Such data shed no light on the possible mechanisms involved in transformation where there is no obvious viral involvement. However, in some animal tumour lines, active *ras* oncogenes coexist with active *myc* genes. Transfection of both *ras* and *myc* into cell lines that are not transformed by either alone, leads to transformation. We can infer that each genes must perform some distinct function necessary for tumour genesis. Such experiments may provide some explanation, at the molecular level, for the multistep nature of carcinogenesis, in that each step may involve the activation of a distinct cellular gene.

The action of oncogenes

The next step in unravelling this puzzle is to find out how gene products of active oncogenes induce and maintain the transformed phenotype. Protooncogenes encode proteins capable of acting in different parts of the cell (see pp. 486–487) and are clearly implicated in all the steps involved in cell division. A striking example is provided by the actions of *ras* oncogenes, which are involved in many human tumours.

The ras *family*

The retroviral homologues of human *ras* genes are the viral oncogenes of the

Harvey (Ha-*ras*) and Kirsten (Ki-*ras*) rat sarcoma viruses. *ras* genes encode 21 kD proteins attached to the inner surface of the plasma membrane by a lipid bond added after translation of the protein. ras proteins are homologues of G proteins and transduce signals in the same way as G proteins. G proteins act as a sort of molecular 'on–off switch' since they can exist in two dynamically interconvertible states, bound to guanosine 5′-diphosphate (GDP) or guanosine 5′-triphosphate (GTP). *Only the GTP-bound form mediates a growth response.* The binding of a growth factor or other mitogen to its receptor leads to GTP being substituted for GDP and activation of the ras protein. The G protein's inherent GTPase activity displaces the GTP and the ras protein becomes inactivated. Mutation of the *ras* gene leads to a loss of GTPase activity and thus the ras proteins are locked into a growth-stimulating mode.

TUMOUR SUPPRESSOR GENES

Genes with products that normally inhibit excessive cell proliferation are known as tumour suppressor genes. Mutation in or loss of these genes results in loss of their growth-inhibiting functions, so that unfettered cell proliferation is more likely to occur. It is this **loss of function** that contributes to oncogenesis, a paradigm whose value has only recently been appreciated.

Many tumours result from multiple genomic events which can include, in a single neoplasm, inappropriate activation of proto-oncogenes and inactivation of tumour suppressor genes.

RECOGNITION OF TUMOUR SUPPRESSOR GENES

Normally functioning tumour suppressor genes inhibit oncogenesis; identification of these genes presents a different set of problems to those encountered in oncogene research.

The existence of tumour suppressor genes can be inferred in a number of ways:

- Tumour formation is suppressed in hybrid cells resulting from fusion of malignant cells and their normal counterparts.
- Alteration or deletion of certain genes is associated with certain hereditary tumours.
- Loss of certain alleles identified by restriction fragment length polymorphisms can be detected in certain tumours (and pretumorous states such as familial adenomatous polyposis coli).
- Cloning of certain suppressor genes has been possible and their activities have been analysed in ex vivo systems.
- Transmission of wild-type suppressor genes into certain tumour cells in culture may restore a suppressed, non-tumorigenic phenotype.

Hybrid cells express a suppressed rather than a transformed phenotype

Hybrid cells resulting from fusion of mouse tumour cells and their non-neoplastic counterparts **express the normal phenotype and lose their tumorigenicity**. With repeated passage, the hybrid cells may lose certain chromosomes or parts of chromosomes and, in this event, revert to the transformed or malignant phenotype.

Reversion of tumour cells to a normal phenotype after hybridization implies that the transformed state correlates with *loss* of certain genetic material, which is restored by the contribution of normal cells to the hybrids.

Association of certain hereditary tumours with mutation or loss of alleles in germline cells

The paradigm for this hypothesis is **retinoblastoma**. This is a rare malignant tumour, affecting 1/20 000 infants and young children. It arises from precursors (retinoblasts) of the photoreceptor cells in the eye, known as cones. Once the retinoblast differentiates fully, it stops dividing and appears no longer to be a target for oncogenic processes. Thus retinoblastoma is not seen in persons older than six years.

The tumour occurs in two epidemiological patterns: sporadic and familial. In the **familial** form the tumours:

- occur early (mean age 14 months)
- are bilateral
- may be associated with a family history of retinoblastoma
- are usually multiple (mean number of tumours – 3).

In such a patient with retinoblastoma who has survived to adulthood and had children, about 50% of the offspring will also develop retinoblastoma. This implies that tumour risk is transmitted from parent to offspring in an autosomal dominant fashion, possibly in the form of a mutated gene. In survivors there is an increased risk for developing second tumours later in life, most notably osteosarcoma.

This is in marked contrast to the sporadic form of the tumour which probably affects no more than 1 in 100 000 children. In **sporadic retinoblastoma** the mean age for tumours to occur is at 30 months, and the tumours are usually unilateral. Survivors show no increase in the risk for developing other tumours.

These epidemiological data were brilliantly interpreted by Alfred G. Knudson in 1971 on the basis of the assumption that a mutated gene in any individual may be acquired through two routes:

1) by **inheritance** from a parent
2) as a result of a **somatic mutation**.

Knudson suggested that the differences in retinoblastoma risk arising from being born into a 'retinoblastoma family' could be explained in the following way (*Fig. 30.8*):

- All retinoblastoma tumour cells carry not one but two mutated alleles of the same gene.
- In familial retinoblastoma, one of the two required mutations is present from conception and must, therefore, be present in *all* cells of the body, including the retinoblasts.
- The second mutation could occur locally as a result of a somatic mutation in one of the already genetically abnormal retinoblasts.
- In sporadic retinoblastoma, *both* the mutations would have to be somatic mutations occurring locally in the retinal cells. The chances of this

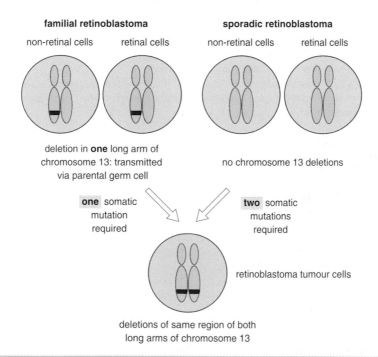

Fig. 30.8   Genetic mutation patterns in familial and sporadic retinoblastoma.

In familial retinoblastoma both retinoblasts and non-retinal cells show a mutation of one of the alleles encoding the RB protein at birth. Such an abnormality must be transmitted in the germ cell from one of the parents. In such circumstances only one further mutational event involving the second allele is required to produce the homozygous mutation required for tumour formation. In sporadic retinoblastoma, neither retinoblasts nor non-retinal cells show any abnormality of either allele of the RB gene at birth. Thus two mutational events, each involving one allele of the RB gene, are required before retinoblastoma occurs.

happening would be much less than is the case for a single somatic mutation. This would then explain the difference in risk.

This 'two-hit' hypothesis for the genesis of retinoblastoma embodies the important point that **both copies** of some gene of major importance must be lost or mutated if a tumour is to develop. In 1981, it was found that retinoblastoma was associated with **loss of part of the long arm of chromosome 13 (13q14)**. *In familial retinoblastoma this abnormality was found not only in tumour cells but in normal cells of all types throughout the affected child's body, whereas in sporadic cases the chromosomal abnormality was found only in tumour cells.*

The gene, which is presumably located somewhere in the deleted portion of chromosome 13, was given the name *RB*. If inactivation of both copies of the *RB* gene is required for tumour formation, it follows that **normal *RB* must have a tumour suppressor function**. This view gains strength from the observation that abnormalities of the *RB* gene, due to either germline or somatic mutations, have been seen in association with both retinoblastoma and osteosarcoma (children with familial retinoblastoma have a much greater risk of developing osteosarcoma during adolescence and early adult life), breast, prostate, bladder and lung cancers.

Loss of function in both alleles of certain genes has now been seen in a variety of hereditary and non-hereditary tumours, some of which are discussed below.

Wilms' tumour

Wilms' tumour is a malignant tumour in which the constituents closely resemble **elements of the embryonic kidney**. Three genomic abnormalities appear to be associated with this lesion in a non-random fashion, these abnormalities being associated with certain 'marker' syndromes. Thus:

1) In the **WAGR syndrome** (Wilms' tumour, aniridia, genitourinary tract anomalies, and mental retardation), there is a deleted region on chromosome 11 (11p13) in which a gene known as *WT-1* has been identified. *WT-1* codes for a nuclear protein believed to exert its suppressor function by regulating transcription.
2) In 15–20% of **sporadic Wilms' tumours**, there is a deletion in the region of 11p15.
3) In some **familial Wilms' tumours**, there is a deletion that does not map to either locus named above.

Neurofibromatosis type 1 (NF-1)

All cases of NF-1 result from the inheritance of a mutant allele. The mutations often appear to arise paternally. Linkage studies suggest that the *NF-1* suppressor gene is located on the long arm of chromosome 17 (17q11.2). As with the mutant *RB* gene, mutated *NF-1* genes are found in all cells throughout the body, so it is interesting that tumour formation is restricted to a few sites.

The *NF-1* gene product is called **neurofibromin**; it shows sequence homology both with mammalian and yeast GTPase-activating proteins. By binding to *ras*-encoded proteins (G proteins), neurofibromin increases the hydrolysis of GTP. Children with NF-1 are also at increased risk of developing neoplastic disorders of the bone marrow such as preleukaemic myelodysplastic syndromes and myeloproliferative disorders.

Familial adenomatous polyposis coli (FAPC)

FAPC is an inherited disorder in which multiple adenomatous polyps develop in the colon in the second and third decades of life. The disorder is inherited in an autosomal dominant fashion, and one or more of the polyps inevitably develops the full phenotype of colo-rectal cancer in later life. Linkage studies show that there is an APC locus, which appears to be deleted from the long arm of chromosome 5 (5q15–22). *This same locus seems to be involved in the genesis of both non-familial colonic adenomas and non-familial colorectal cancer.* Normal APC protein controls transcription by regulating β-catenin bonding to transcription factors TCF-1 and LEF-1. Loss of APC function causes loss of regulation of the transcription factors.

MECHANISMS OF ACTION OF TUMOUR SUPPRESSOR GENES

The products of tumour suppressor genes so far identified include:

- nuclear proteins
- cytoplasmic proteins
- membrane proteins.

Nuclear proteins

The gene products of some tumour suppressor genes, most notably *RB* and *p53* (see pp. 502–504, 504–508), are nuclear proteins, as is the product of the putative Wilms' tumour locus (*WT-1*) on the short arm of chromosome 11 (11p13). Presumably these proteins act normally *either* by regulating the expression of genes or the proteins they encode that are involved in cell proliferation or differentiation, *or* by controlling the biochemical mechanisms that regulate the initiation of DNA synthesis.

The protein encoded at 11p13, believed to be implicated in some cases of Wilms' tumour, is a zinc finger protein; this suggests that it may be a transcription factor. RB and p53 have been studied most extensively and their mode of action is discussed in more detail in a later section.

Cytoplasmic proteins

The *NF-1* gene product, loss of which is implicated in neurofibromatosis, is believed to be a GTPase-activating protein interacting with the p21 *ras* product. It may thus regulate signal transduction pathways concerned with cell proliferation.

Proteins expressed on cell surfaces
The gene known as *DCC* (deleted in cancer of the colon) is located on the long arm of chromosome 18. Its product is a cell surface molecule which belongs to the immunoglobulin gene superfamily and shows homology with neural adhesion molecules. Presumably, it influences the interaction between transformed cells and their neighbours.

HOW DO SUPPRESSOR GENES WORK?

Mechanism of action of the retinoblastoma gene product

The *RB* gene encodes a protein with a molecular weight of 105 kD, known as p105–RB. Its action can best be understood against the background of the normal cell cycle (*Fig. 30.9*). During G1 or G0, the RB protein forms a complex with the transcription factors E2F and DP1. In the presence of this complex, transcription of S-phase genes cannot occur and the cell cycle cannot proceed. The ability of the RB protein to maintain this complex with transcription factors depends on its degree of phosphorylation. RB Phosphorylation is mediated by cyclin-dependent kinases CDK 2 and 4, which are linked with cyclins D and E (*Fig. 30.10*).

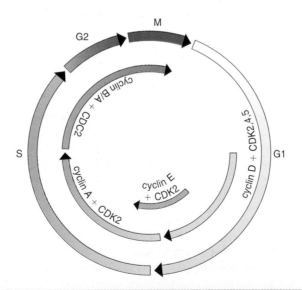

Fig. 30.9   Role of the gene products of *RB* and *p53* in the cell cycle.

The gene products of two important tumour suppressor genes, *RB* and *p53*, act as brakes on initiation of the S phase of the cell cycle and thus prolong the G1 phase. The cycle itself is driven by kinases which act only when bound to proteins known as cyclins and which are therefore known as cyclin-dependent kinases (cdk).

a S phase is initiated by transcription factors E2F and DP1

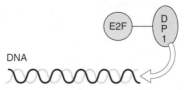

b the gene product of the retinoblastoma gene (RB) binds E2F and DP1 and thus blocks entry to S phase

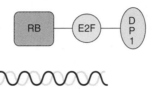

c if the RB protein becomes phosphorylated (P) by the cyclin–cdk complexes E–cdk-2 and D–cdk-4, the bond between RB and E2F–DP1 is broken

S phase transcription is thus free to proceed

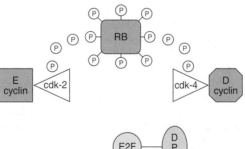

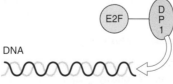

Fig. 30.10 Phosphorylation of the RB protein.

a The S phase is initiated by the transcription factors E2F and DP1. **b** The gene product of the retinoblastoma gene (RB) binds E2F and DP1, and thus blocks entry to the S phase. **c** Phosphorylation of the RB protein breaks the link between RB protein and the transcription factors E2F and DP1. The latter can therefore initiate transcription of S-phase genes and G1 is terminated.

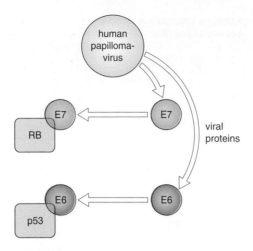

Fig. 30.11 Inactivation of the protein products of tumour suppressor genes by viruses

Both the RB and p53 proteins can be inactivated by protein products of oncogenic human papillomaviruses types 16 and 18. This inactivation of the gene products of two important suppressor genes may explain the oncogenic effect of these strains of human papillomavirus.

Binding of some DNA viral antigens can inactivate RB protein. In 1988 it was shown that p105–RB binds to the E1A transforming protein of adenovirus, to the large T antigen of SV40 virus and to the E7 protein produced by oncogenic strains of human papillomavirus (types 16 and 18) (*Fig. 30.11*). In the case of adenovirus this binding is a prerequisite for transformation, and the site of binding on the E1A protein shows sequence conservation with sites on SV40, polyomavirus, BK virus and human papillomavirus transforming proteins. Interestingly, the E7 proteins of **non-oncogenic human papillomaviruses** bind to p105–RB with much lower affinity.

The *p53* tumour suppressor gene

p53 mutations appear to be the commonest abnormality related to tumour suppressor genes in human neoplasms (*Table 30.3*). Thus far, the only tumour types in which a *p53* mutation has not been found are Wilms' tumour, testicular and pituitary neoplasms, and phaeochromocytomas.

Mechanism of action of p53

The *p53* gene encodes a nuclear phosphoprotein with 375 amino acids. It is known to bind with transforming proteins of certain oncogenic viruses such as the large T antigen of SV40. Complexing the p53 protein with SV40 prolongs the protein's half-life from 6–20 minutes to several hours. This

Table 30.3   Frequency of abnormality of *p53* in common human tumours

Tumour	p53 *mutation (%)*
Lung	56
Colon	50
Oesophagus	45
Ovary	44
Pancreas	44
Skin	44
Stomach	41
Head and neck	37
Urinary bladder	34
Sarcoma	31
Prostate	30
Liver cell	29
Brain	25
Adrenal	23
Breast	22
Endometrium	22
Mesothelioma	22
Kidney	19
Thyroid	13
Haematological neoplasms	12
Carcinoid	11
Melanoma	9
Parathyroid	8
Uterine cervix	7
Neuroblastoma	1

stabilized form of p53 can be identified in cells by immunostaining. *The activity of p53 appears to be controlled by two factors:*

1) the level of the p53 protein, which is very low after mitosis but increases in G1
2) the degree of phosphorylation; like RB protein, p53 becomes phosphorylated during the S phase and it has been suggested that this phosphorylation blocks its suppressor effect.

Normal wild-type p53 can suppress transformation by *ras* oncogenes acting in cooperation with c-*myc* in cell culture systems. This suggests that one function of p53 may be to inhibit the expression of c-*myc*.

Different types of alteration in the *p53* gene occur and the range of activities of the gene product is best looked at in this frame of reference. Tumours may show: **complete loss of p53** or **mutation of the *p53* gene** with production of an abnormal protein. In carcinomas most of the mutations are missense mutations that give rise to an abnormal protein product; in sarcomas, it is more common to find deletions, insertions or gene rearrangements.

Most *p53* mutations are somatic. However, in some families *p53* mutations may be found in the germ cell line. This occurs in a familial neoplastic syndrome known as the **Li–Fraumeni syndrome**, characterized by malignancy (often a sarcoma) appearing at a young age in probands with at least two first-degree relatives with malignant disease (breast, brain or adrenal cortical tumours).

The potency of the *p53* gene product is shown by animal studies. In transgenic mice carrying a mutant *p53* gene, 20% of animals develop tumours by 6–9 months of age. 'Knockout' mice with no *p53* genes develop malignant neoplasms within 3–6 months.

The protein coded for by p53 *stimulates production of another protein* (*Fig. 30.12*).   The p53 protein acts as a transcription factor, 'switching on' the gene responsible for the encoding of another protein with a molecular weight of 21 kD. This gene has at various times been called *cip-1* (cdk interacting protein 1) or *WAF1*.

The protein encoded by this gene in its turn inhibits the activity of enzymes that drive the cell cycle: the cyclin-dependent kinases (cdk) which phosphorylate the RB protein. In this way the complex formed by the RB protein and transcription factors E2F and DP1 remains in being.

p53 *is regulated by the product of an oncogene* mdm-2.   p53 protein is regulated by the protein product of another gene, *mdm-2* (**murine double minute gene 2**). *mdm-2* is a dominant oncogene; it enhances tumour production when overexpressed and its gene product binds to p53 protein and inactivates it so that the *cip-1* gene is not transcribed. Thus some tumours could contain normal amounts of normal (wild-type) p53 protein while overexpressing *mdm-2*. This occurs particularly in sarcomas, in which 5–50-fold amplification of the *mdm-2* gene has been recorded.

KEY POINTS: INACTIVATION OF *p53*

Inactivation of the p53 tumour suppressor gene protein can be due to:

- Mutation of the *p53* gene; this is the commonest situation in human malignancy.
- Degradation of p53 protein by virus-encoded products such as the E6 protein of human papillomavirus.
- Inactivation as a result of overproduction of mdm-2 protein.
- Sequestering of p53 protein in cell cytoplasm so that it cannot act as a transcription factor.

Biological role of p53

Experiments with 'knockout' mice show that *p53* is not required for viability during either fetal or adult life. It seems likely that *p53* plays little or no part in routine growth regulation but is **important in controlling uncontrolled growth such as occurs in malignancy**. It has been suggested that a major function of *p53* is to prevent chromosomal replication when

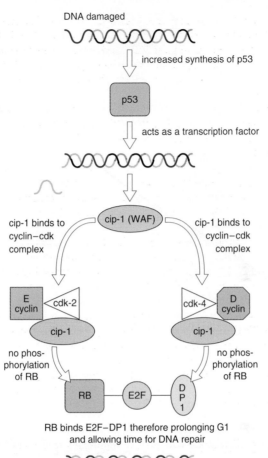

DNA damaged

increased synthesis of p53

p53

acts as a transcription factor

cip-1 (WAF)

cip-1 binds to
cyclin–cdk
complex

cip-1 binds to
cyclin–cdk
complex

E
cyclin | cdk-2

cdk-4 | D
cyclin

cip-1

cip-1

no phos-
phorylation
of RB

no phos-
phorylation
of RB

RB   E2F   D P 1

RB binds E2F–DP1 therefore prolonging G1
and allowing time for DNA repair

Fig. 30.12   Stimulation of production of cip-1 by p53.

p53 prolongs the G1 phase in cells with DNA damage by initiating transcription of a gene
encoding the protein cip-1 (WAF-1). The latter protein prevents phosphorylation of RB protein
by cyclin–cdk complexes (see *Fig. 30.10c*).

DNA has been damaged, and some writers refer to *p53* as 'the guardian of
the genome' (*Fig. 30.13*).

Certainly, the level of p53 protein rises dramatically after irradiation:

- Arrest in the G1 phase in cells with damaged DNA allows time for excision and repair, and thus prevents the transmission of the altered DNA to
  daughter cells.
- In addition, the p53 protein can induce **apoptosis**, which again eliminates
  cells harbouring genomic abnormalities.

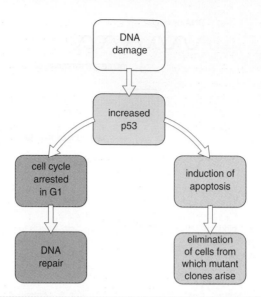

Fig. 30.13   Effects of p53 protein in damaged cells.

In addition to its effect on the G1 phase, p53 protein induces apoptosis in cells with damaged DNA. Both these effects tend to decrease the chances of stem cell mutations being passed on.

The *p16* gene

In 1992 it was shown that the short arm of chromosome 9 contains a susceptibility gene which is mutated in more than half of all malignant melanoma cell lines and which appears to play a significant role in the genesis, in particular, of familial melanoma. Since that time, abnormalities at this locus have been reported in many other tumour types; because the abnormalities include deletions, it has been suggested that another tumour suppressor gene is normally present at this site. Early in 1994 the protein product of this gene was identified and called p16. p16 binds to one of the cyclin-dependent kinases (CDK 4) and thus inhibits its activation by cyclin D1. This is the first tumour suppressor gene product that has been shown to act **directly on the cell cycle**. *p16* deletions have now been shown to be present in 50% of all cancers. Only in two types of tumour, colorectal cancer and neuroblastoma, have *p16* deletions not been found.

Tumour suppressor genes and breast cancer

About 5% of cases of breast cancer are familial. Two-thirds of these are believed to be associated with germline mutations in one of two genes known as *BRCA-1* and *BRCA-2*. The *BRCA-1* gene has now been isolated and localized to the long arm of chromosome 17. It is responsible for about one-third of cases of familial breast cancer and has been found in more than 80% of families in which breast and ovarian cancer occur together. The presence of a zinc finger domain close to the *N*-terminus suggests that the protein may be a transcription factor.

In high-risk families, female carriers of mutated *BRCA-1* genes have an 80–90% lifetime risk of developing breast cancer. It is not known how much risk is attached to mutations in females from families with no documented history of high risk. A frameshift germline mutation (185delAG) is present in about 1% of Ashkenazi Jewish females, and they may be at high risk of developing breast cancer.

The second gene, *BRCA-2*, has not been isolated but has been mapped to the long arm of chromosome 13 close to the location of the *RB* gene. It is probably responsible for the same proportion of cases of familial breast cancer in females as *BRCA-1*, but differs from that gene by being involved in the genesis of familial breast cancer in males as well.

A list of the tumour suppressor genes currently known, their functions and the inherited tumours with which their deletion or inactivation is associated, is given in *Table 30.4*.

MUTATOR GENES

The gene products of normal mutator genes are involved in DNA repair. They were discovered during studies of hereditary non-polyposis colorectal cancer. The first mutator gene, *MSH-2*, was found to have strong homology with the *mut2* gene occurring in bacteria, and is located on the short arm of chromosome 2.

A second gene concerned with DNA repair is *MLH-1*, which is located on the short arm of chromosome 3.

Table 30.4 Suppressor genes, their proposed functions and the inherited tumours that result from their inactivation or mutation

Inherited tumour	Gene	Site	Suggested function
Retinoblastoma Osteosarcoma	RB	13q14	RB gene product binds to two transcription factors, E2F and DP1, and inactivates them. This prevents the cell from entering the S phase from G1. When the RB protein becomes heavily phosphorylated, E2F and DP1 are released and can initiate transcription.
Osteosarcoma Breast cancer Glioma Li–Fraumeni syndrome	p53	17p13	p53 gene product acts as a transcription factor causing transcription of a gene known as cip-1. This encodes a 21 kD protein which binds to cyclin-dependent kinases 2 and 4 and thus inhibits cyclin-dependent phosphorylation of certain targets including the RB protein. The RB–E2F–DP1 complex remains bound together and thus the cell cannot proceed from G1 to S. Mutation of p53 is one of the commonest genomic events in malignant disease. Certain viral antigens may bind with and inactivate p53. Aflatoxin, which can contaminate cereal crops, produces a point mutation in p53 which leads to the production of a mutant gene product.
Polyposis coli	APC	5q21	APC protein communicates between microtubules and certain cell surface proteins.
Nephroblastoma (Wilms' tumour)	WT-1	11p13	WT-1 protein acts as a transcription factor.
Neurofibromatosis type 1	NF-1	17q11.2	The gene product neurofibromin acts as a GTPase-activating protein. It binds to the product of the ras oncogenes and thus increases hydrolysis of GTP bound to these proteins.
Meningioma Acoustic neuroma	NF-2	22q11.1	The gene product is one of the proteins of the cytoskeleton and has been called merlin. Its function is not known.
No inherited tumour but somatic mutations associated with colorectal cancer	DCC	18q21	An adhesion molecule similar to the neural cell adhesion molecules found in the nervous system.
Melanoma	MTS-1	9p21	This is the first suppressor gene product shown to act directly on the cell cycle. It is a 16 kD protein which binds to cyclin-dependent kinase 4 and prevents its activation by cyclin D1. This prevents the cell from progressing from G1 to S phase.
Breast (female) Breast and ovary	BRCA-1	17q	
Breast (female and male)	BRCA-2	13q	
?	MTS-2	9p21	This 15 kD gene product also inhibits the activity of cyclin-dependent kinases.

ONCOGENESIS AND THE MOLECULAR BIOLOGY OF CANCER

- While there are many causes of cancer, the final transforming mechanisms are likely to be small in number and are mediated through alterations in three classes of gene: **oncogenes**, **suppressor genes** and **mutator genes**.
- Cell population homeostasis results from their interaction of the gene products of growth promoting genes (proto-oncogenes) and growth inhibiting genes (tumour suppressor genes).
- Transformation may occur when growth-promoting genes are abnormally **up-regulated** or suppressor genes are abnormally **down-regulated**. In many instances a combination of these is present.
- Activated proto-oncogenes act dominantly and are associated with a gain in function. Inactivated tumour suppressor genes act recessively and are associated with loss of function.
- Gene products of proto-oncogenes act as growth gactors, receptors, signal-transducing factors, DNA-binding proteins or cell cycle proteins.
- Loss of tumour suppressor gene function may be associated with increased risk of certain hereditary tumours (such as **familial polyposis coli** or **retinoblastoma**) or with common sporadic tumours such as breast or colonic carcinoma.

31 Oncogenesis

Epidemiological data indicate that there is no such thing as a single cause of malignancy. As discussed previously, the number of final mechanisms involved in malignant transformation at the molecular level may be rather small.

GENETIC FACTORS

The clustering of certain types of malignancy in some families and the presence of malignant neoplasms as part of some well-recognized inherited syndromes indicate that the individual genotype is important in determining susceptibility to malignant disease. An increase in the liability of an individual to develop a malignant neoplasm may be inherited:

- as part of a clinical syndrome that has diagnostic features of its own apart from the increased risk of malignancy; this makes it possible to recognize those at high risk and to take appropriate measures to reduce the chances of malignancy
- as the only manifestation of a single gene abnormality.

Inherited syndromes associated with an increased risk of malignancy fall essentially into two groups:

1) syndromes with a major, recognizable, chromosome abnormality
2) syndromes apparently determined by a single gene abnormality; these may be associated with an immunological defect, as in **ataxia telangiectasia** (see pp. 185–186), or there may be no identifiable defect in immunity.

CHROMOSOMALLY DETERMINED SYNDROMES

Three such syndromes associated with malignancy have been described:

- Down's syndrome

- Klinefelter's syndrome
- gonadal dysgenesis.

Down's syndrome (mongolism – see pp. 549–551). An increased risk of developing acute leukaemia (myeloblastic:lymphoblastic risk 1:2) appears to be an integral part of the syndrome.

Klinefelter's syndrome (a type of male hypogonadism associated with the presence of an extra X chromosome – see pp. 554–556). Patients with Klinefelter's syndrome show an increased tendency to develop tumours of the male breast.

Gonadal dysgenesis in patients with a female phenotype and a male genotype. Those with gonadal dysgenesis are more likely to develop tumours of the gonads. However, this increased risk may be secondary to the interaction between an abnormal hormonal milieu and an unresponsive target organ rather than a primarily genetically determined type of carcinogenesis.

SINGLE GENE ABNORMALITIES

The syndromes associated with immune deficiencies have been considered already (see pp. 185–195), so only some outstanding examples associated with an increased risk of malignancy and with *no* evidence of an immunological defect are mentioned here.

Xeroderma pigmentosum

This rare condition, inherited in an autosomal recessive fashion, was first described by the famous dermatologist Kaposi in 1874. It is characterized by hypersensitivity to ultraviolet light and by a marked tendency to develop malignant skin tumours during childhood and adolescence. The skin of affected children appears normal at birth, but repeated exposure to sunlight results in a dry scaly skin with many areas of hyperpigmentation. These skin changes are followed within a few years by the appearance of a variety of skin tumours, some of which are malignant, such as squamous carcinoma. It is important for our understanding of this condition to note that **unexposed skin** remains normal. Precise prevalence data are not available, but estimates of the frequency of xeroderma pigmentosum vary from 1 in 65 000–250 000 live births. The condition is most commonly encountered in North Africans. Protection from sunlight, either by suitable clothing or by barrier creams against ultraviolet light, can reduce the risk of tumour development; these are important measures to institute once the condition has been diagnosed.

Lack of the enzymes responsible for excision repair leads to perpetuation of abnormal DNA sequences

The intrinsic defect in xeroderma pigmentosum is of great interest. The main target for ultraviolet light within epidermal cells is DNA. Absorption of photons by DNA results in the formation of several new products, of which the most important are dimers formed by adjacent pyrimidine bases (usually thymine). Normally the abnormal portion of the DNA containing the thymine dimers is excised by an **endonuclease** and replaced by a new length of DNA some 100 nucleotides in length. In xeroderma pigmentosum, the endonuclease responsible for initiating 'excision and repair' is lacking and the UVL-induced change in DNA is permanent.

Other syndromes in which DNA repair is defective, and in which there is an increased risk of malignancy, are **ataxia telangiectasia** and **Fanconi's anaemia** (in which there is an increased risk of leukaemia) and **Bloom's syndrome**, which is also characterized by hypersensitivity to sunlight. In this last condition, unlike xeroderma pigmentosum, the increased risk of malignancy is not confined to the skin. The defect in repair at the molecular level has not been characterized in these three conditions.

These four rare syndromes indicate that **non-reparable alterations to the DNA of a target cell**, however they may be caused, constitute one of the initiating mechanisms of carcinogenesis.

Familial adenomatous polyposis coli and related disorders

Adenomatous polyposis coli, caused by inheritance of an autosomal dominant gene, is rare and accounts for only a small proportion of the deaths due to colorectal cancer. Theoretically, if one parent is affected, half the children may be expected to develop the disease. In practice, the penetrance rate is only about 80%, so that 40% of the children would show features of the disease.

Familial adenomatous polyposis is characterized by multiple polyps in the large gut. The polyps are not present at birth, and appear between the ages of 10 and 20 years. The lesions are distributed fairly evenly throughout the large bowel, but the greatest concentration is to be found in the rectum, which is always involved. In their premalignant phase, the lesions show the features of adenomas on microscopic examination.

Of those who present with symptoms attributable to the polyps, about 65% already have large bowel cancer. The average age at diagnosis in these patients is 40 years (about 20 years younger than in the non-polyposis population). Death as a result of colorectal cancer also occurs at a much younger age in these patients than in the general population. The precise frequency with which patients suffering from polyposis coli develop colorectal cancer is not easy to assess, but some writers maintain that by the age of 60 years 100% of the victims of polyposis will have developed cancer of the large bowel. This gloomy prospect places a heavy burden of decision on the medical attendant of such a patient, because the only means of avoiding malignant transformation of one or more of the polyps is to undertake prophylactic resection of the whole of the large bowel, including the rectum.

Other inherited multiple colonic polyp syndromes are **Gardner's syndrome** and **Turcot's syndrome**.

In Gardner's syndrome, also inherited as an autosomal dominant, there are multiple colonic polyps associated with tumours in skin, subcutaneous tissue and bone. The likelihood of a sufferer developing colorectal cancer is about 100%.

Turcot's syndrome consists of a combination of colonic polyps and brain tumours. It is inherited in an autosomal recessive manner. There appears to be an increased risk of colorectal cancer, but the magnitude of this risk has not been established.

Familial adenomatous polyposis is associated with the inheritance of a malfunctioning *APC* gene, a tumour suppressor gene, on the long arm of chromosome 5 (see p. 501).

INCREASED RISK OF NEOPLASIA WITH NO 'PRECURSOR' SYNDROME

An increased risk of certain neoplasms may be inherited without any recognizable 'premalignant' or 'preneoplastic' syndrome such as polyposis or xeroderma pigmentosum. It is only rarely that these neoplasms occur in a pattern suggesting a major role for inheritance. They include retinoblastoma and phaeochromocytoma. Retinoblastoma and its molecular genetics are discussed on pp. 498–500.

Phaeochromocytoma

This neoplasm arises wherever **chromaffin cells** are present, and is most common in the adrenal medulla. The tumour cells secrete noradrenaline and adrenaline; patients may thus present with systemic hypertension. About 5–10% of these tumours are malignant. Most phaeochromocytomas occur sporadically, but it is thought that 10–20% are familial; these occur in association with one of a number of syndromes.

1) An **autosomally dominant tendency** for phaeochromocytomas to occur. The tumours often occur in childhood and more than 50% are bilateral.

2) **Multiple endocrine neoplasia syndrome type IIa** (Sipple's syndrome), which consists of a combination of **phaeochromocytoma, medullary carcinoma of the thyroid and parathyroid adenoma or hyperplasia**. This syndrome is thought to be inherited as an autosomal dominant with a high degree of penetrance. The phaeochromocytomas occur between the ages of 30 and 40 years and there is an increased tendency for them to be malignant.

3) **Multiple endocrine neoplasia syndrome type IIb.** In this variant there is **phaeochromocytoma, medullary carcinoma of the thyroid and neuromas affecting mucosal surfaces**. It is also transmitted in an autosomal dominant manner.

4) An association between **phaeochromocytoma** and **neurofibromatosis**.

CHEMICAL CARCINOGENESIS

Studies dating back more than 200 years have established that many types of malignant neoplasm occurring in humans are caused by environmental factors. Any such factor which can increase an individual's risk of developing a malignant neoplasm is spoken of as a **carcinogen**, although it might be more precisely referred to as an **oncogen**. Such factors may be chemical, physical or viral. This section is concerned with the first of these.

The history of this field of oncological research starts with the observation in 1775 by Percivall Pott, a noted London surgeon, that there was a high prevalence of cancer of the scrotal skin in chimney sweeps' boys. Anyone who has read *The Water Babies* by Charles Kingsley, a work of more than usually revolting sentimentality, will recall that the hapless children were sent up into the chimneys to sweep them and, consequently, were covered in soot.

Pott's writings were said to have inspired a ruling made by the Danish Chimney Sweepers' Guild in 1778 that its members should bathe daily. The effectiveness of this simple measure is suggested by a study carried out by Butlin a century later, in which he showed that scrotal cancer in chimney sweeps was comparatively rare outside England. Butlin attributed this to the habit of wearing protective clothing and bathing daily.

During the early industrial revolution, a similarly high prevalence of skin cancer was found in association with a number of occupations. Mule spinners in the Lancashire cotton mills, the fronts of whose garments were often soaked with lubricating oils, frequently developed cancer of the skin of the abdomen and scrotum; workers engaged in the extraction of oil from shale appeared to be similarly at risk. All these observations, relatively crude as they were, suggested that **coal tar** or one of its constituents might be responsible for the induction of such skin cancers. This led, ultimately, to the recognition of **polycyclic hydrocarbons** as a group of compounds with considerable carcinogenic potential.

Remote, proximate and ultimate carcinogens: carcinogenicity and mutagenicity

Many of the substances that are called carcinogens on the basis of their ability to produce tumours in certain animal species are not themselves carcinogenic. They become so only after conversion in the body of the host to forms that are more active biologically. In current terminology:

- The parent substance is called a **remote carcinogen** or **precarcinogen**.
- Its metabolites with greater carcinogenic potential are called **proximate carcinogens**.
- The final molecular species that interacts with the host DNA is termed the **ultimate carcinogen**.

This concept is of obvious importance when attempting to identify the carcinogenic potential of new compounds before they are released for use, because the metabolites as well as the parent compounds must be tested for mutagenicity and/or carcinogenicity (see below).

Normal cells transformed by carcinogens show permanent alteration of their phenotypes. This alteration is inherited from generation to generation of the cell line. We can infer from this that a **permanent alteration to the genome** of the transformed cell has occurred. Such an alteration falls within the definition of a **mutation**. It is now known that most of the carcinogenic chemicals so far identified are also mutagens. Not all mutagens are carcinogenic; nevertheless, the demonstration that a given compound is mutagenic sounds a warning that it may also be carcinogenic.

In testing for mutagenicity, the possibility that the test compound may be only a remote carcinogen must be taken into consideration.

Testing for mutagens

Most tests for mutagenicity employ submammalian species. These include bacteria, bacterial viruses (bacteriophages), fungi and insects. All of these are useful because they have relatively small genomes and reproduce themselves quickly.

A commonly used test is the Ames test, in which the effect of the test compound on the histidine-requiring mutant of *Salmonella typhimurium* is assessed (*Fig. 31.1*). Reversion of this strain, produced by a single base-pair substitution or insertion of a single base pair, can be detected quickly and easily. The possibility that metabolic conversion is needed before mutagenicity is expressed can be taken care of by preincubation of the test compound with liver microsomes.

Polycyclic hydrocarbons in relation to carcinogenicity

Despite the recognized association between exposure to coal tar derivatives and skin cancer, it was not until 1915 that the experimental induction of coal tar-related neoplasms in animals was first carried out. By repeated applications of coal tar to the inside of rabbit ears, Yamagiwa and Ichikawa produced skin tumours in the areas of skin on which the tar had been painted. The next step was to be isolation of the substances in the tar that were responsible for the tumours. It was found that the compounds responsible were present in the higher boiling fractions obtained during the fractional distillation of coal tar. The fluorescence spectra of these fractions resembled that of the polycyclic hydrocarbon 1,2-benzanthracene.

This compound is only weakly carcinogenic in the skin-painting model but, using its characteristic fluorescence spectrum as a guide, Sir Ernest Kennaway and his colleagues were able in 1930 to isolate 50 mg of the powerful carcinogen 3,4-benzpyrene as the end-product of the fractional distillation of two tonnes of tar.

3,4-Benzpyrene is a major constituent of cigarette smoke and is also

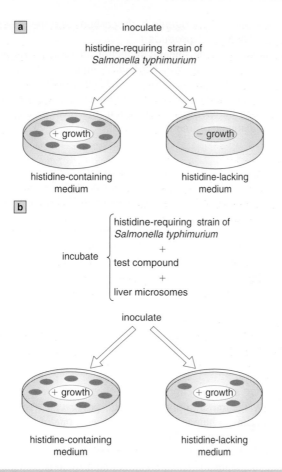

Fig. 31.1 Testing for mutagenicity using bacteria.

a Normal results with a histidine-requiring strain of *Salmonella typhimurium*. **b** The presence of colonies in medium lacking histidine indicates mutation of some bacteria to a state of histidine independence.

present in the exhaust fumes of petrol engines. Many other hydrocarbons have been tested since then. Not all are carcinogenic. Among those that are carcinogenic, there are distinct differences in their ability to induce tumours in experimental animals. Moderate or powerful carcinogenic compounds in this group include:

- 7,12-dimethylbenz(a)anthracene
- 3,4-benzpyrene
- 1,2,5,6-dibenzanthracene
- 3-methylcholanthrene.

The site of application of oncogenic hydrocarbons and the species used affect the type of neoplasm produced

The classical model of experimental induction of tumours by polycyclic hydrocarbons is skin painting, which produces squamous tumours locally. However, the subcutaneous injection of 7,12-dimethylbenz(a)anthracene produces sarcomas in the rat and malignant tumours of the lymphoid system in newborn mice. Intraperitoneal injection in mice produces ovarian tumours; in rats, mammary tumours result.

Mechanisms of action

Carcinogenic hydrocarbons act by binding to host macromolecules within both the cytoplasm and the nucleus. They are activated by mixed-function oxidases to form epoxides which are more water soluble and more reactive than the parent compounds.

The carcinogenic potential of hydrocarbons seems to reside in certain double bonds to which oxygen is added (under the influence of mixed-function oxidases such as **aryl hydrocarbon hydroxylase**). The compounds formed are known as **epoxides**; it is these that appear to have the ability to bind to DNA as well as to macromolecules in the cytoplasm of target cells. This binding tendency is related to the fact that the epoxides are **electrophilic** (positively charged molecules that form covalent bonds with the negatively charged nucleophilic atoms in DNA, RNA and proteins). The greater the degree of DNA binding, the greater the carcinogenic potential of the hydrocarbon.

Cigarette smoking and lung cancer

Almost certainly the most important of the polycyclic hydrocarbons in relation to neoplasms in humans is 3,4-benzpyrene, one of more than 3000 components in cigarette smoke. There is now a vast literature supporting the existence of a direct causal association between cigarette smoking and lung cancer (chiefly of the squamous variety). If one were to regard the risk of a non-smoker developing carcinoma of the bronchus as an arbitrary level of 1, the relative risk to an individual who smokes 20 or more cigarettes per day may be as great as 32. Giving up smoking reduces the chance of carcinoma in that individual: the longer the cigarette-free period, the greater the reduction in risk.

Clearly, not all smokers develop lung cancer (although about 10% do). This raises the possibility that there may be some genetic contribution to the risk of an individual smoker developing cancer. This genetic component may be related to the inducibility of the enzyme **aryl hydrocarbon hydroxylase (AHH)** by the hydrocarbon substrate. It has been reported that differences exist in the inducibility of this enzyme; subjects in whom the enzyme is more readily induced may be at greater risk of developing a smoking-related tumour. Conflicting reports on the importance of AHH inducibility may be due to the fact that AHH measures the sum total of oxidation due to a number of P450 cytochromes and that the conversion of benzpyrene to a carcinogenic metabolite may be a function of only some of these enzymes. High-pressure liquid chromatography shows that benzpyrene is converted to more than 40 metabolites. One of these, a diol epoxide, is highly mutagenic and carcinogenic, and is found covalently bound to cellular DNA.

The ways in which individuals metabolize drugs may also be useful in delineating groups that may be more or less at risk of developing cancer after exposure to carcinogens. In a recent study, most patients with lung cancer were shown to be rapid metabolizers of debrisoquine. The pattern of distribution suggests that this trait is inherited in an autosomal dominant manner.

Lung cancer is not the only neoplasm that appears to be causally associated with smoking: carcinomas of the oesophagus, pancreas, kidney and urinary bladder also seem to be more common in smokers.

Aromatic amines and azo dyes

2-Naphthylamine

As early as 1895, a high prevalence of carcinoma of the bladder was reported in men who had worked in an aniline dye factory in Germany. The causal nature of this association was soon confirmed, and it is now known that several occupations carry an increased risk for the development of bladder cancer. These include aniline dye manufacture, the rubber and cable industry, the manufacture of certain paints and pigments, textile dyeing and printing, and certain categories of laboratory work.

The carcinogens identified in these situations are the **aromatic amines** 2-naphthylamine and benzidine. Only humans and dogs are said to be susceptible to the urothelial effects of the naphthylamine, although bladder tumours have been produced in the rat bladder after naphthylamine feeding in at least one study. In humans bladder cancer occurs on average about 15 years earlier than in the population not exposed to aromatic amines. The average latent period between exposure and the development of bladder tumours is about 16 years. The duration of exposure may be quite short.

The aromatic amines should be classified as **remote carcinogens** because, while it is possible to produce bladder tumours in dogs by **feeding** 2-naphthylamine, the insertion of pellets of this compound directly into the bladder has no such carcinogenic effect. To exert such an effect the amine must be converted into a biologically active form. This is achieved by hydroxylation in the liver, which yields the actively carcinogenic metabolite, 2-amino-1-naphthol. This is normally detoxified in the liver by conjunction with glucuronic acid; the resulting glucuronide is excreted by the kidney. This glucuronide is said to be non-carcinogenic. The susceptibility of human and dog urothelium is explained by the fact that the urothelial cells in these two species secrete the enzyme β-glucuronidase, which splits glucuronic acid from the 2-amino-1-naphthol, thus releasing the carcinogenic molecule (*Fig. 31.2*).

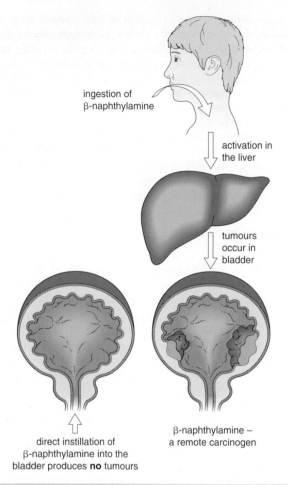

ingestion of
β-naphthylamine

activation in
the liver

tumours
occur in
bladder

direct instillation of
β-naphthylamine into the
bladder produces **no** tumours

β-naphthylamine –
a remote carcinogen

Fig. 31.2   β-Naphthylamine is a remote carcinogen.

Ingestion of β-naphthylamine leads to cancer of the bladder. Instillation of the compound directly into the bladder does not. This indicates that the β-naphthylamine is activated in the course of metabolism and is thus a remote carcinogen.

2-Acetyl-aminofluorene

This amine has excited considerable interest as an experimental model of carcinogenesis. It was developed as an insecticide in the 1940s, but before marketing was found to be carcinogenic. Unlike 2-naphthylamine or benzidine, which appear to produce tumours only in the bladder, 2-acetyl-aminofluorene produces neoplasms in a wide range of tissues including the liver, breast, lung and intestine. As with naphthylamine, this compound is also a remote carcinogen which undergoes hydroxylation in the liver to produce a proximate carcinogen of greater activity. The final step in the production of the ultimate carcinogen is probably esterification to form an *N*-sulphate ester, which is a highly reactive electrophilic compound.

Nitrosamines and nitrosamides

The carcinogenic potential of this group of compounds has excited a great deal of interest since the discovery in 1956 that animals receiving dimethyl-nitrosamine in the diet at a dose level of 50 parts per million developed liver cell tumours after 6–9 months of dosing.

Nitrosamines have the general formula

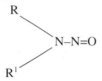

in which one of the R groups is an alkyl radical and the other either an aryl or alkyl radical. In the case of the **nitrosamides**, one R is an alkyl radical and the other an amide or ester. The nitroso compounds have proved to be potent and versatile carcinogens in animals, producing tumours in a wide range of animal species and in many different tissues. An interesting feature of the individual compounds in this large group is their organotropy, many of them showing a marked degree of organ specificity.

In the case of nitrosamines, as with 2-naphthylamine, the parent compound is a remote carcinogen which requires metabolic activation. In the course of this activation, alkylating agents are formed and these bind to both the N7 and the O6 position on guanine. The latter is probably of more significance in so far as malignant transformation is concerned.

Nitrosamines can be formed in the gastrointestinal tract by the interaction of nitrous acid, derived from nitrites, with secondary amines. It has been suggested that the frequency of certain tumours, notably gastric carcinoma, may be related to the dietary intake of nitrites, which are present in large amounts in pickled, salted and smoked foods.

Nitrosamides do not require enzymatic activation to be rendered carcinogenic. Thus, instillation of methyl-nitrosourea into the rat bladder at an appropriate dosage results in the production of urothelial tumours in the majority of instances. An interesting aspect of nitrosamide activity is displayed by the compound ethyl-nitrosourea. When this compound, which has a half-life of only a few minutes, is given to a pregnant rat after the 11th day of gestation, the offspring develop malignant tumours of the brain at about the age of 9 months. Samples of brain taken from the litter at different ages and grown in culture show a stepwise development of the phenotypic evidence of malignant transformation.

Direct-acting alkylating agents

Alkylating agents can bind to DNA without any need for prior activation. This group includes such compounds as mustard gas, β-propiolactone and several agents used in the treatment of malignant disease, such as cyclophosphamide, melphalan and busulphan. While the interaction of these molecules with DNA makes them useful as antitumour agents, this property constitutes a double-edged sword, because they also increase the risk of other neoplasms developing, most notably leukaemia and malignancies of the lymphoid series.

Some naturally occurring chemical carcinogens

The groups of chemical carcinogens considered thus far can hardly be looked on as natural environmental hazards, with the possible exception of nitrosamines derived in the gastrointestinal tract from dietary constituents. The marked influence that geographical factors have on the prevalence of certain neoplasms, such as carcinoma of the liver and oesophagus, suggests that these differences in tumour frequency may be affected by the existence of naturally occurring carcinogens in particular areas.

In relation to carcinoma of the liver, which is comparatively rare in Europe and North America but common in Asia and in certain parts of Africa, an interesting potential candidate for the role of naturally occurring carcinogen is a group of toxins produced by fungi, most notably *Aspergillus flavus*. The toxins derived from this mould, which may contaminate cereal and groundnut crops, are known as **aflatoxins**. Aflatoxins were discovered in 1960 when a large number of poultry fed on groundnut meal imported from East Africa died from extensive liver cell necrosis. When formal toxicological studies were carried out it was found that, at low dose levels, the toxin was capable of producing liver cell carcinoma.

The frequency of liver cell carcinoma is high in those parts of the world where there is a poor, largely agrarian, population that is heavily dependent on cereal crops for subsistence. Such crops may become contaminated by *A. flavus* and, indeed, epidemiological data indicate a positive correlation between aflatoxin consumption and the incidence of liver cell carcinoma. For example, in Thailand, where there was a ninefold difference in aflatoxin intake between two areas of the country, there was a sixfold difference in the frequency of liver cell carcinoma.

It appears that strong synergy exists between aflatoxin and chronic hepatitis B virus infection. Some of the proteins of hepatitis B virus mimic the action of tumour promoters. The resulting large population of dividing cells is more likely to acquire somatic mutations of one kind or another: aflatoxin produces a **point mutation at codon 249 of the *p53* gene**, leading to the production of **an abnormal gene product** (see pp. 485–486).

Occupational carcinogens

The recognition that certain chemicals might be implicated in carcinogenesis stemmed directly from the observations of Pott and others (see p. 517) that certain occupations carried a higher than normal risk for the development of certain neoplasms. A considerable number of occupational hazards of this kind is now known to exist (*Table 31.1*).

While it is impossible to give a detailed account of the 'occupational' neoplasms that have been recognized, a few general points of principle are worth considering.

In general, a neoplasm related to an occupational hazard does not differ from its non-occupational counterpart, either in clinical or structural terms. In some instances there may be associated histological features that may provide a clue as to the occupational aetiology, such as the finding of asbestos bodies in the resected lung of a patient with squamous carcinoma of the bronchus.

Sometimes the clue might reside in the unusual nature of the tumour or in the fact that it is of a type that is unusual at that particular anatomical site. An example of the first is **mesothelioma**, a neoplasm which, as its name implies, arises from the mesothelial cells of serosal linings. Mesotheliomas occur most commonly in the pleura, leading to a tremendous degree of thickening of the visceral pleura.

An example of the second type of situation, in which a tumour unusual at a particular anatomical site is encountered, is **adenocarcinoma of the paranasal sinuses** in hardwood workers. Such a tumour otherwise only occurs rarely at this site.

No general rule appears to operate with respect to the age at which occupationally related neoplasms occur. It appears to be a function of two variables: the age at which exposure begins, and the latent period characteristic of the particular carcinogen. In a study of occupationally related

Table 31.1 Some occupational hazards and their associated neoplasms

Chemical	Neoplasm
2-Naphthylamine	Urothelial malignancy (bladder, ureter, renal pelvis)
Arsenic	Cancers of skin and lung
Asbestos (a fibrous silicate)	Mesothelioma, squamous carcinoma of lung
Ionizing radiation	Cancers of lung and bone, leukaemia
Bischlormethylether	Small cell carcinoma of lung
Nickel	Cancers of lung, paranasal sinuses, larynx
Vinyl chloride monomer	Angiosarcoma of liver
Hardwood dusts	Adenocarcinoma of paranasal sinuses
Benzene	Leukaemia

cancer of the urinary bladder, the mean age at exposure was found to be 29 years and the mean latent period 16.6 years. Thus the tumours became obvious at a somewhat earlier age than is usual for bladder cancer.

CARCINOGENESIS AS A MULTISTEP PROCESS: TUMOUR INITIATION AND PROMOTION

In the late 1940s it was found that painting the skin with compounds such as croton oil, which are not themselves carcinogenic, greatly increased the yield of skin tumours in mice that had previously received a subcarcinogenic dose of the carcinogenic polycyclic hydrocarbon benzo(a)pyrene (*Fig. 31.3*). Croton oil *alone* produced no tumours and, if it was applied to the mouse skin *before* the hydrocarbon, *no* tumour-enhancing effect was noted.

The effect of the benzo(a)pyrene was described at that time as the **initiation of carcinogenesis**, and the enhancing effect of the croton oil was termed **promotion**. For many years this phenomenon was believed to be confined to the mouse skin model, but it is now thought that two-stage or multistage pathways in carcinogenesis exist in respect of a number of neoplasms, including liver, bladder, lung, breast, colon, oesophagus and pancreas.

If the term **promotion**, as originally defined in the mouse skin model, is to have an application in the wider field of carcinogenesis, it is important that common features should be demonstrated in both **operational** and **biochemical** terms between the mouse model and other chemically induced neoplasms.

Chemical carcinogenesis can be regarded, in operational terms, as a series of processes in which a normal cell and its progeny are converted into malignant cells (*Fig. 31.4*).

Initiation

The initiation phase involves a change in the genome of the target cell, this change being inherited by the progeny of that cell. The change in the genetic material, as indicated above, is usually associated with covalent binding of the active form of the carcinogen to DNA.

While high doses of initiating compounds can cause tumours to develop without the assistance of any other factors, a low dose of the initiator will not be expressed in the form of phenotypically altered cells and may induce damage in the genome of only a small number of target cells.

Characteristically, initiation:

- is a very rapid event
- is produced in a dose-related fashion after a single exposure to an initiating carcinogen
- occurs in only a small proportion of the target cell population; the number of cells affected is increased if rapid proliferation of the target cells is taking place.

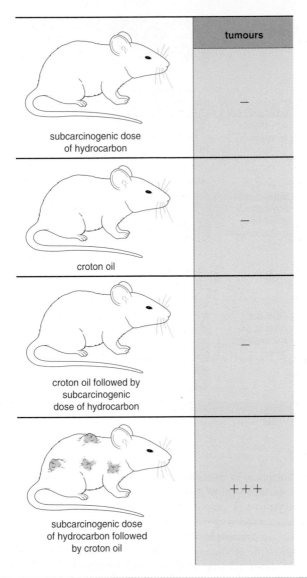

	tumours
subcarcinogenic dose of hydrocarbon	–
croton oil	–
croton oil followed by subcarcinogenic dose of hydrocarbon	–
subcarcinogenic dose of hydrocarbon followed by croton oil	+++

Fig. 31.3   Initiation and promotion of neoplasms in a mouse skin model.

Unless the DNA damage is quickly repaired, and provided the target cell is a 'stem' cell and not a fully differentiated one, the effect on the DNA is permanent and inheritable, even though there is no detectable change in the cell phenotype.

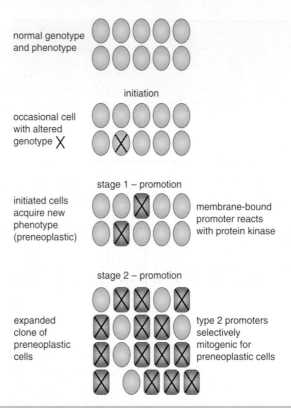

normal genotype
and phenotype

initiation

occasional cell
with altered
genotype X

stage 1 – promotion

initiated cells
acquire new
phenotype
(preneoplastic)

membrane-bound
promoter reacts
with protein kinase

stage 2 – promotion

expanded
clone of
preneoplastic
cells

type 2 promoters
selectively
mitogenic for
preneoplastic cells

Fig. 31.4   Initiation and promotion – a multistep process.

Promotion

The promotion phase in multistep carcinogenesis is brought about by agents that catalyse biochemical events in both normal and initiated cells, leading to an altered pattern of gene expression. In the case of **initiated cells**, this results in the expression of cells with a new phenotype; these cells must be regarded as being **preneoplastic**.

If exposure to the promoter is short-lived, the preneoplastic cells will not increase in number relative to their normal neighbours. The phenotypic changes that have occurred may not be identified easily because only a few cells are affected.

If exposure to the promoting agent is continued, or if the promoter is replaced by another agent capable of causing an increase in cell turnover and hence hyperplasia, there will be a concomitant increase in the number of the initiated and promoted (preneoplastic) cells. A histologically detectable tumour may develop. In the mouse skin model, such a tumour will be a benign papilloma.

It is believed that a further event is necessary for the benign focus of preneoplastic cells to be transformed into an invasive neoplasm. This event will also produce an inheritable change in the genome of affected cells; it may involve either a further biochemical alteration of DNA, some transposition of genetic material, or activation of part of the genome to produce a portion of DNA capable of inducing malignant transformation (an oncogene – see pp. 484–488).

Promotion itself is not a single-stage process

Promotion can be divided into two stages:

1) There is an early phase (stage 1 promotion), which can be brought about by diterpene esters such as 12-*o*-tetradecanoylphorbol-13 acetate (TPA).
2) A later, less specific, phase (stage 2 promotion) occurs, in which other compounds such as turpentine are active.

Specific inhibitors exist for each of these phases. In initiated skin, only a single exposure to promoters that have both stage 1 and stage 2 actions is required for tumours to develop. For the same result, multiple exposures to stage 2 promoters are necessary.

Promotion as a biochemical event

Different biochemical events underlie initiation, stage 1 promotion and stage 2 promotion. Initiating carcinogens react with cellular DNA, while the target for stage 1 promoters is the surface membrane of the cell. High-affinity receptors have been identified for TPA and other promoters on cell surface membranes in many tissues and in many species. The binding of a stage 1 promoter to such a receptor sets off alterations in membrane phospholipid metabolism and in the structure and function of the membrane. The binding site for TPA appears to be the specific calcium- and lipid-binding protein kinase C.

When TPA binds to this enzyme and activates it, phosphorylation of serine and threonine residues in specific cell proteins occurs. *The state of phosphorylation of these proteins is the crucial factor mediating the activity of various hormone and growth factors.* Thus TPA is acting on the cell surface membrane in much the same way as insulin, epidermal growth factor or platelet-derived growth factor, all of which bind to another protein kinase (tyrosine kinase). The effects of TPA on these processes take place very rapidly, but are not by themselves sufficient to bring about tumour development. For this, stage 2 events are also necessary.

Stage 2 promotion is dependent on prolonged exposure to the promoting compound and on sustained cell proliferation, which enables the growth potential of the latent tumour cells to be expressed. Stage 2 promoters induce **enzymes**, the products of which increase the speed of cell division. The enzyme that appears to be particularly concerned is **ornithine decarboxylase (ODC)**, which is the rate-limiting enzyme for the synthesis of certain polyamines that have a role in the synthesis of DNA, RNA and protein. Further investigation has shown that most growth-promoting stimuli (e.g. growth-promoting hormones, epidermal growth factor, partial hepatectomy) induce ODC and also act as stage 2 promoters.

Not all enhancers of tumour development are promoters

Many factors other than stage 1 or 2 promoters can enhance the production of tumours. Some operate by increasing the efficiency with which the active metabolite of an initiating carcinogen is presented to the target cell, whereas others may modify the physiological response of the host to the presence of developing tumour cells. The latter include a wide range of factors, which may be nutritional or may affect immune surveillance mechanisms.

Initiation and promotion occur in tumour formation apart from the mouse skin model

In experimental bladder cancer, saccharin, cyclamates and some metabolites of tryptophan fulfil many of the criteria for a compound to be labelled as a promoter. Induction of ODC in cultured bladder urothelium has been shown after treatment of the cells with saccharin. These data suggest that mechanisms similar to those identified in the mouse skin model may act in this different situation.

The importance of retaining the concept of initiation and promotion in relation to human neoplasms rests chiefly on the realization that a long period of promotion may be part of the natural history of the development of many neoplasms. In some instances, the promotion process may be reversible: this may offer the chance to deploy novel treatment strategies such as the use of retinoids (which inhibit stage 2 promotion) to modify the natural history of neoplasms such as carcinoma of the bladder.

HORMONES AND NEOPLASIA

Recognition of the possibility that the hormonal milieu might play some part in the natural history of cancer dates back to 1895, when Beatson in Glasgow removed the ovaries from a woman with recurrent breast cancer and found that the tumour regressed. This observation suggested that at least some breast cancers were oestrogen dependent; this hypothesis has received considerable support from both human and animal studies.

A single dose of the carcinogen dimethyl-benz(a)anthracene, given either intravenously or via a stomach tube, produces carcinoma of the breast in rats. *If the animal has been ovariectomized before the carcinogen is given, no tumour is produced.* Ovariectomy has a similar inhibiting effect in relation to the tumours produced by the mouse mammary tumour virus. In addition, tumours occurring after administration of dimethyl-benz(a)anthracene regress following ovariectomy. In contrast, if prolactin levels in the rats are raised by giving them drugs of the phenothiazine group, there is an acceleration in the growth of breast tumours. Data of this type suggest that this model of breast carcinoma is hormonally dependent, but do not rule out the possibility that the hormones mentioned may also act as promoters.

Hormones in human breast cancer

A link between ovarian function and human breast cancer is suggested by the increased risk encountered in those who had an early menarche, a delayed first pregnancy (or no pregnancies) and a prolonged period of menstrual activity. It is also true that ablation of ovarian function, whether by surgical, radiotherapeutic or pharmacological means, induces remission, at least temporarily, in a proportion of cases of breast cancer in humans. However, there is at best only conflicting evidence that patients (compared with controls) have high circulating levels of either oestrogen or prolactin.

A relationship has been noted between urinary levels of aetiocholanolone (C19 steroids) and the natural history of patients with breast cancer. When the levels of these steroids excreted in the urine are low, the prognosis is generally, poor; these patients also show a poor response to removal of the ovaries.

Of equal interest has been the recognition of oestrogen receptor sites on certain tumour cells. The oestrogen-binding protein is believed to form part of a two-step process in which oestradiol is bound in the cell and transported to the nucleus. Absence of these receptors from the majority of cells in an individual breast cancer indicates that the response to endocrine therapy is likely to be poor.

Carcinoma of the endometrium

The suggestion that the development of endometrial carcinoma is influenced by oestrogenic steroids is supported by the following data.

Oestrogen-producing tumours of the ovary are frequently associated with endometrial hyperplasia. In some of these patients carcinoma of the endometrium supervenes.

Carcinoma of the endometrium and of the breast occur in the same patient more frequently than would be expected if the association was a chance one.

Administration of oestrogen-containing compounds (hormone replacement therapy) in postmenopausal women is associated with an increased risk of endometrial hyperplasia and carcinoma.

There is an increased risk of endometrial carcinoma in obese females. It is said that 50% of patients with endometrial cancer weigh more than 82 kg (180 lb). This association is believed to be due to the fact that precursor steroids for oestrone, such as Δ-4-androstenedione, are converted in adipose tissue. This conversion rate is twice as high in postmenopausal women as in those still in active reproductive life, and obesity has a marked incremental effect.

Conversion of Δ-4-androstenedione to oestrone is also increased in diabetic females; here too the risk of endometrial cancer is greater than in non-diabetic, age- and weight-matched peers.

It seems likely, therefore, that carcinoma of the endometrium can be regarded as one in which a certain degree of hormone dependency is present and in which oestrogenic steroids may also exert a promotional effect.

Other neoplasms are recognized in which hormones influence the natural history of the disease

Carcinoma of the prostate, like carcinoma of the breast and endometrium, is a neoplasm that has its peak incidence at a time when involution of the tissue could normally be expected. The prostate is clearly a hormone-dependent organ.

Another interesting example of the influence of hormones on tumour genesis is the rather curious **clear-cell adenocarcinoma of the vagina**, which occurred in the daughters of some women given diethylstilboestrol in the course of pregnancy.

PHYSICAL AGENTS IN ONCOGENESIS

ULTRAVIOLET IRRADIATION

The association between skin cancer and exposure to sunlight was reported more than 100 years ago. Epidemiological observations suggesting a role for ultraviolet light as the responsible agent were supported by the induction of skin tumours in rats exposed to ultraviolet irradiation in 1928. Ultraviolet light is a low-energy form of emission and does not penetrate deeply, so the skin absorbs most of the energy and hence is the primary target for this form of carcinogenesis.

Evidence of an aetiological role for sunlight in skin carcinoma is very strong. Most such neoplasms occur in exposed areas. They are relatively infrequent in dark-skinned races, in whom the ultraviolet radiation is filtered out by melanin, and are common in fair-skinned people. The prevalence of malignant tumours of the skin in the fair-skinned appears to be associated with the intensity of solar radiation and is increased in regions close to the Equator. The mechanism responsible for the induction of such neoplasms is likely to be associated with the production of abnormal thymine dimers in the DNA of the epidermal cells and perhaps the lack of efficient excision repair of the abnormal DNA, such as is seen in **xeroderma pigmentosum** (see pp. 514–515).

The most common sunshine-related neoplasms are **basal cell carcinomas**, which may invade locally but almost never metastasize, **squamous carcinoma**, which may both invade the surrounding tissues and metastasize, and **malignant melanoma**, which is often highly malignant and is capable of spreading very widely.

IONIZING RADIATION

It has been recognized since the early part of the century that ionizing radiation constitutes a risk factor for the subsequent development of cancer (see pp. 26–29). In humans this is seen under a number of different circumstances:

- There was an increased prevalence of both leukaemia and skin cancer in radiologists who, during the early days of diagnostic radiology, were inadequately protected.
- There is a greater than normal frequency of leukaemia and carcinoma of the thyroid, breast and lung among the survivors of the nuclear explosions over Hiroshima and Nagasaki.
- There is an increased risk of carcinoma of the thyroid in people who have had irradiation to the neck during childhood.
- There is an increased risk of osteosarcoma following ingestion of bone-seeking radioactive substances.
- A thorium-containing contrast medium, **Thorotrast**, was used to outline the margins of abscess cavities in the 1940s. The prevalence of malignant tumours in patients investigated in this way is about twice as high as would normally be expected, with a sixfold increase in leukaemia and liver neoplasm.

The mechanisms by which ionizing radiation induces malignant transformation are not clear. Irradiation causes free radical generation (see pp. 11–14), and these very active chemical species may react with elements of the target cell genome. Certainly irradiation can produce obvious changes in chromosome morphology and is mutagenic to cultured cells. In at least one model – a virus-induced leukaemia in the mouse – irradiation may activate viral oncogenes and bring about transformation in this way.

FOREIGN MATERIALS

Certain foreign substances are capable of inducing the formation of connective tissue neoplasms when implanted, usually subcutaneously, into the tissues of a variety of animals. The precise physical form in which these foreign materials exist appears to be of fundamental importance in relation to tumour induction. For example, sheets of certain plastics evoke a brisk fibrous tissue response when inserted subcutaneously, which eventually leads to the formation of low-grade fibrosarcomas. If the same plastic sheeting is ground up and then inserted into the connective tissue of the same species, no tumours result. Similarly, if holes are made in the sheeting before insertion, the likelihood of tumour formation decreases; the diminution of risk appears to be associated with the size of the holes. This has been studied using millipore filters as the tumour-provoking agent. If the filter has a pore size greater than 0.22 μm, no tumours appear. The mechanisms involved in this curious form of oncogenesis are not known and there is, as yet, no evidence that the prosthetic materials widely used in surgical practice confer any increased risk of neoplasia.

VIRUSES AND NEOPLASIA

It has been known since 1908 that certain tumours in animals can be caused by viruses. It was recognized at that time that a variety of fowl leukaemia could be transmitted by cell-free extracts of tumour tissue. This discovery was followed by the pioneering studies of Peyton Rous, who found that cell-free extracts of chicken sarcomas produced identical tumours when injected subcutaneously into other chickens.

Viruses that are capable of inducing neoplasms are known as **oncogenic viruses**. Oncogenic viruses are found among both the **DNA** and the **RNA viruses**.

DNA ONCOGENIC VIRUSES

The best-authenticated DNA oncogenic viruses come from three groups:

1) the **papova** group (see p. 312)
2) the **herpes** group
3) the **hepatitis** group.

The papova group

Papillomaviruses

The first virally induced mammalian neoplasm to be recognized was the so-called Shope papilloma, a curious warty lesion on the tails of Kentucky cotton-tailed rabbits. This neoplasm can be passaged in the same way as the Rous sarcoma but, in the case of the Shope papillomavirus, the host response makes a considerable difference to the natural history of an infection. If wild cotton-tailed rabbits are infected with the virus, tumours grow slowly and are usually benign, and free virus can be harvested from the horny layer of infected skin. If, on the other hand, domestic strains of the rabbit are infected, the tumours are rapidly growing, some of them become frankly malignant, and free virus cannot be harvested from the cells. Thus cell-free extracts from tumours in the domestic strain cannot be passaged.

In humans, papillomaviruses are the only ones that have been *proved* without doubt to cause neoplasms. The lesions associated with wart virus infections are the common skin wart, anal and genital warts (**condylomata acuminata**) and cancer of the uterine cervix.

Polyomaviruses

Polyomavirus, a large DNA virus, causes a wide variety of neoplasms in a variety of small animals (mice, rabbits, rats, hamsters) when they are infected in the neonatal period. Adult members of susceptible species are immune unless they have been neonatally thymectomized. This observation suggests an effective degree of T-cell surveillance of cells transformed by the virus. A number of different tumours in various anatomical sites have been described following infection with this virus, hence the name 'polyoma'. There is no evidence of any involvement of polyomaviruses in human neoplasia.

Simian vacuolating virus (SV40)

This virus was discovered in 1960 in the kidney cell cultures used to produce the first polio vaccine. In the course of immunization against poliomyelitis, some thousands of people had also been inoculated with the SV40 virus. Later it was shown that the virus could induce tumours in newborn hamsters and transform human cells in culture. However, no evidence has yet accrued that could lead to this virus being implicated in human neoplasia.

SV40 enters the affected cells through the action of its coat proteins; after uncoating, either the whole or part of the viral genome is inserted into the host DNA. Transcription of the viral DNA takes place in two waves, the earlier messenger RNA being derived from codons responsible for transformation as well as for viral replication.

Herpesvirus in neoplasia

Viruses of the herpes group are certainly responsible for the production of at least one important malignant neoplasm in poultry, and are probably involved in two or more neoplastic diseases in humans.

In chickens, a herpesvirus causes a variety of malignant lymphoma known as **Marek's disease**. Infection with this virus can be economically disastrous unless the birds have been immunized with an attenuated form of the virus, because, unlike most oncogenic animal viruses, the virus of Marek's disease spreads horizontally and is very contagious. Although the cell that undergoes malignant transformation is almost certainly a T lymphocyte, the virus invades epithelial cells in the skin in association with the feather sockets, and is shed from the skin.

ONCOGENIC RNA VIRUSES

The role of the oncogenic RNA viruses as a group is discussed in the section dealing with oncogenes (see pp. 489–493). However, one RNA virus does merit consideration separately – the **mouse mammary tumour virus**. A viral aetiology for breast cancer in the mouse was first proposed following the observations of Bittner in 1936, who studied strains of mice known to have a high prevalence of carcinoma of the breast. Bittner found that the tendency to develop breast cancer could not be ascribed wholly to the genetic make-up of the hybrid strain he was studying and that the **female parent type** was the most important factor. Furthermore, if baby mice from a strain of high prevalence were delivered by caesarean section and suckled by a mother of a low prevalence strain, the young mice did not develop carcinoma of the breast to any appreciable extent when they grew to maturity. Conversely, when the progeny of a low prevalence strain were suckled by a mother of a high prevalence strain, the frequency of breast cancer in these young mice was uncharacteristically high. These data suggested that the oncogenic agent was being **vertically transmitted** via the milk. Confirmation of this hypothesis came when viral particles were demonstrated on electron microscopy of the milk from high prevalence mothers.

In view of the commonness of breast cancer in human females, and the many recorded cases of breast cancer occurring in several members of one family, it is easy to understand why the possibility of a viral aetiology has been enthusiastically canvassed.

Some evidence has come to light that might link the data obtained from the mouse model to the human situation. Particles similar to those seen in the milk of strains of mice with a high cancer prevalence have been identified both in human breast milk and in breast tissue. One report suggests that such particles can be found more frequently in groups of women in whom there is a higher than expected prevalence of breast cancer, such as the Parsee community in Bombay. Serum from some patients with breast cancer has been shown to contain antibodies that bind to the virus-like particles seen on electron microscopy of breast tissue. However, these data are far from conclusive and the case for a viral factor in carcinogenesis of the human breast is not yet proven.

VIRUSES IN HUMAN NEOPLASIA

While viruses are thought to have a causal role in only a few types of human neoplasia, some of them are very common; thus, on a world-wide basis, up to 20% of human cancers may have a viral aetiology. Much of our appreciation of this fact is based on the striking geographical distribution of certain neoplasms and the concordance between this distribution and the prevalence of certain viral infections. Examples include:

- hepatocellular carcinoma and hepatitis B infections
- human T-cell leukaemia virus (HTLV) type 1 infection and adult T-cell leukaemia.

Epstein–Barr virus and neoplasia

Infections by the Epstein–Barr virus (EBV) have been implicated in a number of human neoplastic diseases, some of the most important of which are discussed below.

Burkitt's lymphoma
Burkitt's lymphoma occurs with great frequency in certain parts of tropical Africa, where its distribution is strikingly circumscribed to areas in which malaria is holoendemic (50% of children reaching the age of 7 show evidence of malaria) and where climatic conditions favour the anopheline mosquito.

EBV infection is very common; about 90% of the world's population is believed to be infected. The virus binds to the CD21 receptor on B lymphocytes but can also infect epithelial cells.

If the EBV is as prevalent as epidemiological data suggest, it seems remarkable that Burkitt's lymphoma should, on the whole, be so circumscribed. The data suggest that the difference is to be found in the host response to EBV infection. In view of the fact that malaria is known to be immunosuppressive, it seems probable that African Burkitt's lymphoma represents a malaria-related failure of immune surveillance. This view is strengthened by the observation that people who bear the **sickle cell trait**, and who are thus resistant to malaria, also have a reduced risk of developing Burkitt's lymphoma.

Translocation in Burkitt's lymphoma.   Burkitt lymphoma cells are characterized by a translocation which most commonly involves chromosomes 8 and 14. The breakpoint on the long arm of chromosome 8 is at the site of a proto-oncogene known as c-*myc*. In the course of the translocation the c-*myc* gene comes to lie adjacent to the gene encoding the heavy chain for immunoglobulin and is thus abnormally activated (see p. 486).

Nasopharyngeal carcinoma

An association has also been found between EBV and a curious lympho-epithelial neoplasm found in the nasopharynx. Like Burkitt's lymphoma, this tumour shows a distinctive geographical distribution, being prevalent in China (especially southern China) and some other parts of south-east Asia. The clustering of cases of this tumour, not only within this area but within people originating from it, has been recognized for more than 300 years; indeed, it has led to the disease being termed Kwantung tumour by some, because it is so prevalent in Kwantung province.

On histological examination the neoplasm is seen to consist of two cell lines, one a poorly differentiated epithelial cell and the other a lympho-blastoid cell. EBV can be found in cell lines cultured from both these components, and the patients show high titres of EBV antibodies.

Why should this widely prevalent virus be related to a malignant neoplasm only in a circumscribed geographical area? There is no evidence of an **exogenous modifier** of the host response such as exists in the association between malaria and Burkitt's lymphoma. The possibility remains that a genetic factor may be operating in the case of the nasopharyngeal carcinoma. Support for this view comes from the fact that emigration from the affected areas of Asia does not appear to lessen the risk and that clustering of human leucocyte antigen (HLA) A2 occurs in the people in high-risk areas.

EBV has also been implicated in:

- immunoblastic-type B-cell lymphomas in immunosuppressed individuals (e.g. in those with acquired immune deficiency syndrome)

- Hodgkin's disease (EBV sequences are found in Reed–Sternberg cells in many cases)
- certain rare T-cell lymphomas.

EBV effects on B cells that may be associated with its malignant potential

In human B lymphocytes in culture, infection by EBV results in immortalization of the cell line, an effect that appears to be due to six viral proteins – Epstein–Barr nuclear antigen (EBNA) 1, 2, 3A, 3C, LP, and the virally encoded lymphocyte membrane protein LMP-1. The LMP-1 protein is the only EBV-encoded protein that can transform cells in culture and it is presumably important in EBV-associated malignancy.

Carcinoma of the uterine cervix and human papillomavirus

Epidemiological studies indicate that there is an association between carcinoma of the uterine cervix and the individual level of sexual activity. Virginity, a currently unfashionable state, appears significantly to reduce the risk of cervical cancer; conversely, an early start to sexual activity and widespread distribution of favours increase the risk of subsequent development of squamous carcinoma of the cervix.

Infection with most types of human papillomavirus, of which there are many, usually gives rise to benign and self-limiting epithelial proliferation (e.g viral warts on the hands and feet). Some strains, however, most notably 16 and 18, carry a considerable risk of malignancy, especially in the genital region and most particularly the uterine cervix.

Over 90% of cases of frank cervical cancer and intraepithelial cervical neoplasia show signs of human papillomavirus infection. In young, sexually active women with normal cervical cytology, this frequency drops to about 25%.

The circular, double-stranded DNA, human papillomavirus genome encodes eight major open reading frames (ORFs). Three of these ORFs (E5, E6 and E7) encode proteins that, in cell culture systems, have transforming properties. E6 and E7 complex with and inactivate the p53 and retinoblastoma (RB) proteins respectively (see pp. 504, 506). Thus intracellular expression of viral E6 and E7 proteins has the same effect as somatic mutations of the *p53* and *RB* tumour suppressor genes. E5 encodes a small protein localized chiefly in cell membranes; this appears to function by enhancing the activity of cell surface receptors for growth factors such as epidermal growth factor.

Hepatitis B virus (HBV)

This ubiquitous virus is responsible for one of the more serious varieties of infective hepatitis. The presence of a carrier state (which can be established by identifying the surface antigen of the virus in plasma) can be found in 10–20% of those who become infected with the virus. A significant positive correlation exists between the prevalence of the carrier state and the frequency with which liver cell cancer is seen. In addition, in parts of the world where prevalence of the tumour is high, the carrier rate is about 90% in those with liver cell cancer.

A virus resembling HBV has been found to cause hepatitis in woodchucks, and liver cell carcinoma is not infrequently seen in this species. DNA hybridization techniques have revealed woodchuck virus DNA incorporated within the liver cell genome. Similar observations in respect of the human virus have been made in relation to human cell lines derived from liver cell cancers. These data are strongly suggestive of an oncogenic role for human HBV.

The HBV genome consists of four ORFs: P (encoding reverse transcriptase), C (encoding the core antigen), S (three viral envelope proteins) and X (a transcriptional regulator).

The mechanism by which HBV contributes to malignant transformation is still unknown. Some have suggested that malignancy is due to the repeated cell death and regeneration characteristic of chronic infections. Evidence is beginning to accumulate that the virus may encode some transforming sequences, the current favourite being the X gene.

The X protein functions as a transcription regulator in an unusual and indirect way. It activates protein kinase C and *raf*-1-kinase, both of which play a key role in signal transduction. Thus X expression leads to a signalling cascade which nevertheless requires to be started off by a growth factor–receptor interaction. It has also been suggested that protein X might mimic the function of chemical tumour promoters such as phorbol esters (see p. 529), thus providing a large population of dividing cells in which somatic mutations are likely to become 'fixed'.

Human T-cell leukaemia virus

HTLV-1 infections are rare in most parts of the world. In the USA only 0.025% of the general population are carriers. In southern Japan, the Caribbean, parts of Africa and South America, the prevalence is much higher, reaching 30% in some areas of Japan.

The virus is linked with two diseases:

1) adult T-cell leukaemia; there is a risk that 2% of infected individuals will develop this disorder during their lifetime
2) a neurological disorder – tropical spastic paraparesis.

The chief cellular target is the T helper cell (CD4), about 1–2% of peripheral cells being infected in a typical case.

ONCOGENESIS

- **Genetic factors** are clearly important in some neoplasms. These syndromes may be familial and may represent syndromes with a major chromosomal abnormality (e.g. increased risk of cancer of male breast in Klinefelter's syndrome) or with a single gene abnormality. Some of the neoplasms may be associated with a recognizable 'precursor' syndrome (e.g. xeroderma pigmentosum, ataxia telangiectasia or familial polyposis coli).
- Exposure to a wide range of **chemicals** may increase cancer risk. These include polycyclic hydrocarbons (e.g. tars found in cigarette smoke), aromatic amines and azo dyes and naturally occurring carcinogens such as the toxin in *Aspergillus flavus*.
- Chemical carcinogenesis is a multistep process involving genomic changes (initiation) and changes in the expression of the altered genes (promotion).
- Other factors influencing the risk of cancer include the hormonal milieu (e.g. high oestrogen levels post-menopausally are associated with an increased risk of endometrial cancer), ultraviolet and ionizing radiation, and certain viral infections (e.g. human papilloma virus which is associated with increased risks for cervical cancer).

32 Genetic disorders

A disease may arise because of:

- a genetic abnormality acting alone
- unfavourable environmental factors
- both of the above.

The term 'genetic disorders' covers a set of diseases in which the manifestations are **either wholly or partly due to abnormalities within the genetic material**. These include:

- major chromosomal abnormalities
- single gene defects
- multifactorial disorders
- somatic genetic disorders
- mitochondrial genetic disorders.

Major chromosomal abnormalities. Some of these are associated with highly characteristic clinical syndromes such as Down's syndrome or Turner's syndrome. Such disorders may affect either autosomal or sex chromosomes. Most occur as *de novo* events and are not inherited.

Single gene defects. These are caused either by a mutation in a single allele or in both alleles of a pair. **Single** allele mutations which are expressed clinically are known as **dominant**; mutations that require **both** members of an allelic pair to be affected before the disorder is expressed are known as **recessive**. Either autosomal or sex chromosomes can be affected. Inheritance patterns give valuable clues as to whether the disease is dominant or recessive and whether autosomal or sex chromosomes are involved.

Multifactorial disorders. These are associated with certain congenital developmental disorders and with some common and important conditions including diabetes mellitus, atherosclerosis and its related clinical syndromes, and cancer. Many of these involve interaction between inherited and environmental factors; the relationship between these is complex and poorly understood.

Somatic genetic disorders.   These result from mutations arising in certain somatic cells, largely as a result of exposure to unfavourable environmental factors. Since they affect somatic rather than germ cells, such mutations are not inherited and thus cannot give rise to the disease in the succeeding generation. They are commonly associated with tumour formation and, as in the previous category, often involve interactions between environment and inherited genetic susceptibility.

Mitochondrial genetic disorders.   These are rare. They result from mutations in mitochondrial DNA, which is distinct from the chromosomal DNA lying within the cell nucleus. *These disorders are transmitted only through the maternal line. The pattern of inheritance does not follow Mendelian lines; all the offspring of an affected mother are affected.*

CHROMOSOMAL DISORDERS

THE NORMAL KARYOTYPE

Normal human cells contain 46 chromosomes (44 autosomal; 2 sex chromosomes known as X and Y). The possession of a Y chromosome confers male gender. Thus females are XX and males XY in respect of their sex chromosomes. Each chromosome has a constricted area – the **centromere**. The material above the centromere is known as the p (petit) or short arm and that below the centromere as the q (long) arm. The region at the end of each arm is known as the **telomere**. The position of the centromere (*Fig. 32.1*) serves to divide chromosomes into three groups:

- metacentric
- submetacentric
- acrocentric.

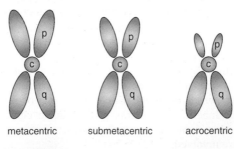

metacentric   submetacentric   acrocentric

c = centromere
p = short arm
q = long arm

Fig. 32.1   Three basic morphological types of chromosome.

Table 32.1 Chromosome types

Type based on position of centromere	Chromosome
Metacentric	1, 3, 16, 19, 20
Submetacentric	2, 4, 5, 6, 7, 8, 9, 10, 11, 12, 17, 18, 23, X
Acrocentric	13, 14, 15, 21, 22, Y

The distribution of the chromosomes in these three groups is shown in *Table 32.1*.

During mitosis chromosomes replicate; each 'daughter' cell possesses the normal diploid number (46 chromosomes). Division in germ cells (meiosis or reduction division) leads to the formation of cells that possess half the normal complement of chromosomes (23 chromosomes – the haploid number). Ova and sperm thus contain one copy of each autosome and, in the case of sperm, either an X or Y sex chromosome. All ova, of course, contain X chromosomes.

Analysis of chromosomes (karyotyping)

The number and morphology of chromosomes may be determined by studying samples of any tissue which may be grown in cell or tissue culture. In many cases blood lymphocytes are used but data are also obtained from amniotic fluid cells, chorionic villus samples, bone marrow, or fibroblasts derived from skin biopsy.

In the case of blood samples, T lymphocytes are induced to transform and proliferate by adding the mitogen phytohaemagglutinin. After 48–72 hours, mitosis is stopped in metaphase by colchicine which interferes with spindle formation by microtubules. Swelling of the cells following the addition of a hypotonic solution separates the chromosomes, and a fixative is then added before drops of the cell suspension are spread on slides.

Preparations are stained with the Giemsa stain which produces a pattern of alternating dark and light bands. This allows the microscopic resolution of 300–500 bands that form the basis for categorizing the different regions of the chromosome. The stained bands are divided into seven groups from the centromere outwards and each band within a group is also numbered.

Thus the nomenclature used to describe a region on a chromosome uses:

- the **number** of the chromosome, e.g. 4
- whether the region is on the **short (p) arm** or the **long (q) arm**, e.g. q.
- the **group** of the band, e.g. 3
- the **number of the band within the group**, e.g. 4.

This region therefore would be called 4q34.

If dividing cells are harvested during prometaphase instead of during metaphase the resolution obtained by staining is greatly increased and up to 1500 bands can be identified.

Gene mapping

Banding techniques are relatively crude. Ordinary Giemsa banding permits resolution of bands containing 4000–5000 kilobases of genomic DNA. Arresting cells in prometaphase improves this by a factor of two but 2000 kb is still much larger than the size of most genes (e.g. the cystic fibrosis gene is 250 kb).

Modern techniques enable mapping of some genes to the correct regions of their chromosomes; more than 2000 autosomal genes and more than 200 X-linked genes have been correctly assigned. Such gene mapping pays useful dividends both in prenatal diagnosis and in the cloning of genes recognized only as a result of gross effects on phenotype.

The methods most commonly used in gene mapping are:

- in situ hybridization
- somatic cell hybridization.

In situ hybridization.   In situ hybridization is used to localize a cloned DNA sequence to a specific chromosome. It depends on the fact that a single strand of the cloned sequence (or probe) will bind to its complementary sequence on a denatured chromosome. The probe can be labelled either with a radioactive marker or a fluorescent dye. The labelled probe is applied to a spread of prometaphase or, better still, interphase chromosomes.

Hybridization can be demonstrated either by autoradiography or by examining the spread in UV light. The use of fluorescent labels carries with it the advantages of technical simplicity and the fact that more than one probe may be used simultaneously provided that each is labelled with a different fluorescent marker. This technique is known as chromosome painting.

Somatic cell hybridization.   Fusion of human cell lines with mouse cell lines results in the formation of hybrid cells that possess both human and murine chromosomes. When these hybrids are passaged they preferentially shed human chromosomes; this occurs in a random fashion. Eventually the hybrids become stable and will maintain their complement of human chromosomes for several passages. The establishment of several different hybrid cell lines provides a panel of cells possessing different complements of human chromosomes. Such hybrids may be used to look for certain human proteins in cell homogenates. If the proteins are present, the cell line must contain the genes which code for them. Examination of the positive cell lines will narrow the possible gene localizations to a few chromosomes and, ultimately, to the chromosome on which the protein is coded.

Alternatively, the hybrid cells may be used to hybridize DNA from the different cell lines to radiolabelled copies of probes which represent the gene, whose location is being searched for.

Genomic imprinting and chromosomes

Our ideas on the transmission of human genetic disorders are largely based on the theory that the parental origin of a mutant gene is irrelevant insofar as the expression of the abnormal phenotype is concerned. Thus in an autosomal dominant disease, affected fathers or affected mothers have a 50% chance of an affected child. There are however some exceptions. *Chromosomes, regions of chromosomes or even specific genes can be influenced in some way during germ cell lineage so that the expression of a phenotypic abnormality depends on the parental origin of the mutant gene or genes. This is known as genomic imprinting.* It may be expressed in the following ways:

- the existence of chromosome sets
- uniparental chromosomes
- deletion of the same regions of either paternally or maternally derived chromosomes, producing different phenotypic effects.

The existence of chromosome sets. In hydatidiform mole the chromosome number is normal but there are two haploid sets of chromosomes derived from the father. In ovarian teratoma, again the chromosome complement is uniparental but both haploid sets are derived from the mother.

Uniparental chromosomes. This term describes a situation in which both copies of an individual chromosome are derived from one parent. This is difficult to establish in humans but has been documented in two cases of cystic fibrosis and short stature, in which both copies of chromosome 7 were maternally derived.

Deletion of the same regions of either paternally or maternally derived chromosomes produces different phenotypic effects. The classic example of genomic imprinting in human genetic disease is embodied in two disorders, cytogenetically identical but clinically distinct:

1. the Angelman syndrome
2. the Prader–Willi syndrome.

Angelman syndrome ('happy puppet' syndrome) is characterized by:

- severe motor and intellectual retardation
- ataxia
- a facies with a large mandible and protruding tongue
- hypotonia.

Patients with **Prader–Willi syndrome** show:

- neonatal hypotonia
- failure to thrive
- obesity
- short stature
- mild to moderate mental retardation.

In about 50% of the cases of each of these disorders there is a deletion of part of the long arm of chromosome 15 (15q11–13). The affected region appears to be the same in both disorders. In Angelman syndrome, the deletion affects the maternally derived chromosome; in Prader–Willi syndrome it is the paternally derived chromosome which is affected.

MAJOR CHROMOSOMAL ABNORMALITIES

Chromosome abnormalities cause some very well-recognized syndromes such as Down's syndrome and Turner's syndrome. They are also important causes of fetal loss: spontaneous abortion occurs in about 15–20% of all pregnancies, and 50% of these abortions are associated with chromosome abnormalities. It is estimated that, overall, about 6% of human conceptions show chromosomal abnormalities.

The frequency of chromosomal abnormality at birth is 5.6/1000. The abnormalities are listed in *Table 32.2*.

ABNORMALITIES IN CHROMOSOME STRUCTURE (*Fig. 32.2*)

Most chromosomal structural abnormalities represent breakage; this may be followed either by loss of genetic material (deletions) or by rearrangement of such material.

Deletions

Losses of chromosomal material cannot be seen on microscopy unless at least 4000 kilobases have been lost; thus the visual identification of a deletion indicates the loss of a great deal of genetic material. This may have crippling effects on development or impair the chances of survival.

Deletion of the short arm of chromosome 5 produces a very characteristic syndrome in the newborn. It is known as the **cri du chat** syndrome because of the typical mewing, kitten-like cry of the affected infants. These children show:

- a round facies
- a small head (microcephaly)
- mental retardation.

Ring chromosome formation

This results from breakages occurring at both extremes of a chromosome with fusion of the truncated ends. It should be regarded as a form of deletion. Usually there is significant loss of genetic material with serious consequences in respect of mental capacity and the chances of congenital malformations.

Table 32.2   Chromosomal abnormalities at birth

Abnormality	Frequency per 1000 births
Abnormal number of sex chromosomes	2
Abnormal number of autosomes	1.7
Structural abnormalities (deletions, translocations, etc.)	1.9

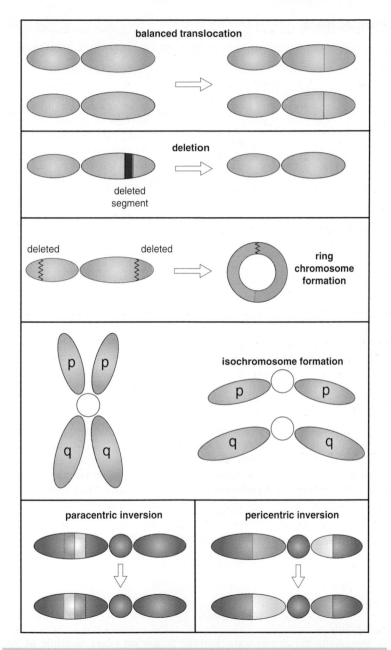

Fig. 32.2 Structural abnormalities in chromosomes.

Translocations

In translocation, a segment broken from one chromosome is transferred to another.

Balanced translocation

In balanced translocation segments break off from two separate chromosomes and are reciprocally transferred. As a result, no loss of genetic material occurs and the affected individual is phenotypically normal. These individuals are, however, at increased risk of producing abnormal offspring since the existence of translocated chromosomal material makes possible the formation of abnormal gametes during meiosis.

Robertsonian translocation

Robertsonian translocation occurs when there is a balanced translocation between two acrocentric chromosomes. The breaks usually affect a long arm in one of the chromosomes and the short arm in the other. The transfer of chromosomal material generally causes the formation of one very large chromosome and one very small one.

Isochromosome formation

Isochromosome formation is the end-result of the loss of either a short or long arm of a chromosome and duplication of the lost material. The isochromosome consists either of two short arms or two long arms.

Inversion

Inversion results from the occurrence of two breaks within a single chromosome. This is followed by 180° rotation of the broken segment which is then reincorporated into the parent chromosome. An inversion that affects only one arm of a chromosome is termed paracentric. If the breaks are on either side of the centromere, the inversion is called pericentric. Most inversions do not have any phenotypic effect but may give rise to abnormal gametes.

ABNORMALITIES IN NUMBER OF AUTOSOMES

Such abnormalities fall into two groups:

- aneuploidy
- polyploidy.

Aneuploidy

In aneuploidy the chromosome number is *not* **an exact multiple of 23**. Aneuploidy may be expressed by the presence of one extra chromosome (**trisomy**) or by the loss of one of a pair of chromosomes (**monosomy**). Aneuploidy may affect either autosomes or sex chromosomes. It is most commonly the result of non-disjunction of chromosomes during meiosis but can also occur as a result of delayed movement of one chromosome during anaphase so that it remains outside the nucleus (anaphase lag).

Polyploidy

In polyploidy there is an additional haploid set of chromosomes to give a total complement of 69 (a multiple of 23). This example of polyploidy (known as **triploidy**) is usually associated with early spontaneous abortion.

Autosomal monosomy

Autosomal monosomy is rare in liveborn children since the amount of genetic information lost is generally too great to permit survival. Liveborn children with monosomies are usually severely handicapped and do not survive for long periods. An exception, however, is monosomy of chromosome 21 which is compatible with survival. It is not without interest that children with monosomy 21 develop severe respiratory difficulties when given oxygen in the course of anaesthesia. This is believed to be related to the fact that the gene encoding superoxide dismutase (which catalyses the conversion of the superoxide anion to hydrogen peroxide) is encoded on chromosome 21.

Autosomal trisomies

Down's syndrome (trisomy 21)

Down's syndrome is the commonest numerical chromosomal abnormality occurring in the newborn. It is also the commonest genetically determined cause of mental retardation.

The overall frequency of Down's syndrome is 1:800 live births but this does not give a true picture of the risk which, to a considerable extent, is related to the **age of the mother** at conception. In women under 20 years at the time of pregnancy, the risk of Down's syndrome is 1:1550; in a mother who is 45 years or more, the risk is 1:28. The rate of increase in risk is very steep after the age of 35 years. Many Down's syndrome conceptions end in spontaneous abortion. In abortions occurring at 12 weeks the abortus of a mother over the age of 45 years shows a Down's syndrome karyotype in 1:13 cases.

Cytogenetics of Down's syndrome. 95% of Down's syndrome infants show trisomy 21. This is due to non-disjunction of chromosome 21, either at the first or the second meiotic division. Where the non-disjunction has taken place at the second meiotic division, the fetus carries two copies of one of the parental chromosomes 21 and one copy of the other parental chromosome 21. The cause of the non-disjunction or why it should be related to maternal age is unknown. In 95% of cases the non-disjunction affects the maternal chromosome 21.

About 4% of cases of Down's syndrome result from a Robertsonian translocation within either the maternal or the paternal germ cell line of

Table 32.3   Risk of recurrence of Down's syndrome in a parentage in which there is translocation of the long arm of chromosome 21

Translocation	Maternal carrier	Paternal carrier
14;21	15%	1%
21;22	10%	5%

the long arm of chromosome 21 to either chromosome 22 or 14. Thus extra genetic material related to chromosome 21 is provided since the fertilized ovum already contains two normal copies of chromosome 21. In most cases, the translocation is present in the germ cell line of one of the parents and is inherited by the fetus. The 'carriage' of the translocation in a parental germ cell line means that there is a distinct risk that more than one child of the marriage may be affected by Down's syndrome (see *Table 32.3*). In other instances the translocation occurs during the formation of the gamete.

In the remaining 1% of cases of Down's syndrome, the cause is a non-disjunction of chromosome 21 in the dividing cells of the zygote. Not all the cells are affected: the fetus contains some cells showing trisomy 21 and others which have the normal chromosome complement. This is known as **mosaicism**. In these circumstances Down's syndrome children tend to be less severely affected than when the non-disjunction has occurred in the germ cell.

The clinical phenotype of Down's syndrome is summarized in *Table 32.4* (see *Figs 32.3* and *32.4*).

The molecular basis of Down's syndrome.   This is still not understood and probably will not be until all the genes on the long arm of chromosome 21 have been correctly assigned and the functions of their gene products worked out. The region which seems to be of functional importance in the expression of the facial, cardiac and neurological manifestations is 21q22.2 and 21q22.3. This is a large region capable of accommodating some hundreds of genes. Genes assigned to this region include:

- GART, coding for an enzyme implicated in purine metabolism
- *ets*-2, a proto-oncogene
- the gene coding for the cell surface receptor of α and β interferons
- the gene encoding the amyloid precursor protein implicated in Alzheimer's disease.

Other trisomies

Several other trisomies have been described. The two commonest of these (though they are much rarer than Down's syndrome) are **trisomy 18 (Edwards' syndrome)**, and **trisomy 13 (Patau's syndrome)**.

Their features are summarized in *Table 32.5*. The combination of malformations in these syndromes is more severe than that in Down's syndrome

Table 32.4 Clinical features of Down's syndrome

System affected	Clinical features
Face	The face tends to be flat with a low bridged nose and oblique palpebral fissure and prominent epicanthic folds (hence the discarded term for Down's syndrome 'mongolism'). The mouth is often enlarged, possibly because of the enlarged protruding tongue. The tongue itself is coarsely furrowed and lacks the central groove.
Hands	There is a horizontal palmar crease, sometimes called a simian crease. The middle phalanx of the little finger is shorter than normal, thus the finger shows inward curving (clinodactyly).
Long bones	Long bones are shorter than normal and the affected individuals are short. Abnormalities of the rib cage and pelvis may also be seen.
Cardiovascular	Approximately 40% of patients with Down's syndrome show congenital cardiac defects. These include endocardial cushion defects, atrial septal and ventricular septal defects.
Haematological	Down's syndrome patients show a marked increase in risk (10–20 fold) of developing acute leukaemia which may be lymphoblastic or non-lymphoblastic.
Immune	Down's syndrome patients show an increased susceptibility to infections especially those of the lung. The mechanism is unknown.
Central nervous system	Most individuals with Down's syndrome show a severe degree of mental retardation, the IQ being about 50. This is associated with a remarkable sweetness of disposition. In those who survive into the forties, virtually all develop the neuropathological features of Alzheimer's disease. It is not without interest that the gene encoding the amyloid precursor protein found in the neuritic plaques of Alzheimer's disease is located on the long arm of chromosome 21 in the region believed to be of significance in bringing about the changes found in Down's syndrome.

and the affected infants seldom survive longer than one year. Many die within the first few weeks of life.

Syndromes associated with aneuploidy of sex chromosomes

Aneuploidy of sex chromosomes is much commoner than in autosomes. This group of disorders is best understood against a background of some general knowledge on the function and expression of sex chromosomes.

The Y chromosome carries little genetic information other than the gene coding for testicular development (*sry* = sex determining region on Y chromosome) and thus the determination of male sex.

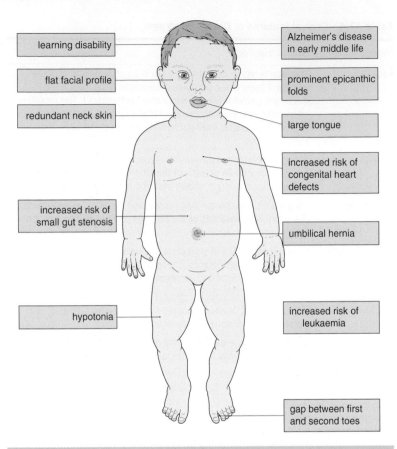

Fig. 32.3   Clinical features of Down's syndrome.

The X chromosome, in contrast, is large and carries much genetic information. Monosomy in respect of X (XO = Turner's syndrome) is certainly compatible with life but its mirror image (YO) leads to a fetus which is not viable.

Since the normal female possesses two X chromosomes she would have a double dose of the genetic information carried on this large chromosome were it not for dosage compensation. This is brought about by inactivation of one X chromosome at about the 16th day of embryonic life; this inactivation occurs in every normal eukaryotic, female, mammalian cell. This process is known as Lyonization (Dr. Mary Lyon described it in 1961). The inactivated X chromosome can be seen on examination of female cells in the form of the **Barr body**. This is a darkly staining small body closely apposed to the nuclear membrane. Since the inactivation is random, it follows that

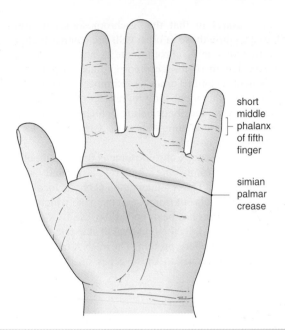

short
middle
phalanx
of fifth
finger

simian
palmar
crease

Fig. 32.4   The hand in Down's syndrome.

Table 32.5   Trisomies 18 and 13

	Edwards' (trisomy 18)	Patau's syndrome (trisomy 13)
Frequency	1:10 000 live births	1:10 000 live births
Chromosome	90% due to non-disjunction; 10% due to mosaicism	80% due to non-disjunction; 10% due to translocation in germ cell line; 10% associated with mosaicism
Clinical features	• Mental retardation • Prominent occiput • Small lower jaw (micrognathia) • Low set ears • Short neck • Overlapping fingers • Congenital heart defects • Kidney and intestinal defects • 'Rocker bottom feet' • Hypertonicity	• Small head (microcephaly) • Mental retardation • Small eye cavities (microphthalmia) • Cleft palate and hare lip • May have more than 5 fingers on each hand (polydactyly) • Dextrocardia and, often, ventricular septal defects • A variety of visceral defects

all females are mosaics in that the X chromosomes in some cells are maternally derived, while those in other cells are paternally derived.

The inactivation of one X chromosome is not total. Many genes distributed along the length of the chromosome are spared and continue to function. This is made clear in Turner's syndrome, in which individuals with an XO karyotype and thus monosomy in respect of X exhibit many abnormalities. In the same way, the abnormalities which result from an individual having more than the normal complement of X chromosomes also indicate that inactivation is never complete.

Inactivation of loci on one X chromosome is brought about by transcription of a gene on the X chromosome which is to be partially inactivated (this is known as acting in cis). The X-inactivation centre is localized to band 13 of the short arm of the X chromosome, and the gene which may be directly responsible for inactivation has been called the XIST (X-inactive-specific-transcript) gene. Its exons show the presence of stop codons, suggesting that this gene does not itself produce protein. The mRNA transcribed from XIST spreads the inactivation signal to those genes on the same chromosome capable of receiving it.

Turner's syndrome

Turner's syndrome results from complete or partial monosomy of the X chromosome in a genotypic and phenotypic female. Several mechanisms exist through which this monosomy may be brought about (see *Table 32.6*). These distinct mechanisms are associated with differing phenotypic severity.

Frequency.   Turner's syndrome is the commonest cause of primary amenorrhoea. The syndrome occurs in about 1:3000 live births. The XO karyotype is probably much more frequent than this figure suggests since the majority of conceptions with this karyotype end in miscarriage.

The clinical phenotype is summarized in *Table 32.7*.

Klinefelter's syndrome

The defining criterion of this syndrome is the presence of more than one X chromosome in a phenotypic male. This arises most commonly when non-disjunction of the X chromosome in the mother gives rise to the karyotype in

Table 32.6   Causes of Turner's syndrome

Frequency (%)	Abnormality
53	Loss of an entire X chromosome, usually the paternally derived one. Karyotype 45X0
17	Complete deletion of the short arm (p) of the X chromosome resulting in the formation of an isochromosome of the long arm. Karyotype 46Xi (Xq)
10	Partial deletion of the short arm
20	Various abnormalities arising from mosaicism

Table 32.7   Clinical features of Turner's syndrome

Affected system	Abnormalities
General bodily appearance	• Short stature, virtually never exceed 5 ft in height • Severely affected infants show peripheral lymphoedema affecting principally the dorsa of the hands and feet • The neck is often webbed. This is due to distended lymphatic channels (cystic hygroma). These later resolve but the neck retains its webbed appearance • The chest is typically broad and the nipples widely spaced • The carrying angle of the forearm is usually increased (cubitus valgus) • Pigmented naevi are common • The posterior hair line is low
Cardiovascular system	There is an increased risk of: • coarctation of the aorta • bicuspid aortic valve and, consequently, aortic stenosis
Genitalia	• The secondary sex characteristics are poorly developed • The gonads develop as ovaries (since there is no Y chromosome present), but do not reach normal size ('streak ovaries'). Both within utero and in the first two years of life, the decline in the number of primordial follicles occurring in all females is much accelerated in girls with Turner's syndrome so that there are no or very few oocytes left by the age of two years. A writer in the *New England Journal of Medicine* has tellingly described this as the menopause occurring before the menarche

the child of 47XXY. More rarely Klinefelter patients may have three or four X chromosomes.

Klinefelter's syndrome is one of the commonest causes of male hypogonadism and one of the commonest chromosomal disorders affecting the sex chromosomes. It occurs in 1:600–850 live births.

In its fully expressed form, Klinefelter's syndrome causes a distinctive bodily appearance:

• The affected males are tall, most of this increased height being due to a disproportionate length of the lower limbs.
• Patients have a eunuchoid appearance with a wide pelvis.
• The testes are atrophic and the penis small.
• The distribution of body hair resembles that of the female rather than the male.
• Gynaecomastia may be present due to high plasma oestradiol concentrations.
• A minority of the affected individuals shows some degree of mental retardation.

The diagnosis can be made easily by finding Barr bodies in the cells of a phenotypic male. Striking testicular changes occur. *It is important to remember that the full-blown syndrome described above may not be present. Hypogonadism and infertility may be the only manifestations of Klinefelter's syndrome.* The risk of carcinoma of the male breast is increased in Klinefelter's syndrome, presumably because of the abnormal hormonal milieu.

XYY syndrome
This syndrome occurs in about 1:1000 male live births. Most affected subjects appear normal but there is a tendency for them to be very tall and to be severely affected by acne. At one time it was suggested that the XYY syndrome was associated with aggressive behaviour and antisocial conduct. In fact only a small proportion of XYY individuals (1–2%) show such behaviour patterns.

'Superfemales': the presence of more than two X chromosomes in a phenotypic female
This syndrome occurs in about 1:1200 female births. The commonest karyotype is 47XXX but cases occur in which there are increases in the X chromosome number beyond this point; in these circumstances there is a considerable risk of mental retardation which appears to increase in severity as the number of X chromosomes increases. All individuals with a 49XXXXX karyotype are likely to suffer from mental retardation.

GENETIC DISORDERS

- Many diseases are due either wholly or in part to abnormalities in the genome.
- They may be:
  - **major chromosomal abnormalities** (e.g. trisomy of chromosome 21 in Down's syndrome)
  - **single gene defects** (affecting either single alleles or both members of an allelic pair)
  - **multifactorial**, in which case three is often interaction between genetic and environmental factors (e.g. diabetes mellitus, atherosclerosis, many cancers).
- Abnormalities of chromosomes may be numerical (as in Down's syndrome or Turner's syndrome) or structural, such as deletions, various forms of translocation, inversion or isochromosome formation. Down's syndrome is the commonest numerical chromosome abnormality occurring in the live newborn (1/800 live births).
- Turner's syndrome (complete or partial deletion of one X chromosome) is the commonest cause of primary amenorrhoea, occurring in 1/3000 live births.
- Klinefelter's syndrome (two or more X chromosomes in the presence of a Y chromosome) occurs in 1/600–850 live births and is one of the commonest causes of male hypogonadism.

33 Single gene defects

More than 4000 single gene defects have been recognized. These are caused by mutations affecting either **autosomes** or **sex chromosomes** and inherited in either a **dominant** or **recessive** pattern.

AUTOSOMAL DOMINANT DISORDERS

These are estimated to occur in 2–9:1000 live births. **The concept of dominance means that a single mutated allele is expressed despite the presence of a normal second allele**. This dictates the features of this group of disorders (*Fig. 33.1*).

KEY POINTS: AUTOSOMAL DOMINANT DISORDERS

- An affected individual normally has one affected parent. There are exceptions since mutations can occur *de novo* in the germ cell of one or other parent.
- Both heterozygotes for the mutation and homozygotes show the phenotypic abnormality. This is usually much more severe in the homozygous state (e.g. in familial hypercholesterolaemia).
- Both males and females are equally affected.
- The disorder shows itself in every generation.
- The marriage between an affected individual and a normal one confers a 1:2 risk of showing the phenotypic abnormality on each child of the marriage.

Penetrance and expressivity

An individual who inherits a dominant mutant may be phenotypically normal. The gene is then spoken of as showing **incomplete penetrance**. For example, if 4:5 of those inheriting the mutant gene are phenotypically abnormal, the gene shows 80% penetrance.

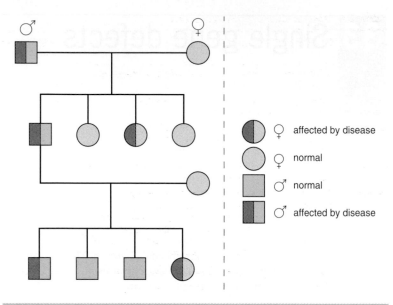

Fig. 33.1 **Autosomal dominant inheritance pattern.**

If *all* those in a sibship who inherit a mutant dominant gene show phenotypic abnormality, but there are differences in the severity of the abnormality, the gene is described as showing **variable expressivity**.

Some important autosomal dominant disorders are listed in *Table 33.1*.

AUTOSOMAL RECESSIVE DISORDERS

The defining criterion of an autosomal recessive disorder is that the disorder only manifests when both alleles at a given locus are mutated (*Fig. 33.2*).

The features of this group of disorders are listed in the key points box.

KEY POINTS: AUTOSOMAL RECESSIVE DISORDERS

- Probands must be homozygous for the mutation.
- The affected individual must have phenotypically normal parents.
- Each parent must be heterozygous for the mutant gene (a carrier).
- Males and females are equally affected.
- 1:4 of an affected sibship will show the phenotypic abnormality.
- The disorder does not occur in every generation.
- Enzyme proteins are frequently affected.
- Penetrance is commonly complete.

Table 33.1 Some autosomal dominant disorders

System	Diseases	Features	Frequency per 1000 births
Blood	Spherocytosis	Anaemia due to premature destruction of red cells	0.2
Lipid metabolism	Familial hyper-cholesterolaemia	LDL receptor defect. Premature atherosclerosis	2
Large gut	Familial polyposis coli	Deletion in chromosome 5; multiple adenomatous polyps with inevitable progression to cancer	0.1
Kidney	Polycystic kidney	Massively enlarged kidney with multiple cysts; progressive renal failure	1.0
Nervous	Huntington's disease	Dementia in middle life associated with involuntary choreiform movements; abnormal trinucleotide repeat in gene on chromosome 4	0.2
	Neuro-fibromatosis	Tumours of nerve sheaths, abnormal skin pigmentation; in Type 1, deletion of gene coding for neurofibromin which interferes with GTP binding by ras proteins	0.33
	Tuberous sclerosis	Skin lesions (sebaceous adenoma); mental retardation, epilepsy, hamartomas in brain and heart	0.08
	Myotonic dystrophy	Delayed muscle relaxation; cardiomyopathy, cataract; diabetes mellitus, etc. Mutation on chromosome 19 is expansion of the copies of a triplet CTG encoding a protein kinase	0.05
Bone	Diaphysial aclasis	Numerous cartilaginous exostoses at ends of long bones	0.5
	Osteogenesis imperfecta	Fragile bones with increased risk of fractures	0.1
	Achondroplasia	Dwarfism; deformity of bone; increased risk of fractures	0.04
	Thanatophoric dwarfism	Severe skeletal deformities; early death	0.08
Connective tissue	Marfan's syndrome	Mutation in gene encoding fibrillin on chromosome 15; long thin limbs, increased risk of aortic dissection	0.1
	Ehlers–Danlos syndromes	Variety of collagen defects giving hyper-extensible joints and increased fragility of tissues	0.05
Ear	Otosclerosis	Deafness occurring from time of adolescence onwards; changes in ossicles of middle ear	3.0
	Dominant early childhood deafness	Deafness from infancy	0.1
Eye	Dominant blindness	Blindness	0.1
Teeth	Dentinogenesis imperfecta	Abnormal development of teeth	0.1
Porphyrin metabolism	Acute intermittent porphyria	Acute abdominal pain and neurological disturbances; dark urine due to presence of porphobilinogen	0.01

The figures quoted in this table are approximations since differences in reported frequency exist. They apply to Europe only.

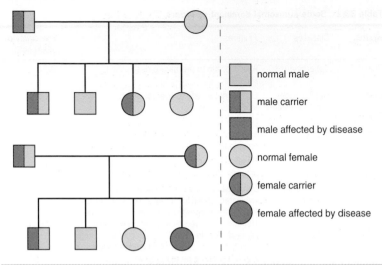

Fig. 33.2 Autosomal recessive inheritance pattern.

Some common autosomal recessive disorders are listed in *Table 33.2.*

X-LINKED DISORDERS

Sex-linked disorders are all related to mutations within the X chromosome. With very few exceptions, the inheritance pattern in these disorders is recessive (*Fig. 33.3*).

The Y chromosome genes are not homologous with those of the X chromosome and thus any deficiency in the male's X chromosome is not counterbalanced by production of normal amounts of normal gene product by the Y chromosome. Thus recessive mutations on the X chromosome are, for all practical purposes, expressed only in males.

If an affected male has children, all his daughters will be carriers of the mutant gene and all his sons will be both genotypically and phenotypically normal.

KEY POINTS: X-LINKED RECESSIVE DISORDERS

- With few exceptions the disorders affect males.
- Unaffected males do not carry the gene and cannot transmit the abnormality.
- The disease is transmitted by unaffected female carriers (who are heterozygous in respect of the mutated gene) to their sons, half of whom are affected.
- Female carriers and affected males can transmit the mutation to their daughters thus creating another generation of female carriers.

Table 33.2 Some important autosomal recessive disorders

Disorder	Features	Frequency per 1000 births
Cystic fibrosis	Defect in chloride transport due to mutation of gene on chromosome 7; viscid secretions, recurrent lung infections, failure to thrive	0.5–0.6
Congenital deafness	Deafness from infancy	0.5
Sickle cell disease	Point mutation on chromosome 6; valine substituted for glutamic acid in haemoglobin; haemolytic anaemia	0.1
Adrenal hyperplasia	Enzyme deficiency leading to block in cortisol synthesis; precocious development of genitalia in males; virilism in females; may have Addisonian crises	0.1
Phenylketonuria	Mental retardation due to accumulation of intermediates of phenylalanine metabolism	0.2–0.5
α_1-antitrypsin deficiency	Chronic liver disease which may present in infancy; emphysema	0.1–0.5
Recessive blindness	Blindness	0.1
Cystinuria	Recurrent renal calculi	0.06
Tay–Sachs disease	Mental retardation and blindness; occurs in Ashkenazi Jews; carrier state can be detected by screening	0.004
Mucopolysaccharidoses	Accumulation of intermediates in macrophages leading to visceromegaly; mental retardation in some disorders	0.03
β thalassaemia	Anaemias, bone deformities, enlarged spleen	0.05
Galactosaemia	Chronic liver disease starting in infancy and leading to cirrhosis and liver failure	0.02
Homocystinuria	Mental retardation; eye, bone and blood vessel abnormalities	0.01
Metachromatic leucodystrophy	Defect in long chain fatty acid metabolism; blindness, intellectual deterioration	0.02
Friedreich's ataxia	Early onset of progressive unsteadiness and dysarthria; skeletal deformities, cardiomyopathy in some cases. Abnormal numbers of copies of triplet GAA in gene X25 on chromosome 9	0.02
Spinal muscular atrophy	Progressive muscle weakness	0.04
Wilson's disease	Involuntary athetoid movements and chronic liver disease associated with abnormal deposition of copper in basal ganglia and liver	0.0033
Some varieties of Ehlers–Danlos syndrome	Various collagen abnormalities; hyperextensible joints and fragility of connective tissues	Not available
Neurogenic muscular atrophy	Progressive muscle weakness	0.01

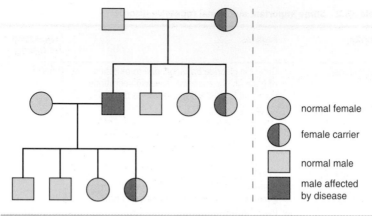

Fig. 33.3   X-linked recessive inheritance pattern.

Some important X-linked disorders are listed in *Table 33.3*.

The fragile X syndrome

This is characterized by:

- severe mental retardation; this occurs principally in males, though 30–50% of female carriers show some degree of intellectual impairment
- a long face with prominent and everted ears
- large testes.

This clinical picture is associated with a non-staining gap on the long arm of the X chromosome (Xq27.3). Special media are required for cell culture before this site shows up on microscopic examination.

Fragile X syndrome is the commonest cause of inherited mental retardation. It has a frequency of 1:1500 males and 1:2000 females. The inheritance pattern originally suggested that this syndrome was inherited as an X-linked dominant syndrome in which penetrance is incomplete. This is an oversimplification since **phenotypically normal males can transmit the condition, not to their children but to their grandchildren**. This strange pattern has given rise to the concept of a **premutation** which needs processing through female meiosis before it can be expressed.

It is now believed that mutation of a gene known as *FMR-1* is responsible for the fragile X syndrome. In affected individuals the striking abnormality in the *FMR-1* gene is an excess number of copies of the trinucleotide CGG (which codes for arginine) in one of the 5′ exons of the gene. In normal individuals the median number of copies of this sequence is 30 (6–54). Phenotypically normal transmitting males and normal female carriers (those with the presumed premutation) have between 60 and 200 copies of the CGG sequence. This number remains stable in the course of male meiosis

Table 33.3 Some important X-linked disorders

Disorder	Features	Frequency per 1000 male births
Fragile X syndrome	Mental retardation; characteristic facies; large testes	0.9
Muscular dystrophy (Duchenne and Becker type)	Progressive muscular weakness more severe in Duchenne type and leading to death in third decade. Complete or partial deletion of gene encoding dystrophin	0.3
Haemophilia A	Excessive post-traumatic bleeding due to lack of clotting factor VIII	0.1
Haemophilia B	Abnormal bleeding due to deficiency of clotting factor IX	0.1
Ichthyosis	Thick skin with excessive keratin due to deficiency of a sulphatase	0.1
Glucose-6-phosphate dehydrogenase deficiency	Haemolysis following ingestion of certain drugs	
X-linked agammaglobulinaemia	Increased susceptibility to infection	
Red/green colour blindness		8
Diabetes insipidus		Not available
Lesch–Nyhan syndrome		Not available
Childhood blindness	Blindness	0.02

but female meiosis leads to a greatly increased number of copies and the development of full blown fragile X syndrome in the sons and daughters of transmitting females. The presence of more than 140 repeats in the carrier indicates a very high risk of the syndrome developing. The fragile X syndrome itself is associated with increases in the number of copies of CGG ranging from 250 to 4000.

Other X-linked disorders

Other inherited disorders characterized by excess copies of trinucleotide sequences include Huntington's dementia and myotonic dystrophy.

X-linked dominant disorders are very rare indeed. They include vitamin D-resistant rickets, in which abnormally large amounts of phosphate are lost in the urine and the bone is inadequately mineralized. The abnormal gene is expressed both in males and females (who receive it from affected hetero-zygous mothers). Fathers with this gene defect can transmit it only to their daughters.

MUTATIONS IN SINGLE GENE DEFECTS

Single gene defects may arise on the basis of the following:

Gene deletions

An example of the effects of deletion of an entire gene is α thalassaemia. Normal individuals have two α-globin genes. If one of these is deleted, there is reduced production of α-globin chains and there is an excess in haemo-globin of β-globin chains (HbH disease). If both α-globin genes are deleted, the fetus cannot make fetal haemoglobin; instead it produces haemoglobin Barts which has virtually no oxygen-carrying capacity. The condition hydrops fetalis is produced and leads to stillbirth or neonatal death. The deletion of a single α-globin gene results from unequal crossing over between homologous chromosomes 16 during meiosis.

Partial gene deletion

If part of a gene is deleted some protein may still be encoded by the remnant, even if this protein is grossly abnormal. This situation is exemplified by the X-linked muscular dystrophies of the Duchenne and Becker types, both of which are caused by mutation in the dystrophin gene. This is the largest gene so far identified; it spans more than 2500 kilobases of genomic DNA and accounts for 1% of the whole X gene.

Duchenne type disease is the more severe of the two. This has been ascribed to the fact that the partial deletion in Duchenne type disease interrupts the reading frame since the deletion causes an **intra-codon break**, thus creating a new reading frame to the 3' end of the mRNA. Most of the deletions seen in the less severe Becker type disease leave the reading frame intact by removing an entire codon or group of codons.

Codon deletion

If a codon or a small set of codons is deleted, the reading frame will not be altered but the protein product of the affected gene will be deficient in one or more amino acids. This is known to occur in several haemoglobin variants, most of which involve the β-globin chain.

An important example of codon deletion is to be found in cystic fibrosis. The commonest mutation here is one where three nucleotides CTT are deleted from exon 10 of the gene encoding a chloride transporter (the cystic fibrosis trans-membrane conductance regulator, CFTR).

Duplications and insertions

While unequal crossing over during meiosis may lead to deletion of whole genes or parts of genes, it can also lead to duplications of genetic material. The effects of such duplications depend on whether disruption of the reading frame occurs or not. In the latter case there is little, if any, effect.

Fusion mutations

Unequal crossing over between non-homologous genes can result in the formation of fusion genes. The commonest example of this occurs in red/green colour blindness which is quite common in males.

There are three pigment genes in humans:

- a blue pigment gene on chromosome 7
- red and green pigment genes situated contiguously at the tip of the X chromosome.

Green colour blindness is about three times as common as red colour blindness. There are several mutational events that lead to colour blindness; one is the formation of fusion genes consisting of parts of each of the red and green pigment genes. This results from unequal crossing over of these genes in the course of meiosis.

Point mutations

Point mutation is defined as **the substitution of one base pair by another in double-stranded DNA**. If a purine is substituted for a purine or a pyrimidine by a pyrimidine, the process is termed **transition**. If a purine is replaced by a pyrimidine or vice versa the process is termed **transversion**. Theoretically, substitution of a base pair should lead to the encoding of a different amino acid. However, because of the degeneracy of the genetic code (see *Tables 33.4* and *33.5*) about one-third of all point mutations are not associated with an alteration in the encoded gene product.

Each amino acid is specified by the codon (triplet of nucleotides) in the mRNA molecule binding with three complementary nucleotides (anticodon) at the tip of a particular tRNA molecule.

RNA is composed of four nucleotides. Thus there must be 64 possible sequences, as shown in Table 33.4. Three of these possible sequences specify the termination of a polypeptide chain rather than coding for an amino acid. These three are known as stop codons. The remainder code for only 20 amino acids. Thus most amino acids are specified for by more than one codon (with the exceptions of methionine and tryptophan which can be specified by only one codon each).

Point mutations may be divided into a number of different classes.

Missense mutations

This is defined as a base substitution leading to the encoding of a different amino acid from that normally specified by that codon. Not all of these have

Table 33.4   The genetic code (mRNA bases)

1st position (5' end)	2nd position U	2nd position C	2nd position A	2nd position G	3rd position (3' end)
U	Phe	Ser	Tyr	Cys	U
	Phe	Ser	Tyr	Cys STOP	C
	Leu	Ser	STOP	Trp	A
	Leu	Ser	STOP		G
C	Leu	Pro	His	Arg	U
	Leu	Pro	His	Arg	C
	Leu	Pro	Gln	Arg	A
	Leu	Pro	Gln	Arg	G
A	Ile	Thr	Asn	Ser	U
	Ile	Thr	Asn	Ser	C
	Ile	Thr	Lys	Arg	A
	Met*	Thr	Lys	Arg	G
G	Val	Ala	Asp	Gly	U
	Val	Ala	Asp	Gly	C
	Val	Ala	Glu	Gly	A
	Val	Ala	Glu	Gly	G

*AUG = a start codon for protein translation.

Table 33.5   Amino acids, their symbols, abbreviations and codons

Amino acid	Abbreviation	Symbol	Codons
Alanine	Ala	A	GCA, GCC, GCG, GCU
Cysteine	Cys	C	UGC, UGU
Aspartic acid	Asp	D	GAC, GAU
Glutamic acid	Glu	E	GAA, GAG
Phenylalanine	Phe	F	UUC, UUU
Glycine	Gly	G	GGA, GGC, GGG, GGU
Histidine	His	H	CAC, CAU
Isoleucine	Ile	I	AUA, AUC, AUU
Lysine	Lys	K	AAA, AAG
Leucine	Leu	L	UUA, UUG, CUA, CUC, CUG, CUU
Methionine	Met	M	AUG
Asparagine	Asn	N	AAC, AAU
Proline	Pro	P	CCA, CCC, CCG, CCU
Glutamine	Gln	Q	CAA, CAG
Arginine	Arg	R	AGA, AGG, CGA, CGC, CGG, CGU
Serine	Ser	S	AGC, AGU, UCA, UCC, UCG, UCU
Threonine	Thr	T	ACA, ACC, ACG, ACU
Valine	Val	V	GUA, GUC, GUG, GUU
Tryptophan	Trp	W	UGG
Tyrosine	Tyr	Y	UAC, UAU

pathological consequences. Important examples of such mutations include sickle cell disease and α_1-antitrypsin deficiency.

Sickle cell disease. GAG (which encodes **glutamic acid**) in codon 6 of the β-globin gene is changed to CTG which specifies the neutral and hydrophobic amino acid **valine**.

α_1-antitrypsin deficiency. GAG (glutamic acid) in exon V of the gene is changed to AAG (lysine) at position 342 of the protein. The resulting protein is abnormally processed within liver cells and secreted only with difficulty by them. It is also not as effective as the more common M protein at combating neutrophil elastase.

Nonsense mutations

A nonsense mutation is one which converts a codon specifying an amino acid to a **stop codon**. The nearer the 5′ end of the gene the mutation occurs, the greater will be the degree of truncation of the protein product.

A nonsense mutation in the second exon of the β-globin gene is one of the common causes of β thalassaemia. A stop codon is produced in place of the mRNA specifying glutamic acid. This leads to a virtual absence of β-globin chains.

Several nonsense mutations are also known to exist in the gene encoding factor VIII in respect of haemophilia A. Patients in whom nonsense mutations are the cause of haemophilia are prone to develop antibodies to the human factor VIII with which they are treated; presumably they produce no endogenous factor VIII and thus recognize the factor VIII given to them as 'foreign'.

Stop codon mutations

This is the exact opposite of a nonsense mutation in that it involves conversion of a stop codon into one encoding an amino acid. This is seen in one of the haemoglobinopathies, haemoglobin Constant Spring, in which the normal stop codon found at position 142 on the α-globin gene (UAA) is altered to CAA which encodes glutamine. The result is an unstable haemoglobin which is associated with the α thalassaemia trait.

Frameshift mutations

Frameshifts can occur as a result of point mutations as well as via partial gene deletions. Such frameshifts occur when either insertion or deletion of a single nucleotide disturbs the reading frame so that a new set of codons is specified near the 3′ end of the gene.

RNA splice mutations

Once transcription has occurred, the original product must have its introns removed for mRNA to be produced in a form suitable for translation. Most normal genes have a dinucleotide GT sequence at the 5′ end of the intron (this is called the **donor site**) and an AG dinucleotide at the 3′ end of the intron (the **acceptor site**). Mutations in the genomic DNA that alter either of these sites cause disturbances in normal splicing, and the resulting mRNA is abnormal and non-functional. Several different splicing mutations have been described in the β thalassaemias. If these mutations are homozygous, no β-globin chains are produced.

Consensus sequence mutations

Splicing defects can also occur as a result of mutations in consensus sequences. These are nucleotide sequences at the borders between introns and exons. At the donor site they include the last three triplets in the preceding exon and the first six in the intron. At the acceptor site they consist of the last ten triplets of the intron and the first triplet of the exon. Several mutations in consensus sequences with consequent defects in splicing have been described in β thalassaemia phenotypes.

Mutations leading to splicing defects can also occur in introns well away from consensus regions. These create new acceptor sites and thus alter splicing.

Transcriptional mutations

Blocks of DNA upstream from the 5′ end of a gene play a significant part in regulating transcription of the gene. Several point mutations have been described in these promoter regions in relation to β thalassaemia phenotypes.

MITOCHONDRIAL DISORDERS

The general characteristics of mitochondrial inherited disorders are described in the introduction to this section.

KEY POINTS: MITOCHONDRIAL GENETICS

- Each mitochondrion contains several copies of a circular chromosome made up of a rather small amount of DNA.
- Mitochondrial DNA encodes a number of protein components of the respiratory chain and oxidative phosphorylation system as well as some special types of RNA.
- The genome contains 2 RNA genes, 22 tRNA genes and 13 protein-coding sequences.
- The genetic code in mitochondria differs in some respects from that which is universal in all other organisms.
- Inheritance of mitochondrial genes in humans occurs entirely through the maternal line.
- Mitochondrial DNA has a high rate of mutations, and the normal population shows considerable variation in respect of mitochondrial genes.

Examples of mitochondrial inherited disorders include:

- Leber's hereditary optic atrophy; this is characterized by late onset bilateral loss of central vision and by disturbances in heart rhythm
- myoclonus with ragged red fibres (MERRF)
- mitochondrial myopathy with encephalopathy, lactic acidosis and stroke (MELAS)
- the Kearns–Sayre syndrome in which there is: paralysis of external ocular muscles (ophthalmoplegia), complete heart block and pigmentary degeneration of the retina.

SINGLE GENE DEFECTS

- Single gene defects, of which more than 4000 are recognized, may affect autosomes or sex chromosomes.
- Expression of the abnormal gene may occur when only a single allele is affected (**dominant**) or may require both alleles to be abnormal (**recessive**).
- The frequency with which individuals inheriting abnormal, dominant genes show an abnormal phenotype is termed the **penetrance** of the gene. Variations in the severity of the phenotypic abnormality are due to variations in gene **expressivity**.
- Important autosomal dominant disorders include familial hypercholesterolaemia, a potent risk factor for premature ischaemic heart disease.
- Important autosomal recessive disorders include cystic fibrosis, sickle cell disease and α_1-antitrypsin deficiency.
- Virtually all sex-chromosome-linked disorders are recessive. They include the fragile X syndrome (a common cause of mental retardation), haemophilia A and B, muscular dystrophy and red-green colour blindness.
- The many genomic events occurring in single gene defects include deletions (complete or partial), codon deletions, duplications and insertions, and point mutations, to name but a few.

Glossary

acinus – the functional unit of a gland; also that part of the lung tissue distal to the terminal bronchiole

adipose – related to fat, fatty; in tissue terms, the collection of cells containing fat

adventitia – the outermost loose layer of connective tissue covering a structure such as a blood vessel or ureter

aetiology – the cause of a disease

allele – one of a pair of genes occupying the same position in an homologous chromosome. The two alleles determine the inheritance of a particular trait. They may be identical (homozygous) or different (heterozygous).

angiogenesis – the process of blood vessel formation

anoxia – absence or severe restriction of the oxygen supply to a cell, organ or individual

apoptosis – programmed cell death involved in many situations both physiological and pathological. It is regulated by the transcription of certain genes and is associated with a characteristic set of morphological cell changes.

asystole – failure of the left ventricular muscle of the heart to contract. This leads to absence of a cardiac output.

atrophy – a shrinkage in the size of cells, organs and tissues. This may leads to loss of function.

caudad – directed posteriorly, i.e. away from the head

cephalad – directed anteriorly, i.e. towards the head

coagulation – clotting of a fluid to form a jelly-like mass; typical of blood, in which coagulation is a vital process in stopping bleeding

commissure – a joining together

desquamation – the shedding or peeling of the most superficial layer of a surface; most commonly applied to skin

diathesis – an inherited or inborn tendency to develop a certain disease

dimer – a chemical species (in the context of pathology often a protein) which consists of two identical molecules joined together

diploid – having two sets of chromosomes (the normal mammalian state)

distal – in anatomical terms, further away from a point of reference

diuresis – the passage of a larger than usual volume of urine

dysplasia – an abnormal development of a body tissue; also applied to cells showing nuclear abnormalities suggesting partial expression of a neoplastic phenotype

dystonia – a state characterized by abnormally increased muscle tone

effusion – an abnormal collection of fluid in a body cavity, e.g. the pleural or pericardial cavity

embolism – obstruction of a blood vessel by an abnormal mass formed elsewhere in the circulation and transported to its point of impaction

epitope – the part of an antigen eliciting a specific antibody response

eukaryotic – a cell with a well-defined nucleus bounded by a nuclear membrane and dividing by mitosis

exudation – the process by which water, electrolytes and plasma proteins escape from small blood vessels into the extravascular compartment; a characteristic occurrence in acute inflammation

fibrillation – abnormally rapid and ineffective contraction of muscle fibres, especially in the heart

fibrosis – the formation of fibrous, tissue, usually as a reaction to chronic inflammation or the presence of certain neoplasms, or in the replacement of cells which are not capable of regeneration

fistula – an abnormal passage between two internal organs (e.g adjacent loops of bowel, bowel to urinary bladder, bladder to vagina), or between an internal organ and the external surface of the body

gangrene – strictly speaking, the combination of tissue necrosis with infection by putrefactive microorganisms; also used to describe necrotic tissue showing blackish discolouration not necessarily accompanied by infection (as in diabetic gangrene affecting the lower limb)

genome – the total complement of genes in an individual

homeostasis – the maintenance of a 'steady state' in respect of physiological function, at both cell and system level, in the face of environmental variation

hyperaemia – a state in which there is an increased inflow of blood into an organ or tissue

hyperkeratosis – an increase in the thickness of the horny layer (stratum corneum) of the epidermis

hyperplasia – an increase in the number of cells in a given cell population; this cell proliferation, unlike that occuring in neoplasia, is regulated by normal feed-back mechanisms

hypertrophy – an increase in the size of individual cells in the absence of any increase in number. This usually represents an increase in work load (e.g. left ventricular hypertrophy in individuals with raised systemic blood pressure)

hypoxia – a reduction in the supply of oxygen to cells and tissues

impaction – the lodgement of some abnormal mass in a hollow muscular tube causing blockage of the lumen

infarct – an area of tissue necrosis caused by interruption of the blood supply to the affected region (ischaemia)

interstitial – describes the spaces lying between the formed elements of an organ or tissue (e.g. the spaces between the nephrons in the kidney)

intima – the innermost layer of a blood vessel and, thus, that part whose surface is in contact with flowing blood

ischaemia – the pathophysiological state in which the blood supply of an organ or tissue is reduced below its metabolic needs

lamina – a thin layer in tissues, often consisting of a mixture of fibrillar proteins

ligand – an organic chemical species binding to a complementary site on another molecule

liquefaction – the conversion of solid material into liquid; in pathology often refers to death of tissue accompanied by the activation of proteolytic enzymes; occurs in the brain especially following ischaemic necrosis

lumen – the interior space of a tubular structure (e.g. the lumen of a blood vessel providing a conduit for blood)

lysis – the breakdown of cells or tissues brought about by enzymes

metaplasia – a change in cell populations from one fully differentiated form to another fully differentiated form (e.g. columnar epithelium lining a bronchus may be replaced by squamous epithelium as a result of cigarette smoking)

micelle – a grouping of amphipathic molecules arranged so that hydrophobic groups are on the inside of the aggregate and hyophilic ones are on the outside

microvasculature – the small delivery vessels in the circulatory system comprising arterioles, capillaries and venules

mitosis – the process by which cells divide, giving rise to two daughter cells, each of which has a normal chromosome and DNA content

multimer – a molecule formed of two or more identical sub-units joined together

mural – pertaining to thrombus: a thrombus attached to the inner lining of the blood vessel and projecting into the lumen without occluding it

necrosis – death of tissue within a circumscribed area (as in myocardial infarction)

occlusion – blockage of the lumen of a hollow muscular tube

oligomeric – of a biological set made up of a small number of units

oncogene – a gene whose products are implicated in causing neoplastic transformation

ontogeny – the processes involved in the biological development of an individual

opsonization – the process by which the binding of certain protein molecules to the surfaces of microorganisms renders them more readily phagocytosed

organization – the set of processes by which persisting inflammatory exudate, dead tissue, thrombus, etc., are converted to scar tissue

papule – a small palpable skin lesion with a diameter of less than 1.5 cm

pathogenesis – the biological steps involved in the production of a disease

pathognomonic – a special characteristic of a given disease, the presence of which is indicative of that disease

perfusion – the passage of fluid through the vessels of an organ; most commonly applied to blood flow through an organ or tissue

phagocytosis – the set of processes by which material is engulfed within specialized cells, either to be held there or to be destroyed. This is a pivotal mechanism in the body's defence against pathogenic microorganisms.

phosphorylation – the addition of phosphate to an organic compound, often a protein or amino acid

plaque – in vascular pathology, the archetypal raised lesion in atherosclerosis, consisting of a mixture of lipid and newly-formed connective tissue; in neuropathology, a localized area of demyelination in the brain or spinal cord seen typically in multiple sclerosis

ploidy – the number of chromosome sets in a cell nucleus (e.g. diploid, when there are two such sets)

proband – the member of a family in whom a trait or an inherited disease is first observed and through whom the rest of the family is brought under observation

proximal – in anatomical terms, near the point of reference from which observations are being taken; thus, in the arm, the humerus is regarded as being proximal, the radius and ulna distal

stenosis – narrowing of a hollow muscular tube

stricture – abnormal narrowing of a hollow muscular tube, often by scar tissue; frequently applied to the gastro-intestinal tract

stroma – the supporting framework of an organ or tissue; the connective tissue, often reactive, which surrounds the cellular elements of a tumour

thrombosis – the formation of an abnormal intravascular mass from the constituents of flowing blood; it involves activation both of platelets and the coagulation pathway

thrombus – an abnormal intravascular mass formed from the constituents of flowing blood

transfection – the introduction of foreign DNA into cultured cells

Index